BLANCHE STURGEON

CHECK·UP

ENGLISH THROUGH MEDICAL READINGS

WITH ANSWER BOOK

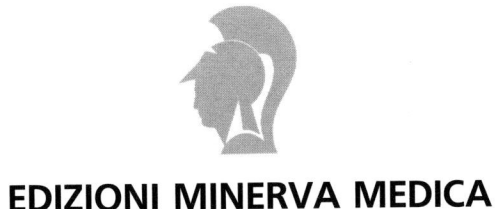

EDIZIONI MINERVA MEDICA

GEORG THIEME VERLAG

The original edition of this volume
has been published by:
© EDIZIONI MINERVA MEDICA – TORINO (ITALY) 1992

ISBN 3-13-134501-2

Sole distribution rights GEORG THIEME VERLAG
Rüdigerstraße 14, D – 70469 Stuttgart, Germany.

Dedicated to the memory of Mr. Francesco Ponzoni

Unit	Contents of Text	Text-based Exercises	Extension Exercises
1	Percutaneous Automated Diskectomy	word check comprehension prepositions	compound words opposites expression with *back*
2	Sharing materials in human genetics	word check comprehension sentence building adverbs	should/shouldn't ought to phrasal verbs with *to run*
3	A device that can save cardiac patients	word search comprehension	nouns from verbs irregular verbs phrasal verbs with *to be*
4	A crippling orthopaedic disease	word check comprehension	past/present participles idiomatic expressions with *to be*
5	An award to a molecular biologist	double noun expressions sentence reconstruction	names of specialists adverbs
6	Deciphering the genetic code; gene therapy	comprehension adjectives prepositions	word substitution nouns from verbs
7	Mapping chromosomes and sequencing genes	word check comprehension nouns	adjectives phrasal verbs with *to come*
8	Growth-hormone therapy	word check comprehension sentence building	idiomatic expressions with *to come*
9	Verbal pain descriptors	comprehension mixed verbal forms	synonyms nouns from verbs

Grammar Point	Writing	Speaking	Idioms
The Future Will or going to?	Describing the diskectomy technique	Doctor/Patient dialogue Asking questions	The cure is worse than the disease
The Future Using the Present Continuous	Writing about the Human Genome Project	Discussing data sharing Interview	His patients loved him for his bedside manner
The Future Using the Simple Present	Diagram completion Describing the structure and action of the heart	Doctor/Patient dialogue Asking questions	The patient thanked the doctor from the bottom of his heart
Comparatives than	Writing a summary	Doctor/Patient dialogue	She's just had a brain wave
Relative Clauses who/that	Describing a process Word forming	Presentation/ Interview	I really put my foot in it
Simple Past/Present Perfect	Writing information	Discussing genetic engineering	This will hurt me more than it hurts you
The Passive	Writing instructions for sequencing genes	Describing: process, structure and function	He managed to find his feet
Understanding Incomplete Sentences	Writing about hormones and endocrine glands	Asking questions Doctor/Patient dialogue	He got a dose of his own medicine
Past Perfect	Describing differences: Involuntary/voluntary responses	Describing the structure and function of neurons Doctor/Patient dialogue	After his speech, doctor Spencer was given a big hand

OUTLINE OF PROGRAMME: language structures and exercises

Unit	Contents of Text	Text-based Exercises	Extension Exercises
10	Purifying peptides	word check prepositions verbs	prefixes not only… but also
11	Major surgery on a fetus	word check sentence reconstruction	using commas to separate clauses adjectives with "less" phrasal verbs with *to do*
12	An "uncommon" neurological disorder	word check comprehension opposites	verbs from nouns phrasal verbs with *to put*
13	Atherosclerosis: reversing the damage	word check asking questions prepositions	nouns from verbs idiomatic expressions with *to do*
14	Heart Tests/Test for non-A, non-B hepatitis virus	word check comprehension	revision of idioms phrasal verbs with *to get*
15	The physical effects of stress on healthy hearts	word check comprehension nouns	revision of phrasal verbs the Past Perfect with *just* and *when*
16	A book that helps plan exercise programmes for patients with special needs	word check adjectives verbs from nouns	do/does/did in affirmative sentences idiomatic expressions with *to get*
17	The factors causing diabetes	comprehension adverbs/prepositions	reflexive pronouns phrasal verbs with *to look*
18	Immunology: a rapidly progressing field	word check synonyms/nouns	describing body systems

Grammar Point	Writing	Speaking	Idioms
Present Perfect Continuous for/since	Form Filling Letter Writing	Summarizing Doctor/Patient dialogue	Take this medicine it will do the trick
So/Such	Describing fetal surgery	Discussing fetal therapy	Her new car cost her an arm and a leg
Future Perfect/ Future Perfect Continuous	Basic terminology in pathology	Spelling Defining	He's got two left feet
Past Continuous	Writing about blood vessels/heart attack	Explaining the benefits of a NordicTract	He's pulling your leg
Past Perfect Continuous	Writing notes	Doctor/Patient dialogue	She has a heart of gold
Question Tags	Stress Test	Doctor/Patient dialogue	You've got a nerve!
Conditionals – type 1	What specific patients *can* and *can't* do Writing an application	Guidelines for Exercise Training after Cardiac Transplantation	On the morning of the examination he got cold feet
Conditionals – type 2	"The Doctor Answers"	Preventive therapy for diabetes	He has a sweet tooth
Conditionals – type 3	Sentence completion	Describing drug therapy for colon cancer	He's got nothing between his ears

Unit	Contents of Text	Text-based Exercises	Extension Exercises
19	The immune system's response to infection	word check comprehension asking questions	defining having+past participle
20	Difficulties in creating new vaccines	word check comprehension nouns from verbs	actives to passives idiomatic expressions with *to look*
21	Reverse genetics	opposites prepositions	asking questions with perhaps
22	Report on smoking raises new worries	word check correcting sentences prepositions	I think so I don't think so expect/suppose
23	Training the mind but neglecting the body	word search comprehension adjectives/nouns	idiomatic expressions with *to make*
24	Fitness pays	word check sentence reconstruction nouns/adverbs prepositions	the verb *tend* there were+number revision of idioms phrasal verbs with *to make*
25	Telephoning for specialist information	mixed verbal forms	revision of phrasal verbs uncountable nouns negative/affirmative interrogatives

Grammar Point	Writing	Speaking	Idioms
Variations of conditionals	Describing the components of the immune system.	AIDS risk	As he was feeling very generous, he offered to foot the bill
Want+Indirect Object	AIDS: causes and symptoms	Doctor/Patient dialogue	He's got a skeleton in the cupboard
Wish+Past Tense	DNA/RNA Transcription	The human Telomere	He's got pins and needles in his feet
Used to/to be used to	Writing about the report on smoking	Transdermal Nicotine Patch Doctor/Patient dialogue	He's got eyes in the back of his head
Verb+Infinitive	Letter writing	Fighting colon and breast cancer with vitamin D	He has skin like a rhinoceros
Verb+Gerund	Fitness Questionnaire	An objective measurement of fitness	She has a big mouth!
Comment Tags	Anagrams Writing questions	Telephoning	He had to sit down as his feet were killing him

No one wants to read yesterday's news. This is especially true in the rapidly progressing medical field. Members of the medical profession able to read medical articles in English, have an advantage when it comes to keeping up-to-date with the latest breakthroughs and techniques.

Try this test. Take any medical article. Read it carefully and underline the words you do not know. The result will be interesting and unexpected. The words best understood will be the medical terms. The words which prove to be the greatest obstacle to comprehension will probably be other types: nouns, adjectives, verbs and idiomatic expressions.

It is in order to try to offer practical assistance in solving these problems that I have proposed a global approach to the subject. The student will find his reading skills improved through vocabulary explanations, comprehension exercises, the explanation and use of phrasal verbs and idiomatic expressions. Not only will the student find exercises designed to improve his writing skills but also exercises which will give him practice in speaking.

Each of the 25 Units is based on a specific medical article. The exercises that make up the unit are based on the vocabulary and language structures found in the article.

Text-Based Exercises help to extend the student's vocabulary and assist in the comprehension of the text.

Extension Exercises develop the expressions and language structures found in the text.

The Grammar Point is not intended to be exhaustive. It is a grammar revision with "check-up" exercises intended to give further practice in the use of the particular rule or structure.

Writing exercises are of various types. Often, the student will be asked to put into his own words the information he has read in the article and use the vocabulary he has studied.

Speaking exercises are often dialogues, interviews or presentation of information. The students will usually work in pairs or groups.

Memory Tests are to be completed at the end of every unit.

Check-Up is a global approach to English through medical readings suitable for medical students, doctors and other members of the medical profession. The subject matter has been chosen bearing in mind recent breakthroughs and the present continuing research in the medical field.

I hope the students who use *Check-Up* will find it both interesting and enjoyable.

Yet another book about Medical English: so what?

Well, to put a simple answer bluntly: we ought to have an ever-increasing command of English because the latter is fast becoming *the* international language of science. I should like to include research and development and teaching in my statement, too. The consequences of these developments are clearly visible in the natural sciences and in medicine. Thus, all the leading journals – such as NATURE, NATURE GENETICS, CELL, THE JOURNAL OF CLINICAL INVESTIGATION, THE AMERICAN JOURNAL OF PHYSIOLOGY, THE NEW ENGLAND JOURNAL OF MEDICINE, to quote only a rudimentary few – are in English. Nowadays anyone needing a review of the most recent information in a given field will doubtless resort to a computerized literature search that understands but one language: English. Finally, our medical students go abroad by the hundreds; they will have to be able to communicate orally and to read textbooks in those countries, and this will most often be accomplished in English. Taken together it is fair to say that English is now a "must" (to steal an ad slogan from Cartier) for anyone interested in the essentials of present science and/or medicine.

It is for these very reasons that Georg Thieme Verlag is to be commended for placing "Check-Up" within easy reach of German physicians, students and scientists. "Check-Up" is an inspiring compilation of well-written recent articles taken from several corners of modern medicine. It is of course possible to criticize the present selection as being "trendy"; but then any selection will always be subject to some kind of selection bias. It could also be said about the didactic chapters of "Check-Up" that they were too reminiscent of how we were taught at age 15 in grammar school – at least this is how I feel about them. True also that "English through Medical Readings" is necessarily focused on articles about some more abstract issues in medicine rather than on lively case presentations, case histories or case discussions. Therefore it covers only a certain albeit important aspect of medical English. However, let us be realistic: there is only so much any book can do.

The presentations in "Check-Up" certainly make for pleasant study. Anyone wishing to improve his or her reading skills in English will no doubt enjoy "Check-Up" as a useful assist to his or her purposes.

Dresden, März 1994

Peter Gross, Prof. Dr. med.,
Schwerpunktprofessor für Nephrologie
Universitätsklinikum Carl Gustav Carus

CONTENTS

Unit

Spelling differences

American	*British*
anemia	anaemia
anesthesia	anaesthesia
behavior	behaviour
catalog	catalogue
center	centre
color	colour
favorably	favourably
favorite	favourite
fiber	fibre
harbor	harbour
labor	labour
meter	metre
a mold	a mould
neighbors	neighbours
program	programme
traveled	travelled

Abbreviations

coll.	colloquial
etc.	etcetera
esp.	especially
fig.	figurative
i.e.	that is
inf.	informal
n.	noun
pl.	plural
p.p.	past participle
p.t.	past tense
sl.	slang

UNIT 1

Percutaneous Automated Diskectomy

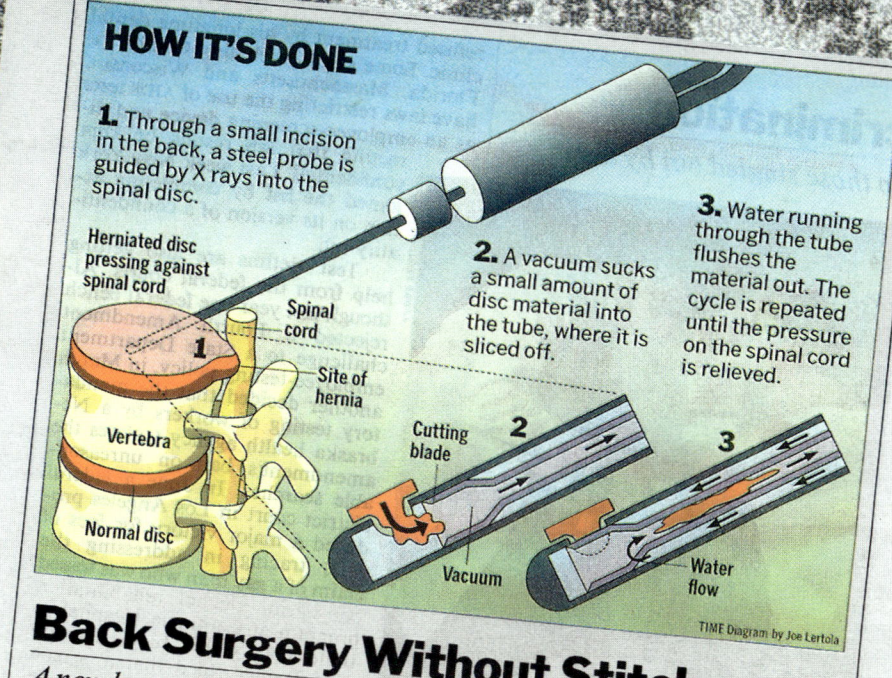

HOW IT'S DONE

1. Through a small incision in the back, a steel probe is guided by X rays into the spinal disc.

Herniated disc pressing against spinal cord

Spinal cord

Vertebra

Normal disc

Site of hernia

Cutting blade

Vacuum

2. A vacuum sucks a small amount of disc material into the tube, where it is sliced off.

3. Water running through the tube flushes the material out. The cycle is repeated until the pressure on the spinal cord is relieved.

Water flow

TIME Diagram by Joe Lertola

Back Surgery Without Stitches

A novel operation for ruptured disks saves patients money and pain

Lower back pain, as prevalent as the common cold, is the price human beings pay for walking upright. In most cases, simple treatments like bed rest, exercise and pain-killers bring relief. But many sufferers are not so lucky. If one or more of their spinal disks—pulpy masses that cushion pairs of vertebrae—rupture and press on nerve roots, the pain that radiates from the back and down the legs can be excruciating and disabling. For many the only treatment is surgical removal of part of the blown disk, a major operation called a laminectomy that requires general anesthesia, the dissection of muscle and removal of bone.

Now there is a new and far less traumatic option for some disk patients. Known as percutaneous automated diskectomy, it is an outpatient procedure performed under local anesthesia through a tiny (2 mm long) incision in the back. Developed by Radiologist Gary Onik and Neurosurgeon Joseph Maroon of Allegheny General Hospital in Pittsburgh, the operation breezed through its clinical trials and has been performed on some 15,000 patients around the country—at approximately one-third the cost of conventional surgery.

The relatively simple operation is similar to arthroscopic surgery, in which damaged tissue is removed, typically from knee joints, through a hollow tube. In the diskectomy technique, a stainless-steel tube, guided by X ray, is slipped into the incision until the tip of the instrument rests against the disk. Next the surgeon threads a combination cutting-suction device the diameter of a pencil lead down the cannula, pushes it gently into the center of the disk and steps on a floor pedal. Suction draws disk material, which has the texture of crab meat, into a porthole near the probe's tip. There it is neatly sliced off with a tiny pneumatically driven guillotine-like blade that slides back and forth. After each cut, the probe is flushed of disk tissue, which is sucked out and collected in a bottle.

The procedure usually takes less than an hour and requires no stitches. Patients walk out of the hospital with only a Band-Aid over the incision. Recalls Sheila Aronoff, who had the surgery at Allegheny General last year: "I could feel the pain start to leave while I was in the recovery room. Except for those whose jobs require physical labor, the vast majority of patients are back at work in a week or two. Discomfort is rare: most patients need only a non-narcotic analgesic, if anything. Says Onik: "The biggest problem is keeping them from doing too much too soon because they feel so much better." Another important advantage is that the operation can be repeated or followed by a laminectomy if necessary. But when the more drastic operation is performed first, reoperation is much more difficult because of the scar tissue and adhesions that often form around the nerve roots, causing chronic pain and loss of flexibility.

Despite its high marks, the new operation can be less successful than a laminectomy and is not for everyone. Onik says it works only for a "contained" rupture—a disk that has become distended but has not yet broken through the fibers that hold its contents in place. Moreover, 12% to 15% of Onik's patients require a second operation, usually a laminectomy, because X rays failed to reveal that the tissue had already burst out of the disk and lodged against a nerve. An additional 10% experience only partial relief but are not in enough pain to want another operation.

Still, Onik and others who perform the minisurgery are enthusiastic about its proven success in nearly four out of five cases. "It's made it possible for me to reduce the number of laminectomies I do by 70%," observes Nashville Back Specialist G. William Davis, who claims that he has done more of the new operations than any other surgeon. "The savings in pain and money are enormous."

—By John Langone.

disk = disc

Reported by Suzanne Wymelenberg/Boston

VOCABULARY

Study the meaning of the following words and expressions as used in the text. The number refers to the line where the word first appears.

3 upright
  - erect
7 pulpy
  - of or like pulp
8 to cushion
  - to protect with soft material
11 excruciating
  - extremely painful
13 blown (fig.)
  - destroyed
22 tiny
  - small
26 breezed (coll.)
  - passed through without difficulty
26 a trial
  - a test
27 some
  - considerable
34 hollow
  - having the interior empty
39 to thread
  - to pass cautiously through
39 a device
  - a mechanical tool
48 to flush
  - to clean by a rush of water
53 a Band Aid
  - a small, waterproof sticking plaster
84 to fail
  - to be unsuccessful
86 to lodge
  - to attach firmly
88 to be in pain
  - to have pain

TEXT BASED EXERCISES

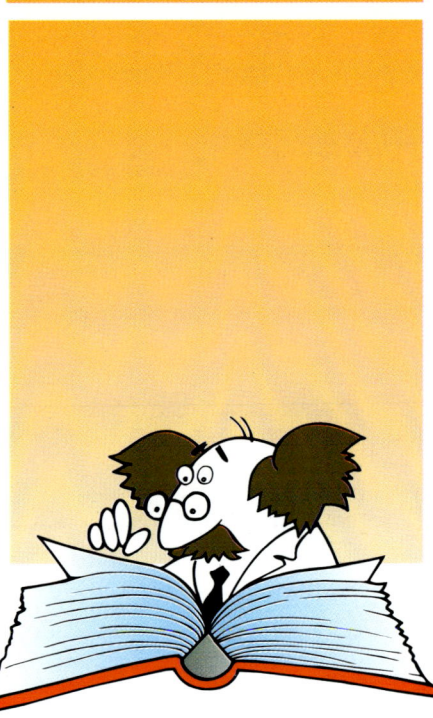

1 WORD CHECK

Explain what you understand by the following expressions.

title stitches.
  5 pain-killers.
 20 an outpatient procedure
 26 clinical trials.
 29 conventional surgery.
 45 a probe.
 57 recovery room.
 71 scar tissue.
 73 chronic pain.

2 COMPREHENSION

Answer the following questions.

1 In the writer's opinion, what is the price human beings pay for walking upright?
2 What are the treatments used to solve the problem for the majority of sufferers?
3 What causes the severe pain which passes from the back down the legs?
4 What is the difference between a laminectomy and a percutaneous automated diskectomy?
5 How does the cost of the new treatment compare with the cost of conventional surgery?
6 What is arthroscopic surgery?
7 In the diskectomy technique, how far into the incision is the tube inserted?
8 What are the benefits of the new procedure?
9 In doctor Onik's opinion, what mistake do patients often make because they find themselves free of pain after the operation?
10 Why is it more difficult to perform the new operation, if a laminectomy is first performed?
11 What does Onik mean when he says that the new operation is not for everyone?
12 Why do 12-15% of Onik's patients require a second operation?

3 REPHRASING

Rewrite the following sentences, replacing the words *in italics*, with words or expressions from the text which have the same meaning.

e.g. But many *people who suffer* are not so lucky.
But many *sufferers* are not so lucky. (line 6)

1 Now there is a new and far less *distressing* option for some disk patients.
2 The procedure is performed using *anesthesia only on the area being operated*.
3 *A cut* is made in the back.
4 The procedure has been *carried out* on some 15,000 patients.
5 It is neatly sliced off with a tiny pneumatically driven *blade like a guillotine*.
6 The vast majority of patients *return to work* in a week or two.
7 It *is successful* only for a "contained" rupture.
8 Moreover, 12% to 15% of Onik's patients require a second operation because X rays *were unsuccessful in revealing* that the tissue had already burst out of the disk.
9 An additional 10% experience *some relief but not complete relief*.
10 Back specialist G. William Davis, claims he has done more of the new operations than any other *doctor who performs surgery*.

4 NOUNS

Fill in the blanks with one of the following *nouns*.

- ✔ treatments
- ✔ incision
- ✔ surgery
- ✔ operation
- ✔ technique
- ✔ instrument
- ✔ procedure
- ✔ tissue
- ✔ X ray
- ✔ relief
- ✔ stitches
- ✔ cases
- ✔ joints
- ✔ probe

1 The .... usually takes less than an hour and requires no ....
2 The relatively simple .... is similar to arthroscopic ...., in which damaged .... is removed, typically from knee ...., through a hollow tube.
3 In most .... simple .... like bed rest, exercise and pain-killers bring ....
4 In the diskectomy ...., a stainless-steel tube, guided by ...., is slipped into the .... until the tip of the .... rests against the disk.

5 After each cut, the .... is flushed of disk tissue, which is sucked out and collected in a bottle.

5 PREPOSITIONS

Fill in the blanks with a suitable *preposition*.

1 Percutaneous automated diskectomy is performed .... local anesthesia.
2 A tiny incision is made .... the back.
3 The operation has been performed .... some 15,000 patients.
4 A stainless-steel tube is slipped .... the incision.
5 The surgeon threads a combination cutting-suction device .... the cannula.
6 He pushes it gently .... the center .... the disk and steps .... a floor pedal.
7 Scar tissue and adhesions often form .... the nerve roots.
8 It works only .... a disk that has become distended but has not yet broken .... the fibers.
9 X rays failed to reveal that the tissue had already burst out .... the disk and lodged .... a nerve.
10 The back specialist reduced the number .... laminectomies he does .... 70%.

EXTENSION EXERCISES

6 COMPOUND WORDS

Make similar *compound words* that correspond to the following descriptions.
e.g. A blade that looks like a guillotine; a guillotine-like blade.

a An object that is shaped like a heart.
b An analgesic that is not a narcotic.
c A device that saves labour.
d A drug that kills pain.
e A disease that threatens life.
f An action that is like a pump.
g An effect that will only be seen over a long term.
h Foods that are rich in calcium.

7 OPPOSITES

The opposite of *successful* is *unsuccessful*. Give *the opposite* of the following words.

lower	advantage
lucky	partial
majority	enthusiastic
usual	reduce
comfort	success

8 PREFIXES WITH NOUNS

When the prefix *re* is added, *operation* (69) becomes *reoperation*. Give the nouns formed with the

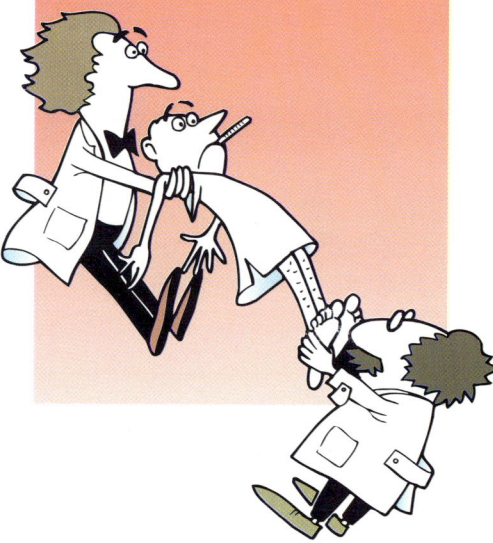

words below when the prefix *re* is added.
e.g. conversion → reconversion.

✓ construction
✓ development
✓ investigation
✓ publication
✓ distribution
✓ formation
✓ orientation
✓ production
✓ organization
✓ insertion

9 PREFIXES WITH VERBS

Now add the prefix *re* to the following verbs. Make a sentence

with each of the newly-formed words. Use any suitable verbal form.
e.g. write → rewrite.

✓ make
✓ consider
✓ construct
✓ issue
✓ join
✓ mould
✓ double
✓ trace

10 EXPRESSIONS WITH BACK

47 *Back and forth* means repeatedly moving from one place to another and back again. Read the following descriptions which all contain the word *back*. Find the expressions below which correspond to the descriptions.

1 An issue of a periodical, or newspaper, earlier than the current one.
2 A distant isolated place, far from centres of civilization.
3 A position of little importance, power or responsibility.
4 Someone who criticizes the actions or decisions of others which do not concern him.
5 With the back where the front should be and vice versa.

a a back seat
b a back-seat driver
c a back number
d back to front
e the back of beyond.

THE FUTURE

When do I use *WILL* or *GOING TO*?

1   We use *both* will and going to, in order to express what we think will happen in the future.

e.g.   *student to friend*: "Do you think you'll pass the Histology exam?"
friend: "I must. If I don't, I'm never going to be a doctor."

In these examples *will* and *going to* are interchangeable. However, there are some occasions when only *one* form is possible.

2   *WILL*
This form is constructed with will (contracted to 'll) + the infinitive without to.
We use will, when we *decide to do something at the time of speaking*. The speaker has not decided before.

e.g.   *doctor to nurse*: "Nurse, I need some bandages."
nurse: "I'll get them immediately."

3   *GOING TO*
This form is constructed with the Present Continuous of the verb to go + the infinitive with to.

We use going to when we have *already decided to do something*. The action has

GRAMMAR POINT

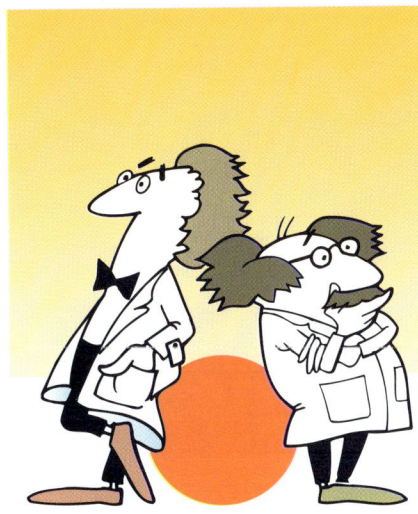

usually been planned or prepared.

e.g.   I'm going to be a doctor.

This form can express the subject's *intention*.

e.g.   I'm going to graduate next year.

It can also be used to make a *prediction*.

e.g.   If you don't hurry, you're going to be late.

11   GRAMMAR CHECK

Read the sentences below. *Offer to help.* Use the first person singular in the contracted form (I'll). Use a suitable verb and an object pronoun.

e.g.   *A*: My car's broken down
B: I'll fix it.

1   The telephone's ringing.
2   I can't find the case notes.
3   Mike wants to learn to drive.
4   She doesn't understand the lesson.
5   We haven't got time to visit Mary.
6   I'd like a cup of tea.
7   He needs some help.
8   They must be told.

12   GRAMMAR CHECK

Answer the following questions using the *going to* form. Use the word or words in brackets to answer the question. Begin each answer with "No".

e.g.   *A*: Is he going to visit Oxford? (York)
B: *No, he's going to visit York.*

1   Are they going to be neurologists? (cardiologists)
2   Is he going to fail the exam? (pass)
3   Are you going to study tonight? (football)
4   Is she going to marry John? (George)
5   Are they going to be late? (on time)
6   Are you going to watch the film? (a book)
7   Is Tony going to come alone? (brother)
8   Are they going to keep their old car? (a new one)

WRITING

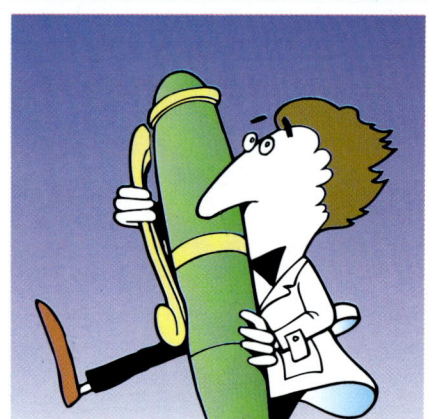

13 RECONSTRUCTION

Write *a short summary* to describe how a diskectomy is performed. The following words will help you.

outpatient - local anesthesia - incision - back - tube - guided - X-ray - combination cutting-suction device - floor pedal - suction - sliced off - guillotine-like blade - the probe - flushed - disk material - sucked out - cycle - pressure - relieved - no stitches

Notes

SPEAKING

14 DOCTOR/PATIENT DIALOGUE

Work in pairs.
Conduct the following doctor/patient dialogue. One student takes the part of the doctor, the other the patient.

A patient suffering from lower back pain, visits his G.P. The doctor asks questions and the patient describes his symptoms. The doctor suspects a herniated disk. The patient is worried that he might need a major operation. The doctor explains the possible operations for this condition.

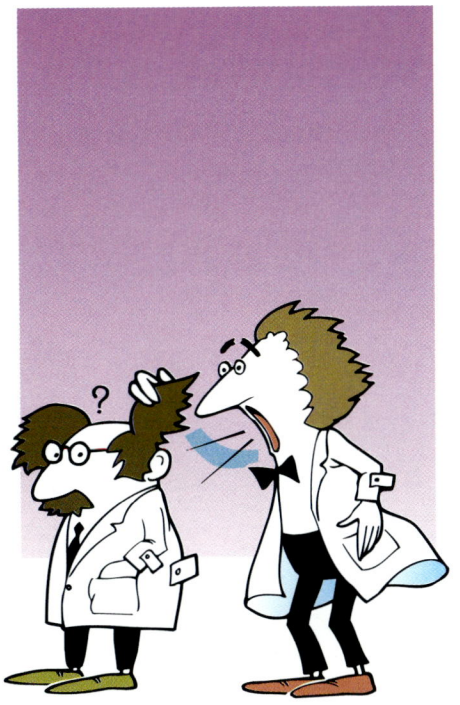

15 ASKING QUESTIONS

Group work.
One student takes the part of Sheila Aronoff, the patient who had surgery at Allegheny General last year. The other students should ask her questions about the operation from the patient's point of view.

e.g. How long after the operation were you able to return to work?

UNDERSTANDING IDIOMATIC ENGLISH

Idioms form a rich part of English at all levels. In order to communicate effectively with native speakers, an understanding of idiomatic English is important. This is not the difficult task that perhaps you always thought it was. You will find an idiomatic expression at the end of every unit. Look at the illustration, but don't be deceived. The illustration often depicts the literal and not the idiomatic meaning. *Explain* the meaning of the idiom. *Learn* it by heart. Then try to *remember* it and *use* it.

> The cure is worse than the disease

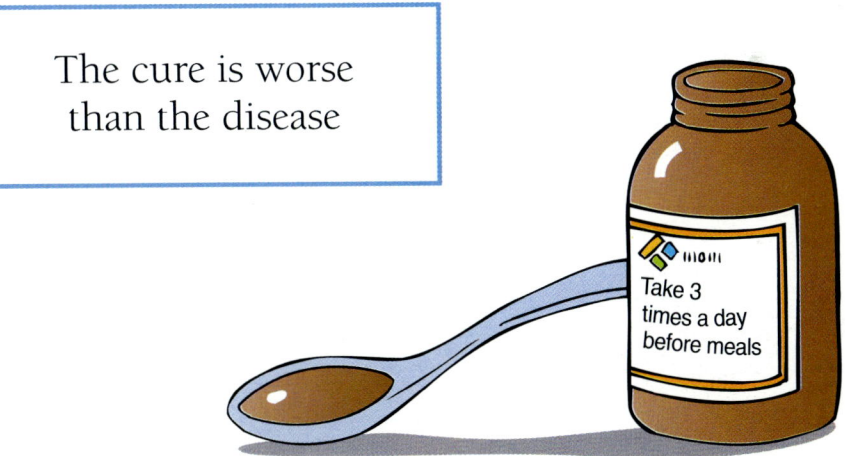

UNIT 2

Sharing materials in human genetics

Genome Project: An Experiment in Sharing

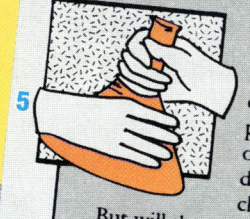

The Human Genome Project is in many respects a gigantic experiment in data sharing. Around the world, investigators are working on pieces of the same puzzle. And whether the project succeeds will depend in large measure on these investigators making available their data and materials—cell lines, probes, and clones—to their colleagues and competitors.

But will they do it voluntarily, or do they need a nudge—or a kick? While sharing may be the norm in, say, immunology or bacterial genetics, human genetics has always been intensely competitive. So should the National Institutes of Health and the Department of Energy, which both fund the genome project, promulgate rules to govern access to data and sharing of materials? And, whether they are formal or informal, what should the rules be? Some of the issues the genome project raises are brand new. Everyone agrees, for example, that materials should be available at the time of publication, but much of the information generated in the genome project will never be published, at least not in a conventional sense.

A DOE committee has drafted some guidelines, which have yet to be formally endorsed. They stipulate that data and materials must be publicly available 6 months after they are generated or characterized. But at NIH, James Watson, who heads the genome project, is shying away from setting rules. "I hope groups will form their own rules. We are very loathe to impose rules on anyone, unless we are forced to," he says.

Watson's laissez-faire attitude is not shared by Walter Gilbert of Harvard University. He thinks that rules are clearly in order, and that NIH ought to get on with drafting them. "In my view, the genome center should take a stronger position that materials should be available," he says.

But, like Watson, Maynard Olson of Washington University, a member of the NIH genome advisory committee, is leery of rules. "We are talking about such a vast amount of data and potentially so many biological reagents. If you take a rule-based approach to this venture, then following close on its heels will be a large bureaucracy to enforce it," he says. Instead, "What you would like to do is change the culture."

And that is just what is starting to happen, says Watson, who speaks of a "much greater spirit of cooperation." He points to the new collaborative plans to map chromosome 21 as evidence that the community will develop its own ways of sharing data. Because of its known role in Down syndrome and its suspected role in Alzheimer's disease, chromosome 21 has generated a vast amount of interest. Lots of groups are already hard at work constructing maps of the chromosome—first developing a series of landmarks spaced along the chromosome, and then a collection of ordered DNA fragments. But the maps all these groups generate will be essentially useless unless they pool their data and adopt a common language. For that reason, David Cox, a chromosome 21 mapper at the University of California at San Francisco, called together 30 of the major groups in early April. As Cox hoped, they pooled their data and agreed to a common set of landmarks, or DNA markers, to guide their efforts.

But that was "pretty ho-hum" compared with what happened next, says Cox. To his surprise, these highly competitive groups also agreed to a collaborative venture to obtain a complete set of overlapping fragments or clones, using the very large yeast artificial chromosome (YAC) clones developed by Maynard Olson and his colleagues at Washington University (see article on p. 956). David Patterson of the Eleanor Roosevelt Institute for Cancer Research is getting a complete set of these YAC clones and, provided NIH kicks in some funds, he will run a screening service for anyone who wants to participate. Investigators will send their DNA probes, or a bit of sequence that will identify the probe, to Patterson, who will then search the YAC library for the corresponding clone. In return, the clone "becomes the common property of the entire group," says Cox.

"There are lots of ways the plan could crash and burn," says Cox, who admits that "paranoia is still alive and well." A few people, for example, said they would not send their sequences to Patterson because he might use them for his own ends. "As if he would have time," laughs Cox. Still, Cox is optimistic: "I think it will work. The cooperation is truly remarkable. People aren't fighting to sequence the same small piece of DNA and pull out the same clone."

If the chromosome 21 plan becomes a model, Watson's hands-off approach to setting rules could be proved right—at least for mapping data.

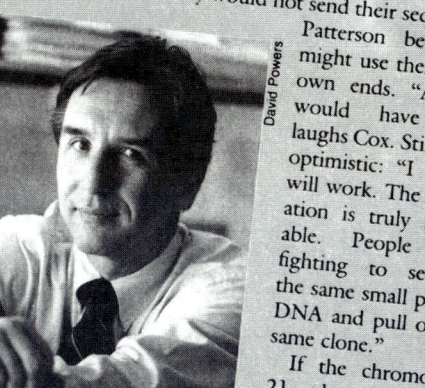

David Powers

The 21 club. *Mapper David Cox helped push plan for chromosome 21.*

But, as Watson himself concedes, establishing guidelines for sequencing data may be trickier. The issue, at bottom, is how long an investigator gets to ponder the long-sought information in private. "There is no problem about holding onto it for a reasonable time. If you have worked out the sequence, you want the fun, the pleasure, of looking at it," says Watson. But how long is reasonable? Watson has just set up a sequencing subcommittee to advise the genome center on it.

The issue is clearly contentious. "It is unacceptable to get the sequence and then immediately release it," says Craig Venter, an NIH researcher who is one of a handful of biologists embarking on large-scale sequencing—working out 5 million bases or so. It could take several years to sequence that long a stretch, and Venter thinks researchers should have another year to characterize the DNA before making the sequence public. Still others argue that they should be able to hang onto the data until they are done, period.

But some researchers regard even a year as far too long. "My view is that if government pays for it, it can perfectly well demand the sequence be deposited promptly," says Gilbert, who is on the committee Watson has established. He thinks sequence data should be made public within 3 months and suggests that such a requirement be written into grants and contracts.

The debate will likely continue for some time. But in forcing researchers to confront the issues in the first place, the genome project is already beginning to break down some of the intense competitiveness among human geneticists. ■ **LESLIE ROBERTS**

GLOSSARY OF TERMS

Anonymous DNA: a length of DNA of unknown gene content.

Chromosome bands: alternating light- or dark-staining sections along a chromosome that are visible by light microscopy after staining procedures are used.

Chromosome walk: a method of aligning pieces of DNA by consecutive hybridizations in which probes corresponding to one end of a cloned piece of DNA are used to identify the next clone in line.

Contig: a set of overlapping pieces of DNA that span an uninterrupted stretch of the genome.

Cosmid: a piece of DNA (35 to 45 kb) cloned into a vector that usually consists of *cos* sequences required for packaging the DNA into a bacteriophage, an origin of replication, and a drug resistance marker.

Genetic linkage map: a map that shows the relative position of loci on the basis of frequency of recombination events. Units are in centimorgans (cM) where, over small distances, 1 cM is equivalent to a 1% chance of recombination.

Physical map: a map in which the distances between landmarks such as clones, restriction endonuclease sites, or specific loci are expressed in kilobases.

Polymerase chain reaction (PCR): a technique that involves repeated cycles of DNA denaturation, renaturation with short lengths of DNA (primers) separated by up to 4 kb, and polymerase-mediated replication. This results in an exponential increase in the number of copies of the sequence between the primers.

Polymorphic marker: a locus at which there is normal sequence variation within the population that is inherited and occurs with a frequency of >1%.

Polytene chromosome: a giant chromosome consisting of many identical, slightly condensed strands of chromatin held together in parallel and in register.

Yeast artificial chromosome (YAC): a cloning vector in which sections of yeast chromosomes needed for initiation of DNA synthesis and stability are used to replicate large (>100 kb) pieces of DNA.

GENOME

RECENT ADVANCES IN

Chromosome	1	2	3	4	5	6	7	8	9	10	11
Number of genes											
Estimated	4150	3950	3200	3050	2900	2750	2700	2250	2200	2200	2200
Mapped	236	131	72	84	82	115	128	59	63	75	142
Disease-related	43	18	16	22	15	14	16	15	17	11	33
Number of polymorphic markers											
Total	158	99	333	148	202	165	196	88	50	91	265
PCR-based	13	15	12	14	13	12	12	11	9	4	20
Kilobases of sequence	450	558	104	181	142	471	381	167	177	158	655

This table is a depiction of the current progress on the mapping of the human genome as of 28 July, 1991. There are an estimated 3,000 megabases (Mb) of DNA sequence in the human genome, containing an estimated 50,000 to 100,000 genes. Since the publication of The Human Genome Map 1990 [*Science* 250, 262a (1990)], 359 new mapped genes and 673 new polymorphic markers have been added to the map.

The estimated number of genes is based on the estimated total number of genes in the human genome, distributed proportionally according to the relative size of each chromosome [J. C. Stephens *et al.*, *Science* 250, 237 (1990)]. The number of genes mapped is the number of genes that have been localized to the chromosome. The number of disease-related genes is based on locus entries that are referenced in V. McKusick, *Mendelian Inheritance in Man* (Johns Hopkins Univ. Press, Baltimore, MD ed. 9, 1990). Polymorphic markers include genes and anonymous DNA segments. They are useful in genetic linkage studies for the localization of genes to specific regions within a chromosome. The number of polymerase chain reaction (PCR)-based polymorphic markers is the subset of polymorphic markers that can be detected by PCR. PCR-based markers obviate the

MAPS

HUMAN GENE MAPPING

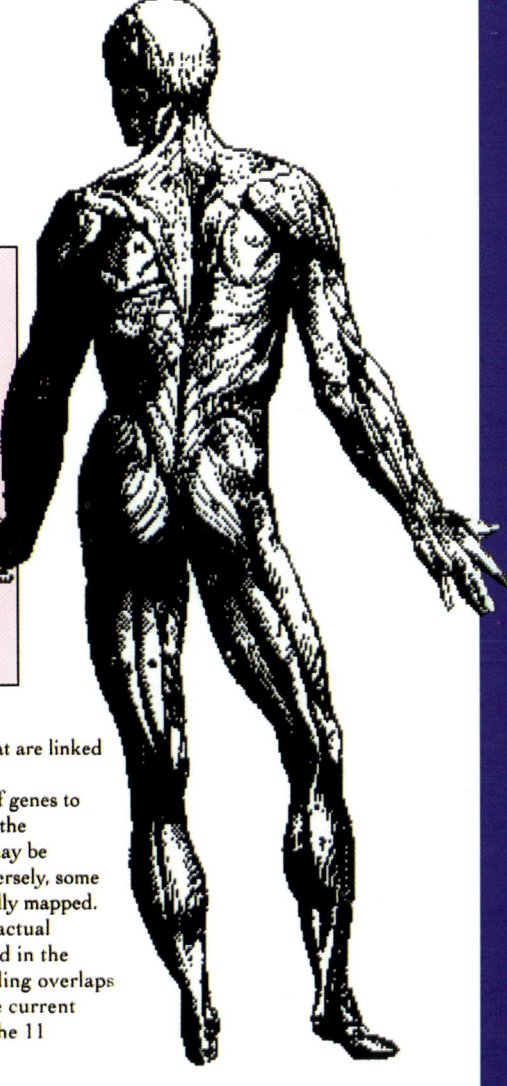

12	13	14	15	16	17	18	19	20	21	22	X	Y
2050	1800	1750	1650	1400	1350	1250	1150	1050	900	950	2350	1000
117	28	65	59	71	121	22	104	42	39	71	202	16
17	6	12	12	12	18	4	20	11	4	18	93	1
69	58	54	55	130	192	35	73	57	71	124	255	25
10	4	8	5	8	20	2	12	31	10	4	24	0
416	82	260	102	309	623	94	266	124	51	141	441	19

need to distribute cloned probes for linkage or other molecular studies. Kilobases of sequence that are linked to known loci are based on analysis of information obtained from GenBank, Los Alamos, NM.

There are some caveats to these analyses. For example, comparison of the estimated number of genes to the number of genes currently mapped to a particular chromosome may not be a precise index of the completeness of a map on a given chromosome. In some cases, large portions of a chromosome may be physically mapped, although the genetic content of those regions has yet to be established. Conversely, some chromosomes for which a large number of genes have been described are not extensively physically mapped. In addition, some chromosomes may have a higher density of genes than others. Finally, the actual amount of sequence available for each chromosome is likely to be less than the amount stated in the table, because the amounts given are based on the total amount of sequence reported, including overlaps in sequence data, rather than only the unique sequences. Further information regarding the current status of the human genome map will be presented in the Perspective (P. Pearson *et al.*) in the 11 October, 1991 issue of *Science*.

TEXT BASED EXERCISES

VOCABULARY

Study the meaning of the following words and expressions as used in the test.

9   a nudge
    - a push with the elbow
10 a kick
    - a violent forward movement of the foot
17 brand new
    - completely new
21 to draft
    - to make a preliminary sketch
25 to shy away from
    - to want to avoid
26 to loathe
    - to detest
34 leery
    - cautious
37 heel
    - posterior part of the foot
48 a landmark
    - a feature by which one can recognize a locality
50 to pool
    - to put into a common fund
71 alive and well (inf.)
    - living and active
75 ends (fig.)
    - purposes
93 trickier
    - more difficult to deal with
107 to hang onto (inf.)
    - to keep; to retain
109 far
    - much
114 a grant
    - a gift of money given to further a specified aim

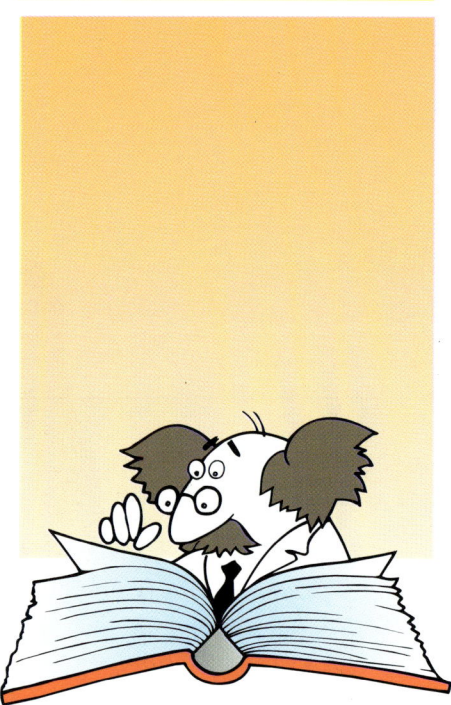

1 WORD CHECK

Explain the following expressions in your own words.

5   in large measure
9   voluntarily
36 a rule-based approach
37 close on its heels
64 provided NIH kicks in some funds
75 his own ends
89 hands-off approach
94 long-sought
103 large-scale sequencing
116 in the first place

2 COMPREHENSION

Read the following sentences and choose *the most appropriate* answer as applied to the text.

1 *The success of the Genome Project will largely depend on investigators*:
   a working on pieces of the same puzzle.
   b data sharing.
   c working in various places around the world.
2 *James Watson*:
   a is in charge of the project.
   b is the one who has drafted the guidelines.
   c advises the committee on forming rules.
3 *Walter Gilbert thinks that rules are*:
   a not necessary.
   b very necessary.
   c to be avoided.
4 *Maynard Olson believes*:
   a making rules will be closely followed by a large bureaucracy.
   b avoiding making rules will free the project from a large bureaucracy.
   c they could make rules, but it wouldn't be immediately that they would have to deal with a large bureaucracy.
5 *Chromosome 21 has generated a vast amount of interest because*:
   a it has a role in Down syndrome and Alzheimer's disease.

b it has a suspected role in Down syndrome and Alzheimer's disease.

c it has been proved that it has a role in Down syndrome and it is thought that it might have a role in Alzheimer's disease.

6 *David Patterson will:*

a ask for a screening service to be set up.

b suggest that the NIH provides funds for a screening service.

c organize a screening service if the NIH provides funds.

7 *Cox admits that the project could fail because:*

a it will not help in the treatment of paranoia.

b some people are suspicious of what Patterson is doing.

c Patterson has too little time to run the project properly.

8 *Cox thinks that the project will work because the cooperation is:*

a excellent.

b good enough.

c sincere.

9 *The fundamental issue facing sequencing data is:*

a how long the investigator should keep the information to himself.

b how long the investigator should spend on searching for the information.

c if the investigator should be allowed to keep the information to himself.

10 *The sequencing data issue is:*

a totally unacceptable.

b clearly impractical.

c causing disagreement.

3 SENTENCE BUILDING

Make *complete sentences* with one phrase from each of the three columns. Refer back to the text, if necessary.

1	2	3
Around the world, investigators	argue	a complete set of these YAC clones
A DOE committee	ought to get on with	a sequencing subcommittee to advise the genome center on it
Watson	is getting	rules on anyone, unless we are forced to
Still others	has drafted	pieces of the same puzzle
We are very loathe to	are working on	that they should be able to hang onto the data until they are done, period
David Patterson of the Eleonor Roosevelt Institute for Cancer Research	has just set up	some guidelines
He thinks that rules are clearly in order and that the NIH	impose	drafting them

4

A BIT OF (66) tells us that a small piece or portion of the sequence can be sent. It is not necessary to send all of it.

Fill in the blanks with the words and expressions below as used in the text.

✔ some
✔ the entire group
✔ lots of groups
✔ a common set
✔ pieces
✔ a vast amount

a Investigators are working on .... of the same puzzle.

b They pooled their data and agreed to .... of landmarks.

c Chromosome 21 has generated .... of interest.

d In return, the clone becomes the common property of ....

e .... are already hard at work.

f The Genome Project is already beginning to break down .... of the intense competitiveness among human geneticists.

5

Fill in the blanks with the words below.

- ✔ role
- ✔ view
- ✔ interest
- ✔ issues
- ✔ guidelines
- ✔ debate
- ✔ approach
- ✔ sequence
- ✔ experiment
- ✔ venture

1 Some of the .... the Genome Project raises are brand new.
2 These highly competitive groups also agreed to a collaborative ....
3 The .... will likely continue for some time.
4 The Human Genome Project is a gigantic .... in data sharing.
5 Watson's hands-off .... to setting rules could be proved right.
6 A DOE committee has drafted some ....
7 Because of its known .... in Down syndrome and its suspected .... in Alzheimer's disease, chromosome 21 has generated a vast amount of ....
8 My .... is that if government pays for it, it can perfectly well demand the .... be deposited properly.

6   ADVERBS

Fill in the blanks with the *adverbs* below as used in the text.

- ✔ promptly
- ✔ essentially
- ✔ perfectly
- ✔ highly
- ✔ intensely
- ✔ clearly
- ✔ truly
- ✔ publicly

a Human genetics has always been .... competitive.
b They stipulate that data and materials must be .... available 6 months after they are generated or characterized.
c But the maps all these groups generate will be .... useless unless they pool their data and adopt a common language.
d To his surprise, these .... competitive groups also agreed to a collaborative venture to obtain a complete set of overlapping fragments or clones.
e The cooperation is .... remarkable.
f The issue is .... contentious.
g "My view is that if government pays for it, it can .... well demand the sequence be deposited ....," says Gilbert.

7   PREFIXES

Join the words in column B to their respective prefixes in column A in order to form complete words as used in the text.

A	B
in	front
in	committee
co	tense
con	formal
sub	searchers
con	acceptable
in	agents
re	operation
re	tracts

EXTENSION EXERCISES

8 SHOULD/ OUGHT TO

Change the following sentences. Replace *SHOULD* by *OUGHT TO*.

e.g. He *should* study.
He *ought to* study.

1 Materials should be available at the time of publication.
2 In my view, the genome center should take a stronger position.
3 Venter thinks researchers should have another year to characterize the DNA before making the sequence public.
4 Still others argue that they should be able to hang onto the data until they are done.
5 He thinks sequence data should be made public within 3 months.

9 SHOULDN'T

Use *should not* (shouldn't) to comment on the following statements. Change the form of the verb *in italics*. Make any other changes necessary.

e.g. Watson *is* leery of rules.
Watson *shouldn't be* leery of rules.

a A DOE committee *has drafted* some guidelines.
b David Cox *called* together 30

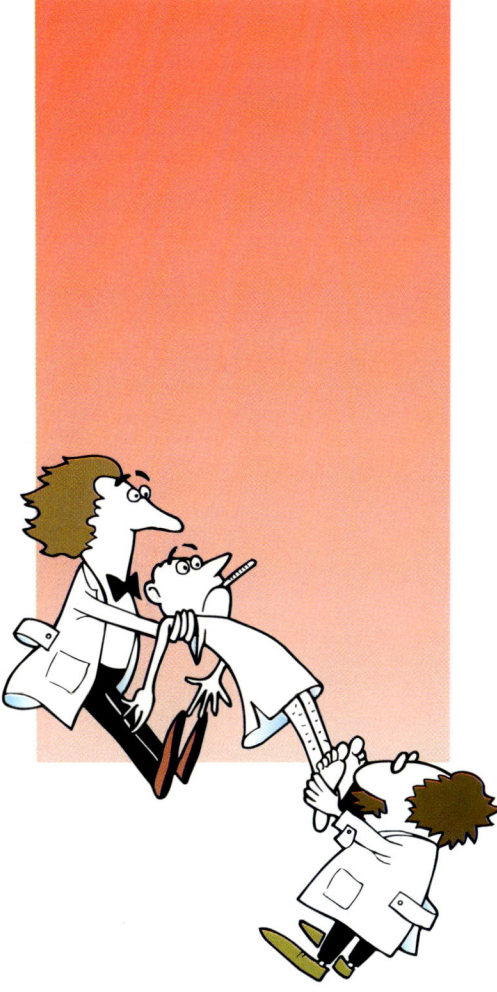

of the major groups early in April.
c David Patterson *is getting* a complete set of these YAC clones.
d The clone *becomes* the property of the entire group.
e He *suggests* that such a

requirement be written into grants and contracts.
f The community *will develop* its own ways of sharing data.
g They *pooled* their data.

10

Some *nouns* end in "FUL".

e.g. 102 a *handful* of biologists

A handful means as much as the hand can hold, a small amount.

Fill in the blanks using each of the words only once.

✓ spoonful	✓ plateful
✓ armful	✓ fistful
✓ mouthful	✓ glassful
✓ cupful	✓ bowlful

1 When I saw her, she was carrying an.......................... of books.
2 A....................... of sugar helps the medicine go down.
3 She drinks a .... of tea for breakfast.
4 Mario eats a .... of spaghetti for lunch every day.
5 Her husband took a .... of her cake and realized that she had forgotten to add the sugar.

6 A .... of dollars.
7 The dog drank a .... of water.
8 She wasn't used to drinking wine. After her first .... she felt very light-headed.

PHRASAL VERBS

Phrasal verbs are very common in English. In fact, they are much used.

A PHRASAL (or composite) verb, is a verb followed by a *preposition* or an *adverb*. The meaning of the verb changes according to the preposition or adverb used.

e.g.   *To set up*

64 He will *run* a screening service for anyone who wants to participate.

To set up has a different meaning from *to set off*, *to set down* and *to set aside*.

Here are some guidelines to help you learn these verbs.

1 Don't be afraid of them. With practice in their use, they will help you to a better understanding of the written and spoken English of native speakers.
2 Study the verbs carefully. Compare them and try to understand the different meanings.
3 Try to recognize them in written and spoken English.
4 Try to use them.

11 PHRASAL VERBS WITH RUN

64 He will *run* a screening service. In this sentence run means to organize or operate.

Study the meanings of the verbs below. They are all formed with the verb to RUN.

Phrasal verb	Meaning
to run down (1)	to speak ill of someone
to run down (2)	discharged (clocks etc.)
to be run down	to be in poor health after an illness etc.
to run into	to collide with a vehicle
to run into/across	to meet someone accidentally
to run out of	to have nothing left; to have used up a supply
to run over (1)	overflow
(2)	drive over accidentally
(3)	check; revise
to run up against	to meet with difficulties

Complete the following sentences using the above verbs in an appropriate form. Add any additional words necessary.

1 The tin is empty. I have ....
2 Jack was in hospital for six weeks. He's at home now but he's very ....
3 If you fill the glass too much, the liquid will ....
4 Peter doesn't like his colleague. He is always ....

5 I was reversing out of the hospital car park when ....
6 She didn't see the old man crossing the road until he was in front of her car. She just managed to avoid ....
7 I've got a lot of notes to read for my exam tomorrow. I'll have to stay at home tonight and ....
8 I hadn't seen Bill Scott for years. I was at the conference in Milan last week when I ....
9 I got into my car and turned on the ignition. The car didn't start. The batteries were ....
10 The new procedure is very easy. I don't expect we'll ....

THE FUTURE

Using the Present Continuous

The Present Continuous Tense is formed with the Present Tense of the verb to be + the present participle:

e.g. I *am* arriving tomorrow.

The Present Continuous can express a definite arrangement in the *near future.*
However, *the time must be mentioned or understood* so as not to be confused with the present.

GRAMMAR POINT

12 GRAMMAR CHECK

Put the verbs in brackets into the appropriate form of the *Present Continuous.*

1 He (take) his medical exams in June.
2 My brother (come) out of hospital tomorrow.
3 The teacher is ill. He (not give) the Chemistry lecture this afternoon.
4 Mr. Carter (have) his operation at four o'clock.
5 David (start) a new job in the Casualty Department next week.
6 The doctors (meet) to discuss Mr. Baxter's case later today.
7 I (go) to the dentist on Monday.
8 I want to finish early today as I (have) lunch with my wife at Mario's.
9 "You (do) anything tomorrow evening?"
"Yes, I (study) for my examinations."
10 Doctor Wallace (expect) an important telephone call at half past five.

13 GRAMMAR CHECK

Ask questions about the future using *the Present Continuous* and the word *when.*

e.g. He is leaving on Wednesday.

　　　When is he leaving?

1 Their findings are being published next week.
2 They are drafting the guidelines tomorrow.
3 He is meeting the major groups in April.
4 We are sending our DNA probes next week.
5 The debate is taking place tonight.
6 The project is starting in a few weeks.
7 The issue is being discussed on Monday.

WRITING

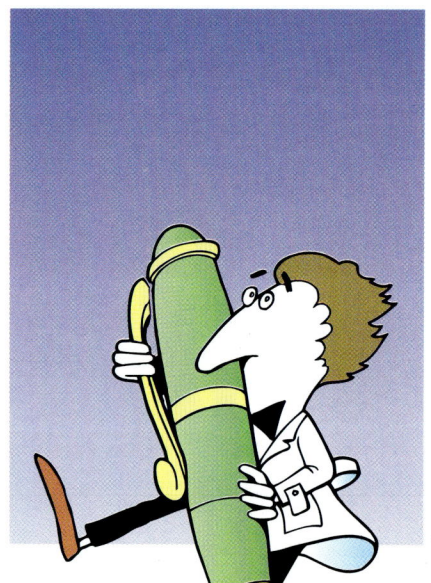

14 PARAGRAPH RECONSTRUCTION

Write three paragraphs under the headings given. The paragraphs should consist of complete sentences formed from the words below.

THE HUMAN
GENOME PROJECT

- data sharing.
- on the same pieces of puzzle.
- making available their data.
- voluntarily/ a nudge.

- human genetics/ intensely competitive.

RULES

- NIH/DOE/ fund the Genome/ rules.
- issues/ brand new.
- DOE/ guidelines.
- James Watson/ shy away from.
- Walter Gilbert/ rules in order.

EVIDENCE OF COOPERATION

- Watson/ collaborative plans to map chromosome 21.
- essentially useless unless they pool.

Notes

SPEAKING

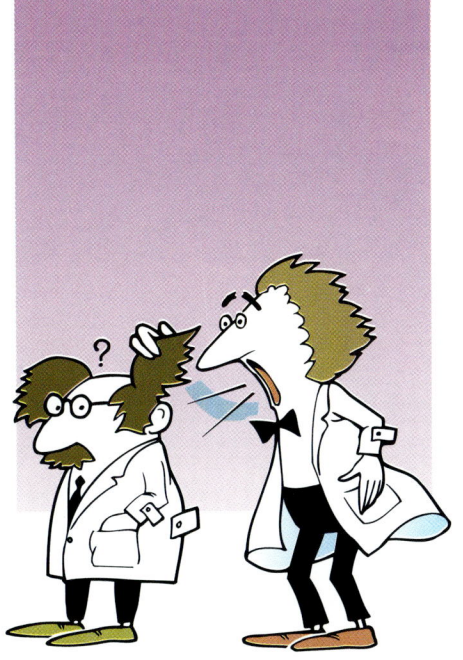

15 DATA SHARING

Group work.
You are attending the meeting called by the chromosome 21 mapper, David Cox, to discuss the issues of pooling data and adopting a common language. One student takes the part of Cox. The other students should put forward some of the different opinions held by the other researchers and interested parties.

e.g.- Formal/informal rules.

- The genome center should/shouldn't take a stronger position
- Government has/hasn't the right to demand the sequences be deposited

16 INTERVIEW

Group work.
After the meeting called by David Cox, a press conference is held. One student takes the part of Cox. The other students take the parts of journalists who write for scientific magazines. They should ask key questions.

e.g. Do you think the project will succeed?
Will the guidelines drafted by the DOE committee be formally endorsed?
Do you think that James Watson is right in shying away from setting rules?

UNDERSTANDING IDIOMATIC ENGLISH

Explain the idiom.

His patients loved him for his bedside manner

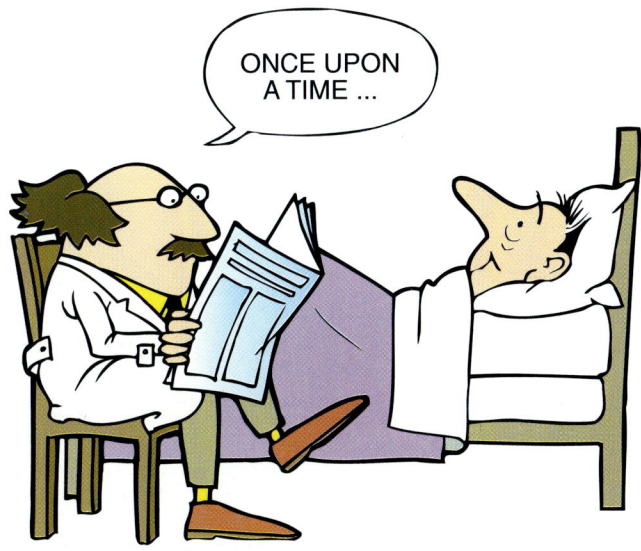

ONCE UPON A TIME ...

UNIT 3

A device that can save cardiac patients

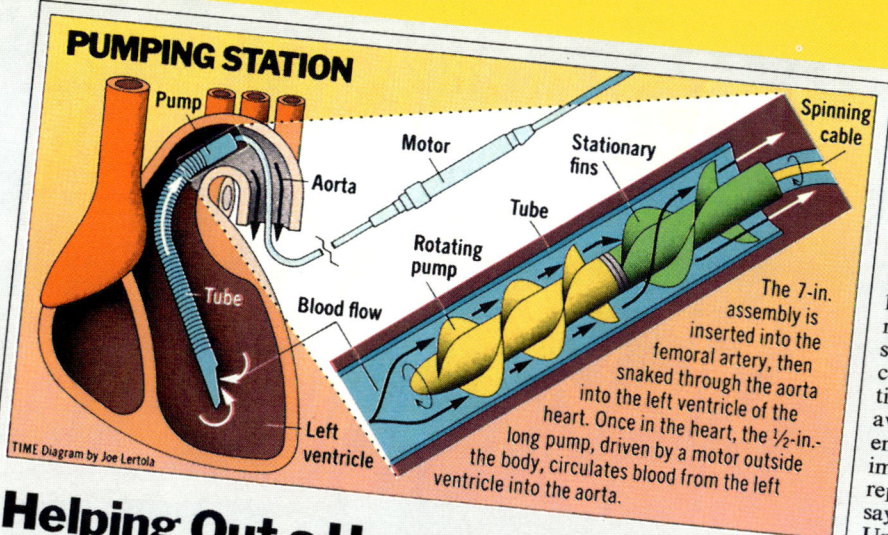

PUMPING STATION

Pump

Motor

Aorta

Stationary fins

Tube

Spinning cable

Rotating pump

Tube

Blood flow

Left ventricle

TIME Diagram by Joe Lertola

The 7-in. assembly is inserted into the femoral artery, then snaked through the aorta into the left ventricle of the heart. Once in the heart, the ½-in.-long pump, driven by a motor outside the body, circulates blood from the left ventricle into the aorta.

Helping Out a Heart in Texas

Dramatic debut for a device that can save cardiac patients

Doctors have long suspected that the heart could heal itself even when damaged by a heart attack or during surgery—if only there were a way to let it rest. For more than 20 years, researchers have been trying to develop implantable pumps that temporarily take over part of the heart's job. Some half a dozen such devices are now available, most of them experimental, bulky and requiring risky open-heart surgery. But at a medical conference last week in Reno, O. Howard Frazier, director of the transplant program at the Texas Heart Institute in Houston, described the first successful use of a radically different newcomer. It is a tiny, disposable pump that can handle most of the heart's workload and that can be inserted in 20 minutes without major surgery.

Frazier first tried the device last month on a patient who was near death after a heart transplant. Working from an incision in the patient's groin, the surgeon threaded a 7-in. assembly made of a tube connected to a miniature, propeller-like pump through the patient's arteries and into his left ventricle, the main pumping chamber of the heart. The stainless-steel pump, driven by a slender cable linked to a motor outside the body, took on the work of the ailing ventricle. Spinning 25,000 times a minute—about four times as fast as a sports-car engine—the pump drew a steady stream of blood out of the chamber and into the aorta, the main vessel carrying blood to the body. Afterward, Frazier exulted, "This is really an astonishing device."

Within days, the patient's condition improved, and his transplanted heart began to beat strongly on its own. The dramatic case marked the debut of the Hemopump, an experimental device just ¼ in. wide and ½ in. long, manufactured by Nimbus Medical Inc., of Rancho Cordova, Calif. Although a second patient given the pump died, the cause was apparently unrelated to the device.

Allan Lansing, director of Humana Heart Institute International in Louisville, expects to begin further tests soon on the Hemopump, which was approved for human trials by the Food and Drug Administration last March. "I'm impressed," says Lansing. "If this pump does work, it could be of enormous benefit to many patients." Eventually, he says, it could be available in coronary-care units and emergency rooms to treat heart attacks immediately after they occur. "It won't replace anything that is now available," says Heart Surgeon Jack Copeland of the University of Arizona Health Sciences Center in Tucson. "But it will add a dimension to what we can do for patients."

The pump's inventor, Richard Wampler, 39, a California physician, took his inspiration from pumps he saw in deep wells ten years ago in Egypt. The pump's continuous flow of blood and the resulting continuous spinning motion and the resulting continuous flow of blood from the heart represent a departure from the natural pulsating action that most other devices try to mimic. Some researchers at first feared that the whirling blades would destroy blood cells and that the body would be unable to tolerate the nonpulsating blood flow. So far, the problem has not materialized. Another potential drawback: small as the pump is, it may be too large to use in women and children or in patients with narrowed arteries.

If the device works in future tests, Wampler and Frazier estimate, it might eventually be used in as many as 150,000 people a year. With a $3,000 price tag, the whirring little pump may be the ultimate rarity in medical technology: a bargain.   —By Denise Grady.

Reported by Andrea Dorfman/New York and Richard Woodbury/Houston

VOCABULARY

Study the meaning of the following words and expressions as used in the text.

2   to heal
    - to cure
7   to take over
    - to assume
8   half a dozen
    - six
10 bulky
    - taking up a lot of space
10 risky
    - dangerous
15 newcomer
    - one who has just arrived
17 to handle
    - to assume; to take on
23 groin
    - meeting-point of abdomen and thigh
29 slender
    - thin
29 a cable
    - an insulated conductor for conveying energy
29 to link
    - to join; to connect
31 to ail
    - sick, suffering from a disease
31 to spin
    - to turn rapidly round and round
75 to whirl
    - to rotate rapidly
78 so far
    - until now
79 a drawback
    - a disadvantage

TEXT BASED EXERCISES

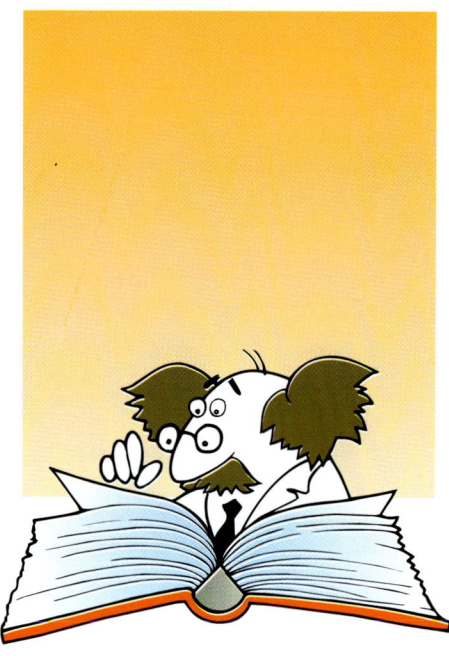

1   WORD SEARCH

Find *a word or expression* from the text which has the following meaning.

a   A cardiac arrest.
b   An operation which transfers an organ from a doner to a recipient.
c   An amazing tool.
d   A heart that has been transplanted.
e   A tiny disposable device that can assume the heart's workload.
f   Hospital departments where coronary cases are treated.
g   The continuous movement of blood through the body.
h   Cutting tools that turn rapidly.
i   Arteries which have become narrow.
j   A ticket that shows the cost.

2   COMPREHENSION

Read the following statements. Say whether they are *TRUE* or *FALSE*. Correct the false statements.

1   The Hemopump will permanently take over part of the heart's job.
2   The new device is very different from other such devices presently available.
3   The device drew blood out of the left ventricle.
4   It took a long time for the patient's condition to improve.
5   The Hemopump is rather large.
6   If the pump does work, it will greatly help many patients.
7   Most other devices try to copy the natural pulsating action of the heart.
8   Some researchers were convinced that the whirling blades would destroy blood cells and that the body would be unable to tolerate the nonpulsating blood flow.
9   The pump may be too small to use in women and children.
10 The device is very costly.

3 NOUNS FROM VERBS

Study this sentence.

1 Doctors have long *suspected* that the heart could heal itself even when damaged by a heart attack or during surgery - if only there were a way to let it rest.

Suspected is the past participle of the verb *to suspect*.

Suspicion is the noun formed from this verb.

Give *nouns* related to the verbs below.

Verb	Noun
to risk	
to bleed	
to insert	
to occur	
to treat	
to devise	
to save	
to test	
to improve	
to tolerate	
to invent	
to beat	

EXTENSION EXERCISES

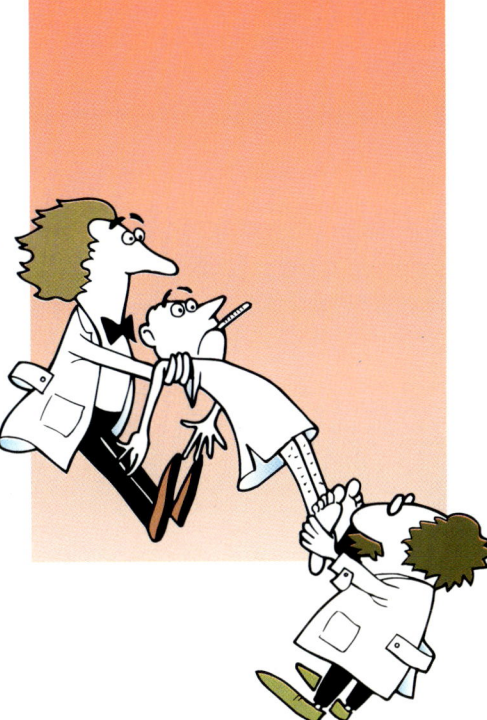

4 VERBS

The cardiac sphincter *prevents* the backflow of blood.

The following verbs describe different actions. Choose the appropriate verb, *in the correct form*, to complete the sentences.

✓ support

✓ rebuild

✓ emulsify

✓ receive

✓ reconvert

✓ close

✓ absorb

✓ open

✓ contract

✓ increase

✓ contain

✓ measure

1 A sphygmomanometer .... the force of the blood within the arterial walls.
2 After physical exercise, the pulse rate ....
3 The left auricle .... blood from the lungs.
4 Proteins .... tissues.
5 The liver .... some of its glycogen when necessary.
6 Bile .... fats.
7 Villi .... digested proteins and sugars.
8 Valves .... to allow blood to be pumped from the left auricle into the left ventricle then .... to prevent the backflow of blood

when the left ventricle
....

9 The red corpuscles ....
   an iron compound known as
   haemoglobin.

10 The back muscles ....
   the spine.

5 IRREGULAR VERBS

34 The pump *drew* a steady
   stream of blood out of the
   chamber and into the aorta.

Drew is the irregular past of to
draw.

Give the irregular past of the
following verbs.

e.g. seek → sought

- ✔ bind
- ✔ bleed
- ✔ deal
- ✔ fight
- ✔ freeze
- ✔ grow
- ✔ hurt
- ✔ kneel
- ✔ lead
- ✔ stick

6 PHRASAL VERBS WITH BE

Study the meanings of the verbs
below. They are all formed with
the verb *TO BE*.

Phrasal verb	Meaning
to be away	to be away from home
to be back	to have returned
to be for	to be in favour of
to be in	to be at home or in a place
to be in for	to be about to encounter (usually unpleasant)
to be out	not to be at home etc.
to be out of	to be temporarily without
to be over	to be finished
to be up	to expire, finish, come to an end
to be up to	to be someone's responsibility or duty

Complete the following sentences.
Add the missing part of the phrasal
verb.

1 Dr. Brown wasn't ....
   His secretary said I'd find him
   at his surgery if I called back
   about three o'clock.

2 When the meeting's ....
   we'll look for a good
   restaurant and have lunch.

3 Professor Philips is ....
   on holiday this week. He
   won't be .... until
   Friday.

4 I must renew my subscription
   to the Lancet. I think it's
   .... at the end of the
   month.

5 We haven't any two-inch
   bandages. We are ....
   .... them at the moment.

6 Patient: "I want to go home,
   nurse."
   Nurse: "You'll have to wait
   until the doctor does his
   rounds.
   It's really ....
   him when you can leave."

7 I've been sneezing all day. I
   think I'm ....
   a cold.

8 The chief isn't ....
   trying the new treatment on
   his patients until he has more
   information.

9 Patient phoning to surgery:
   "I'd like to speak to doctor
   Jenkins please."
   Secretary: "I'm sorry that isn't
   possible at the moment.
   He's .... on a call."

GRAMMAR POINT

THE FUTURE

Using the Simple Present
The SIMPLE PRESENT can be used to express *a definite future arrangement*. The time *must* be expressed.

e.g. The new hospital wing *opens* on Monday.
(The new hospital wing is opening on Monday is also possible but it is less formal).

RULE: *learn by heart*

ONLY *ONE* FUTURE VERB PER SENTENCE IN ENGLISH

e.g. I'll call you when I get back.

    FUTURE   *PRESENT*

N.B. The future is *not* used in the part of the sentence following the word when.

Notes

7 GRAMMAR CHECK

Put the verbs in brackets into the correct form. Use *will/won't,* a *Present Simple* or *a Present Continuous.* Sometimes, more than one answer is possible.

1 Doctor, "When I've read the case notes, I (be) ready to examine the patient".
2 "When you (see) Doctor Wilson, tell him that Doctor Davidson (look for) him".
3 His parents (be) very angry if he (not pass) the examination.
4 "I (phone) you as soon as they (tell) me when I (get) out of hospital."
5 "If you (come) at three o'clock, I (try) to see you."
6 Sister to Nurse: "Don't forget to give Mr. Jackson his injection before he (go) to sleep.
7 The hospital board (meet) tomorrow.
8 Doctor to Patient: "Take this medicine. When you (return) in six weeks you (feel) much better."
9 Bill: "When you (know) if you've got the job, Derek?" Derek: "They (tell) me as soon as they (decide):
10 The examination (start) at ten o'clock.

WRITING

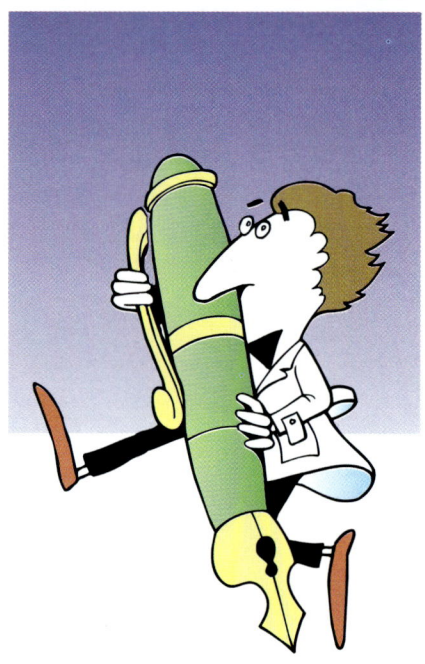

8 DIAGRAM COMPLETION

Study the diagram of the heart. Write the words below on the diagram.

right auricle
left auricle
pericardium
aorta
right ventricle
left ventricle
tricuspid valve
mitral valve
pulmonary arteries
pulmonary veins
superior vena cava
inferior vena cava

9 STRUCTURE AND ACTION OF THE HEART

Describe the structure, function and action of the heart using the words in exercise 8. Here are some more words to help you.

STRUCTURE: four-chambered; a hollow muscle; specialized cardiac muscle fibres.

FUNCTION: muscular pump; carbon dioxide, oxygenated; deoxygenated; the Pulmonary circuit; the Systemic circuit.

ACTION: pumping-action; rhythmic contractions of the muscles.

N.B. When describing the flow of blood, remember that the verb pass can be followed by different prepositions to describe different directions.

e.g. to pass *into*; to pass *from*; to pass *through*; to pass *out of*.

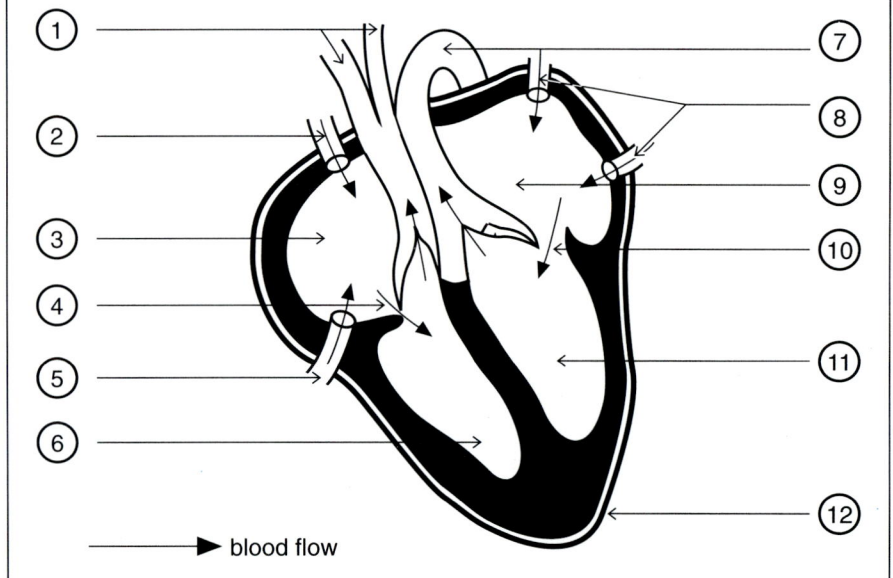

blood flow

SPEAKING

10 DOCTOR/PATIENT DIALOGUE

Work in pairs.
Conduct the following doctor/patient dialogue.

A patient who is overweight, unfit and a heavy smoker, comes to you for advice. Give him some practical suggestions on how to modify his lifestyle in order to reduce the risk of a heart attack.

Use the *imperative* in some sentences, e.g.: eat; don't eat.

Use *you must/you mustn't.*

Use also *should,* e.g.: you should; you shouldn't.

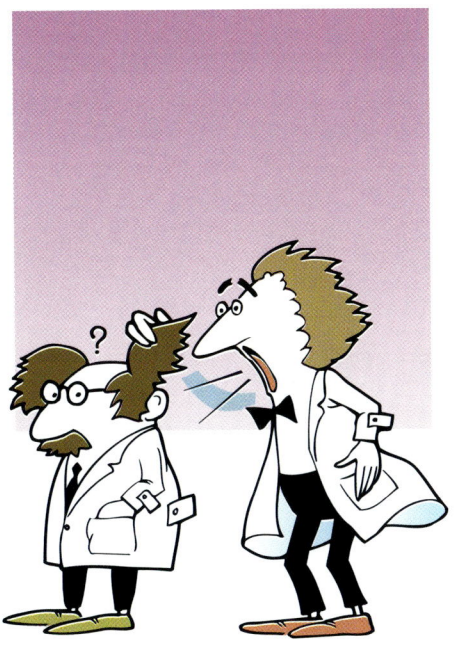

11 ASKING QUESTIONS

Group work.
Howard Franzier, director of the transplant program at the Texas Heart Institute in Houston, attends a medical conference to describe the first successful use of the Hemopump. One student takes the part of Franzier, the other students should ask him questions after his description.

e.g. How long does it take to insert the pump?
How wide is the device?
How long is it?

UNDERSTANDING IDIOMATIC ENGLISH

Explain the idiom.

The patient thanked the doctor from the bottom of his heart

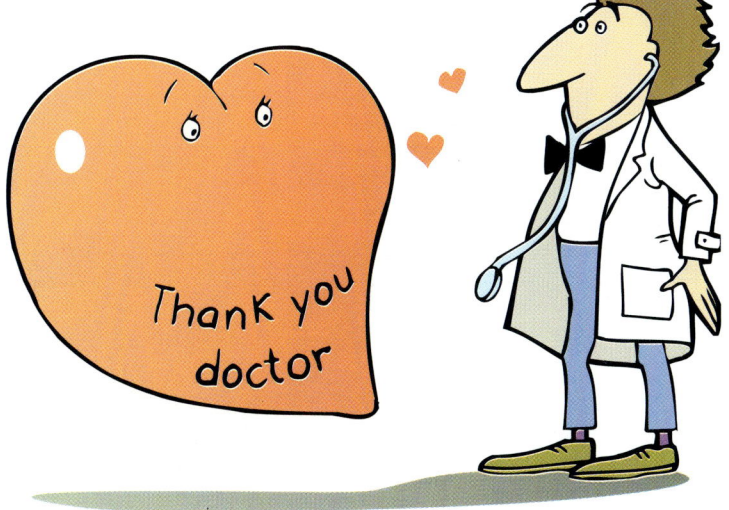

UNIT 4

A crippling orthopaedic disease

Lumbar Spinal Osteotomy in Ankylosing Spondylitis

Michael J. McMaster, M.D., F.R.C.S.
Edinburgh Scoliosis Unit
Princess Margaret Rose Hospital
Fairmilehead, Edinburgh, EH10 7ED, UK

ABSTRACT

Lumbar spinal osteotomy in patients with ankylosing spondylitis can be a difficult and potentially dangerous operation with a high incidence of serious complications. However, the majority of these problems can be overcome by a modification of the original Smith-Petersen technique and by the use of a compression device to provide a slow and finely controlled closure of the osteotomy and rigid internal fixation.

INTRODUCTION

1 Ankylosing spondylitis when allowed to run its own course can on occasion present as one of the most crippling diseases seen by the orthopaedic surgeon. The characteristic spinal deformity is a flattening of the
5 normal lumbar lordosis, and an increasing thoracic kyphosis with the head and neck thrust forwards. Occasionally there is increasing flexion at the cervico-thoracic junction. Eventually, as the disease progresses, the entire spinal column from the sacrum to the occiput
10 becomes ankylosed by bone in this deformed position.

Reprint Address:
Michael J. McMaster, M.D., FRCS
Edinburgh Scoliosis Unit
Princess Margaret Rose Hospital
Fairmilehead, Edinburgh, EH10 7ED, UK

At this stage, the patient is bent forward and forced to look at the ground. This ugly posture is not only functionally disabling but is also psychologically disturbing.

Smith-Petersen, Larsen and Aufranc recognised the
15 plight of these unfortunate patients and in 1945 introduced the operation of spinal osteotomy, by which the spine is hyperextended in the lumbar region enabling the patient to see straight ahead. Since their paper, relatively few surgeons have attempted the operation
20 /1-6, 8-11/ and many have reported a high incidence of major complications. The reported mortality rate has been as high as 10 percent and neurological complications, up to and including paraplegia, have occurred in as many as 30 percent of the patients.

25 The main indication for the operative correction of the severely flexed posture in a patient with ankylosing spondylitis is difficulty in seeing straight ahead with the field of vision limited to the area around the feet. However, before proceeding to surgery it is important to
30 assess the contribution of all levels of the spine from the occiput to the sacrum as well as the hips to the flexed posture. Frequently, all of these regions are affected but some are more deformed than others. Severe flexion contracture of the hips can often be corrected by total
35 hip replacement and this may be sufficient by itself to allow the patient to see straight ahead. A spinal osteotomy is indicated only if the hips are not significantly deformed or if, after hip operations, the patient is still unable to see straight ahead. The thoracic cage is
40 usually the most flexed region but osteotomy at this level does not help because the ankylosed thoracic cage

prevents extension of the spine. A thoracic deformity is best overcome by the creation of a compensatory lumbar lordosis by means of a lumbar osteotomy (Figs. 1 and 2). Ideally the lumbar spine should be extended until the patient can see straight ahead. The centre of gravity of the upper body should then lie just behind the site of the osteotomy helping to maintain the correction.

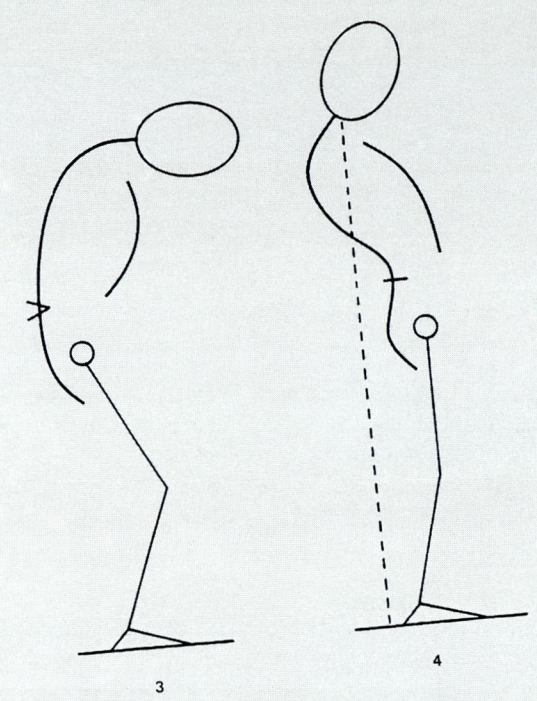

Fig. 3 and 4: If the major spinal flexion deformity is at the cervico-thoracic junction, an attempt to correct this by means of an extension osteotomy in the lumbar spine may unbalance the patient.

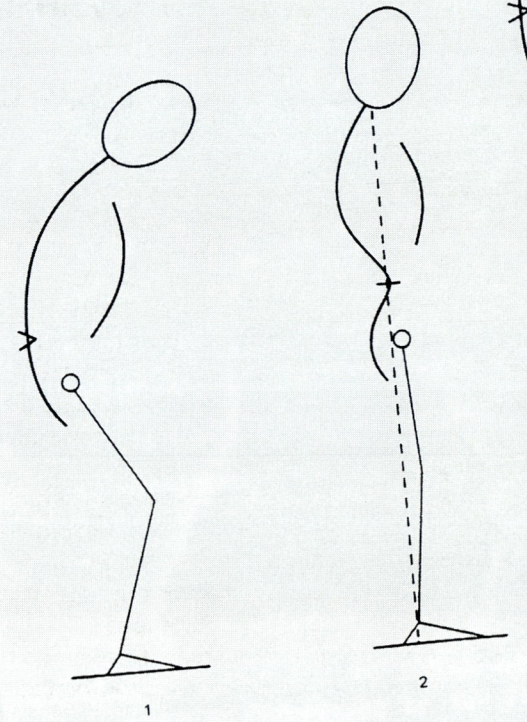

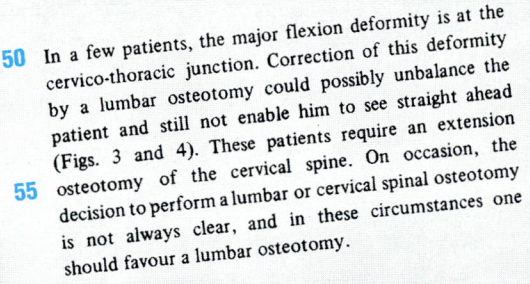

Fig. 1 and 2: The flexion deformity in the thoraco-lumbar spine is overcome by creating a compensatory lumbar lordosis.

In a few patients, the major flexion deformity is at the cervico-thoracic junction. Correction of this deformity by a lumbar osteotomy could possibly unbalance the patient and still not enable him to see straight ahead (Figs. 3 and 4). These patients require an extension osteotomy of the cervical spine. On occasion, the decision to perform a lumbar or cervical spinal osteotomy is not always clear, and in these circumstances one should favour a lumbar osteotomy.

TEXT BASED EXERCISES

VOCABULARY

Study the meaning of the following words and expressions as used in the text.

3 to cripple
   - to disable; seriously handicap
3 a disease
   - an illness
4 to flatten
   - to make flat
6 to thrust
   - to push forcefully
9 entire
   - whole, complete
11 stage
   - point of development
11 to bend
   - to curve, to incline
13 to disable
   - to incapacitate
16 a plight
   - a difficult or unpleasant position or situation
18 to enable
   - to make able
24 to occur
   - to be found; to happen
32 as well as
   - in addition to
33 to affect
   - to attack
40 unable
   - not able
44 to overcome
   - to conquer
49 a site
   - area, position
52 to unbalance
   - to throw out of balance

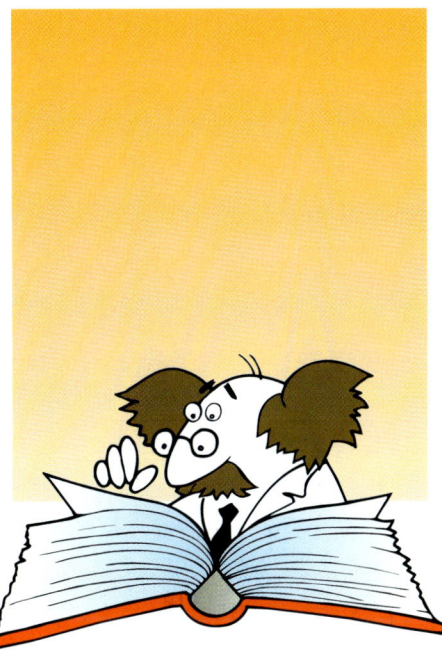

1 WORD CHECK

Explain what you understand by the following expressions.

1   Ankylosing spondylitis.
2   When allowed to run its own course.
3   An orthopaedic surgeon.
10 This deformed position.
11 Forced to look at the ground.
17 Spinal osteotomy.
23 Neurological complications.
24 Paraplegia.
36 Hip replacement.
40 The thoracic cage.

2 COMPREHENSION

Ask questions to which the following are the answers.

1   Ankylosing spondylitis.
2   A flattening of the normal lumbar lordosis and an increasing thoracic kyphosis.
3   The entire spinal column from the sacrum to the occiput becomes ankylosed by bone in this deformed position.
4   It can also be psychologically disturbing.
5   An operation by which the spine is hyperextended in the lumbar region.
6   It enables the patient to see straight ahead.
7   Relatively few.
8   As many as 30 percent of the patients.
9   When the patient's field of vision is limited to the area around the feet.
10 Yes, frequently. But some are more deformed than others.
11 By total hip replacement.
12 Only if the hips are not significantly deformed or if, after hip operations, the patient is still unable to see straight ahead.
13 By the creation of a compensatory lumbar lordosis by means of a lumbar osteotomy.
14 When the major flexion deformity is at the cervico-thoracic junction.
15 One should favour a lumbar osteotomy.

3

Try to fill in the missing words without referring back to the text. Refer back only to check your answers.

Ankylosing spondylitis, when allowed to (1) .... its own course, can on occasion present as (2) .... of the most (3) .... diseases seen by the orthopaedic (4) .... The characteristic (5) .... deformity is a (6) .... of the normal lumbar lordosis and an (7) .... thoracic kyphosis with the head and (8) .... thrust (9) .... Occasionally, there is increasing flexion at the cervico-thoracic (10) .... Eventually, as the disease progresses, the (11) .... spinal column from the sacrum to the occiput becomes ankylosed (12) .... bone in this deformed position. At this (13) .... , the patient is (14) .... forward and forced to look (15) .... the ground. This ugly posture is not (16) .... (17) .... disabling (18) .... is (19) .... (20) .... disturbing.

4

Join a word from column A with a word from column B to form an expression as used in the text.

A	B
hip	cage
serious	column
thoracic	forward
lumbar	replacement
spinal	posture
bent	ahead
ugly	complications
straight	osteotomy

5 NOUNS FROM VERBS

Give *nouns* formed from the verbs below as used in the text.

e.g. to operate → operation

Verb	Noun
to contribute	
to complicate	
to deform	
to extend	
to correct	
to decide	
to create	
to replace	
to indicate	
to modify	

6

Fill in the blanks with one of the following words as used in the text.

✔ rate

✔ spine

✔ deformity

✔ patients

✔ kyphosis

✔ junction

✔ closure

✔ posture

✔ complications

a a slow and finely controlled ....
b an increasing thoracic ....
c these unfortunate ....
d a high incidence of major ....
e the reported mortality ....
f the severely flexed ....
g the major flexion ....
h the cervico-thoracic ....
i an extension osteotomy of the
j cervical ....

7 OPPOSITES

Give the *opposite* of the adjectives and adverbs in the list below.

- ✓ forward
- ✓ superior
- ✓ forwards
- ✓ internal
- ✓ inward
- ✓ internally
- ✓ inwards
- ✓ posterior
- ✓ upward
- ✓ upper
- ✓ upwards
- ✓ inner

8 PAST / PRESENT PARTICIPLES

Both *present participles* and *past participles* can be used as adjectives.
Present participle adjectives are ACTIVE.

e.g. An excruciating pain.

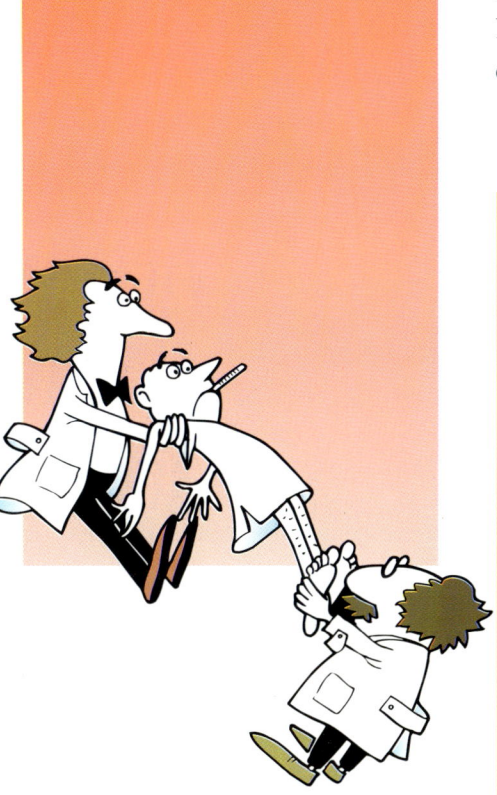

This means that the pain has this *effect*.

Past participle adjectives are PASSIVE.

e.g. A transplanted heart.

This describes the result of an action.

If an adverb is present in the phrase, it goes in front of the participle.

e.g. A *correctly*, functioning valve.

Change the expressions below by inserting a present or past participle in front of the nouns.

e.g. Arteries that have become narrow;
narrowed arteries.

a disease that is crippling	....
a position that is deformed	....
an illness that threatens life	....
an immune system that has been weakened	....
a spine that has been severely damaged	....
news that is disturbing	....
a posture that disables functionally	....
factors that affect health	....
a disease related to smoking	....
a technique that is widely used	....

35

9 IDIOMATIC EXPRESSIONS WITH BE

Idiomatic expressions are much used in English and can be found in Medical English as in any other form of written and spoken English. You have already met some idiomatic expressions in Unit 2.

e.g. To be close on its heels.
To have a hands-off approach.

The guidelines for studying idiomatic expressions, are the same as those for studying phrasal verbs. Turn back now to Unit 2 and re-read the suggestions before beginning the exercise.
Study the following expressions. They are all formed with the verb *TO BE*.

Idiomatic expression	Meaning
to be afraid that	to be sorry to have to say
not to be a blind bit of use	not to make the slightest difference or effect
to be made that way	to have it in one's nature to be or do something
to be touch and go	to be in a situation in which death or disaster etc. will only be or has only been narrowly avoided
to be off one's food	to lose one's appetite
to be glad to see the back of (someone or something)	to be glad to see someone or something for the last time
to be dog tired	to be extremely tired
to be dead right	to be absolutely right
to be cruel to be kind	to say or do something painful that a greater good may come from it
to be a dab hand	to be skilful or experienced at doing something

Read the following sentences. Replace the part of the sentence *in italics* with one of the above idioms in the correct form.

1 I'm *sorry to have to tell you that* you'll need an operation in order to solve the problem.

2 I couldn't work in surgery and stand for long hours under the heat of the strong lights. *It's not in my nature.*

3 When I first went to work on the wards, I was hopeless at giving injections. At home, I used to practise on an orange and eventually *I was very good* at it.

4 You could try complaining but I don't think it will *change anything*.

5 The patient's relatives waited in the hospital all night for news of any change in his condition. It was *uncertain if he would deteriorate or improve*.

6 I don't know what's wrong with me. I usually have a good appetite but I have *hardly been able to eat anything* for the last few days.

7 Derek had been in hospital for ten weeks. He was grateful for the attention and care he had received but he was very *pleased to be leaving the hospital*.

8 I was on night duty last night and I was called out three times for emergencies. I can't wait to go home and go to sleep. I'm *exhausted*.

9 Nurse to Patient: "Now I know you don't want this treatment Mr. Smith but you need to have it. I'll have to *cause you some pain if we want you to get better*."

10 The doctor suspected his patient had a rare disease. When the results of the tests arrived he saw that *his suspicions had been perfectly correct*.

COMPARATIVES

There are three degrees of comparison.

AFFIRMATIVE

old

new

useful

COMPARATIVE

older

newer

more useful

SUPERLATIVE

oldest

newest

most useful

ONE-SYLLABLE ADJECTIVES
- form the comparative and superlative by adding ER or EST.

ADJECTIVES OF 3 OR MORE SYLLABLES
- form the comparative and superlative by placing more and most in front of the affirmative.

GRAMMAR POINT

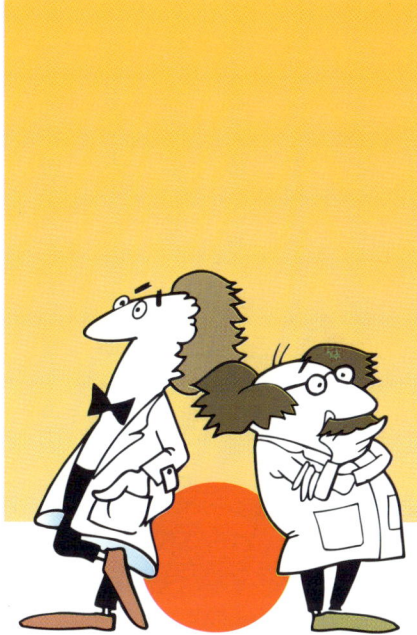

ADJECTIVES OF 2 SYLLABLES
- follow one of the above rules. Although the adjectives ending in ful
(e.g. helpful) usually take more or most
(e.g more helpful, most helpful).

10 GRAMMAR CHECK

When a comparison is made the word *THAN* is used.

e.g. All of these regions are affected, but some are *more deformed than* others.

Change the following sentences as in the example.

e.g. All of the operations were difficult.
All of the operations were difficult, but some *were more difficult* than others.

1 All of the sufferers are bent.
2 All of the cases are unfortunate.
3 All of the conditions were serious.
4 All of the diseases could be life-threatening.
5 All of the machines are expensive.
6 All of the clinical trials have been successful.
7 All of the tissues have been damaged.
8 All of the procedures are painful.

11 GRAMMAR CHECK

Give the comparative and superlative of the following adjectives.

e.g. easy/easier/easiest

✓ serious
✓ good
✓ young
✓ little
✓ bad
✓ slow
✓ many
✓ difficult

WRITING

12 WRITING A SUMMARY

Write *a short summary* of the article on Lumbar Spinal Osteotomy in Ankylosing Spondylitis. Divide the summary into three paragraphs. The following phrases will help you.

Ankylosing spondylitis
- run its own course
- crippling disease
- spinal deformity
- thoracic kyphosis
- entire spinal columns
- functionally disabling/ psychologically disturbing

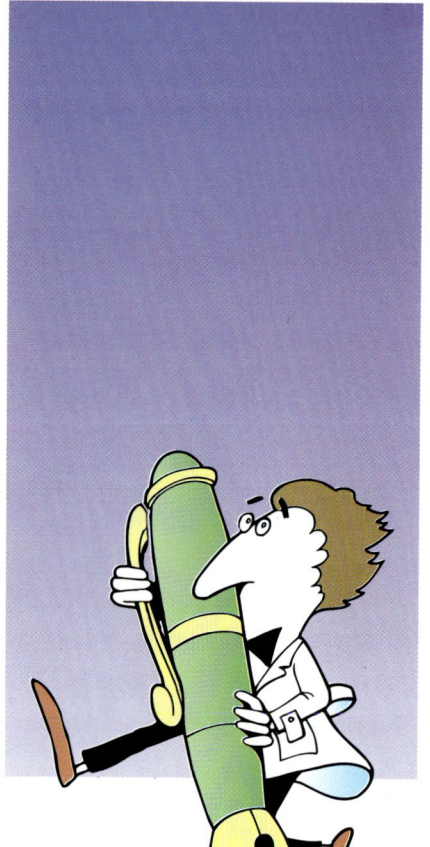

The operation of spinal osteotomy
- hyperextended
- few surgeons
- high incidence of major complications
- neurological complications/ paraplegia
- 30% of the patients

Before proceeding to surgery
- the contribution of all levels of the spine
- severe flexion contracture of the hips/total hip replacement
- indicated only if the hips are not significantly deformed
- thoracic deformity/compensatory lumbar lordosis
- an extension osteotomy of the cervical spine
- lumbar or cervical spinal osteotomy not clear/favour a lumbar osteotomy

Notes

SPEAKING

13 DOCTOR/PATIENT DIALOGUE

Work in pairs.
Conduct the following
doctor/patient dialogue.

A patient needs to strengthen his
back. Describe a few easy exercises
he can do at home which will
help. Describe the exercises using
short, simple sentences.

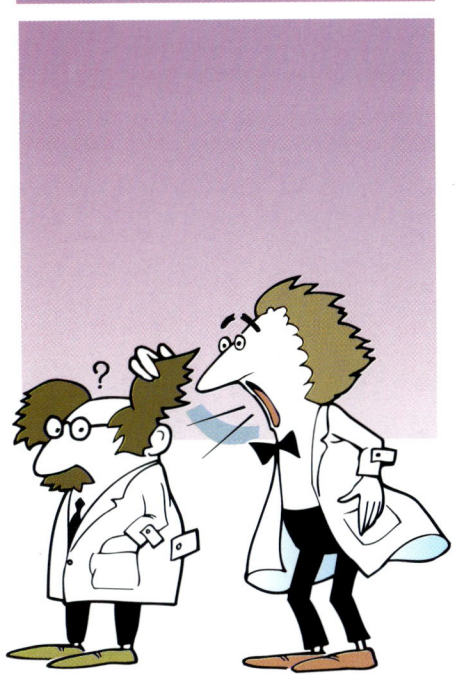

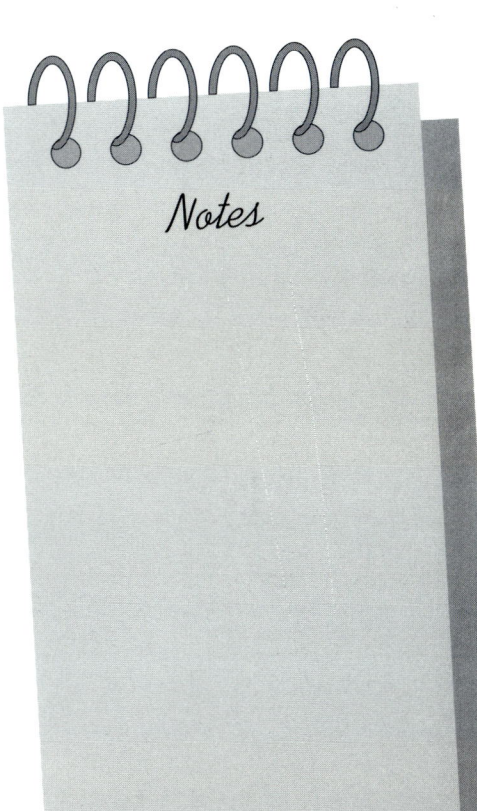

Notes

UNDERSTANDING IDIOMATIC ENGLISH

Explain the idiom.

She's just had
a brain wave

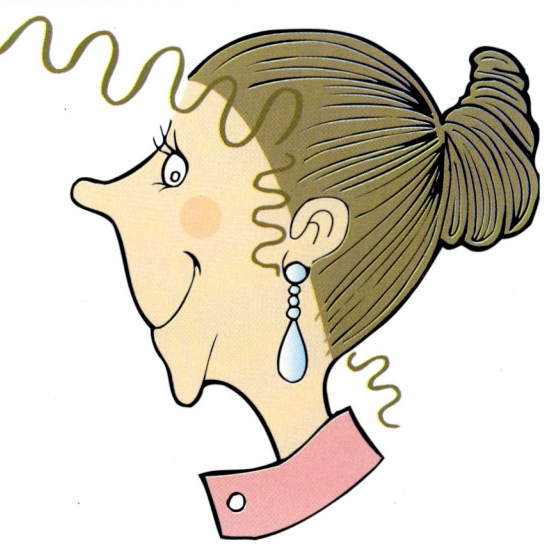

UNIT 5

An award to a molecular biologist

We Congratulate Dr. Elizabeth Blackburn For Discovering A Basic Truth About Life.

The discovery made by Dr. Elizabeth Blackburn and her research group is another chapter in one of the great stories of modern science: the unveiling by molecular biology of the way life works at the most basic level.

Dr. Blackburn has identified a key enzyme that is necessary for chromosomes to make copies of themselves before cell division.

She accomplished this by studying chromosome ends. Their biological properties make these ends notoriously difficult to study. But Dr. Blackburn, who is professor of molecular and cell biology at the University of California at Berkeley, overcame all obstacles.

For this, Dr. Blackburn has received the 1990 Award for Molecular Biology from the National Academy of Sciences at its award ceremony in Washington.

Monsanto Company is proud to be the sponsor of this award, which is given yearly by the Academy to an outstanding scientist. We join with the Academy in congratulating Dr. Blackburn for her remarkable achievement.

Monsanto

VOCABULARY

Study the meaning of the following words and expressions as used in the text.

3   to unveil
  - to remove a veil; to reveal
10   notoriously
  - having a widespread, bad reputation
15   an award
  - a prize given for merit
19   outstanding
  - prominent, remarkable
22   remarkable
  - worthy of notice

1   DOUBLE NOUN EXPRESSIONS

Find *double-noun expressions*. Choose one word from column 1 and one from column 2.

Column 1	Column 2
pain	ends
cell	ceremony
chromosome	biology
cell	department
research	killers
award	flow
outpatient	transplant
blood	room
heart	division
emergency	group

TEXT BASED EXERCISES

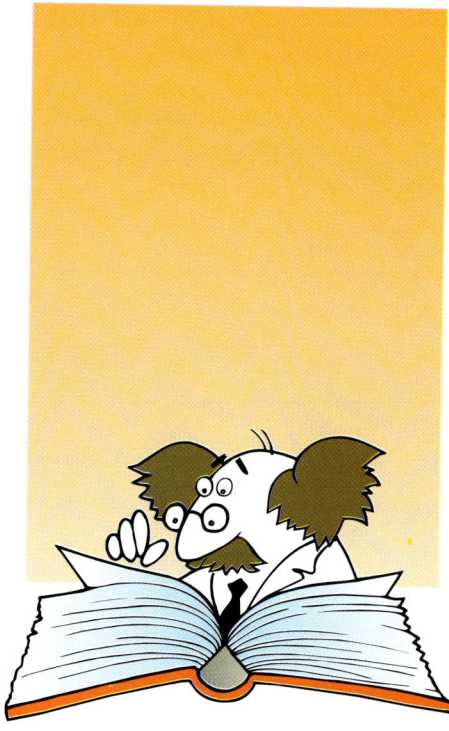

Notes

2   SENTENCE RECONSTRUCTION

Rearrange the words below, and add additional words, in order to make complete sentences.

e.g. *We: Dr. Elizabeth Blackburn : basic truth : life: congratulate.*
We congratulate Dr. Elizabeth Blackburn for discovering a basic truth about life.

1   Discovery : Dr. Elizabeth Blackburn : research group : was made by.

2   Dr. Blackburn : a key enzyme : chromosomes : copies : cell division : to make : has identified : necessary : themselves.

3   She : chromosome ends : studying : accomplished.

4   Biological properties : ends : notoriously difficult : make : to study.

5   Dr. Blackburn : obstacles : all.

6   Dr. Blackburn : professor : molecular and cell biology : University : California : is.

7   Dr. Blackburn : 1990 Award : Molecular Biology : National Academy of Sciences : has received.

8   Monsanto Company : proud : sponsor : award : is.

9   Award : yearly : Academy : outstanding scientist is given.

10   We : Academy : Dr. Blackburn : remarkable achievement : congratulating : join.

EXTENSION EXERCISES

3

Put suitable adjectives after the following adverbs and make complete sentences in your own words.

e.g. Notoriously.

Their biological properties make these ends *notoriously difficult* to study.

a Relatively.
b Intensely.
c Radically.
d Functionally
e Highly.
f Exceptionally.
g Psychologically.
h Extremely.

4 SPECIALISTS

Give the word that refers to the specialist who works in the following fields.

e.g.   biology → biologist

✔ neurology
✔ immunology
✔ psychology
✔ paediatrics (pl. n.)
✔ surgery
✔ cardiology
✔ radiology
✔ pathology
✔ physiotherapy
✔ psychiatry

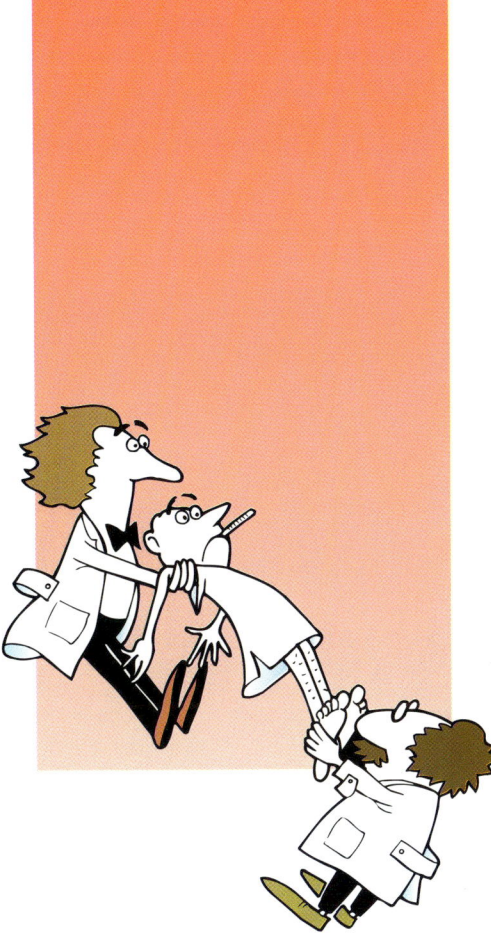

5 ADVERBS

Yearly is an adverb formed from the noun *year*. Give the adverbs formed from the following nouns and make complete sentences to show their meaning.

e.g. Year .... yearly.
The National Academy of Sciences makes the award *yearly*.

a Every hour ....
b Every day ....
c Every week ....
d Every month ....

6 PREPOSITIONS + VERBS

Verbs placed immediately after prepositions must be in the gerund form. Complete the sentences below in your own words.

e.g. She accomplished this by ....
She accomplished this by studying chromosome ends.

1 I'm looking forward to ....
2 He's absorbed in ....
3 Is she interested in .... ?
4 Mary's really fond of ....
5 There's no point in ....
6 They are fed up with ....
7 He had thought of ....
8 They're not keen on ....
9 I'm sorry for ....
10 Did you have difficulty in .... ?
11 This is a device for ....
12 She is very good at ....
13 What about .... ?
14 In spite of ....
15 We're tired of ....

7

Say what the following refer to in the description below.

1 While a cell is growing, this is in a resting stage so far as reproduction or division is concerned.
2 23 pairs or 46.
3 When the cell is ready to divide, this material comes together.
4 A small body that attracts a set of chromosomes to each end of the dividing cell.
5 This appears between the centrosomes.
6 The chromosomes duplicate themselves to form pairs of these.
7 This becomes constricted by the cell membrane.
8 These appear around each new nucleus.

Notes

8

Fill in the blanks with the following words as used in the text below.

- ✔ material
- ✔ mitotic
- ✔ hereditary
- ✔ stage
- ✔ species
- ✔ full-grown
- ✔ generation
- ✔ daughter
- ✔ around
- ✔ again
- ✔ once
- ✔ pass

The cell membrane between the (1) .... cells is completed. Nuclear membranes appear (2) .... each new nucleus.
The chromosome (3) .... breaks up and becomes dispersed (4) .... more.
Each daughter cell goes into the resting (5) .... in which it grows and the (6) .... stages will start (7) .... in division of each (8) .... daughter cell.
Thus the body cells of a (9) .... retain their characteristic number of chromosomes from (10) .... to generation, and (11) .... on (12) .... characteristics.

Study the following description and answer the questions in exercise 7.

MITOSIS

While a cell is growing, its nucleus is in a resting stage so far as reproduction, or division, is concerned. When the cell is ready to divide, the network of nuclear material breaks up into little pieces known as chromosomes which are not apparent in the resting cell. Each species of plant and animal has a characteristic number of chromosomes in the nucleus of each of its body cells which is always the same for the   5
specific species. For example, man's chromosome count is 23 pairs, or 46.

The following phases outline the process of mitosis:

1 When the cell is ready to divide, the chromosomal material comes together to form the number of chromosomes characteristic of the species of plant or animal of which the dividing cell is a part.   10
2 A small body, the **centrosome**, divides into two equal parts, each of which migrates to opposite poles of the cell. The centrosome attracts a set of chromosomes to each end of the dividing cell.
3 A spindle of ray-like fibres of protoplasm appears between the centrosomes.
4 The chromosomes duplicate themselves to form pairs of **chromatids** and become   15
arranged at the equator of the spindle.
5 The chromatids separate from each other, one member of each pair moving to the two poles of the nucleus.
6 The cell cytoplasm becomes constricted by the cell membrane.
7 The cell membrane between the daughter cells is completed. Nuclear membranes   20
appear around each new nucleus. The chromosome material breaks up and becomes dispersed once more. Each daughter cell goes into the resting stage in which it grows and the mitotic stages will start again in division of each full-grown daughter cell. Thus the body cells of a species retain their characteristic number of chromosomes from generation to generation, and pass on hereditary characteristics.   25

GRAMMAR POINT

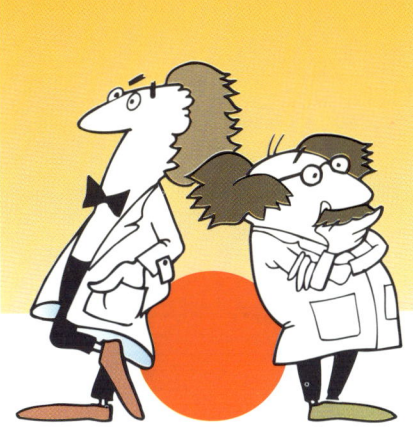

RELATIVE CLAUSES (WHO/THAT)

A *clause* is part of a sentence. A relative clause explains which person or thing the speaker refers to.

Study this sentence.
The man who was injured in the car accident is still on the critical list.
Who was injured in the car accident is a relative clause.

THAT is used when talking about *things.*

e.g. "Where are the case notes that were on the table?"

WHO and THAT are used when talking about people.

e.g. The doctor that (or who) won the award overcame all obstacles.

WHO must be used in clauses supplying additional information where there are commas at the beginning and end.

e.g. Dr. Blackburn, who is professor of molecular and cell biology at the University of California at Berkeley, overcame all obstacles.

Find the sentence in column 2 that completes the sentence in column 1.
Make them into *one sentence* using a relative clause.
Make any changes necessary.

e.g. An anaesthetist is a doctor. He administers anaesthetics to patients before surgery.

An anaesthetist is a doctor who administers anaesthetics to patients before surgery.

Column 1	Column 2
A neurologist is a specialist.	He deals with the skin and its diseases.
An aspirin is a tablet.	He treats mental and nervous disorders.
These are the results of the tests.	It records the action currents in the heart.
A dermatologist is a specialist.	He deals with the structure and functions of the nervous system.
Rabies is a disease.	They were carried out yesterday.
A cardiologist is a specialist.	He deals with children's diseases.
The Lancet is a medical magazine.	It can be found in all chemist shops.
A paediatrician is a specialist.	He deals with the heart and its diseases.
An electrocardiogram is a test.	Humans can catch it from infected dogs.
A psychiatrist is a specialist.	It informs the medical profession of new techniques and breakthroughs.

WRITING

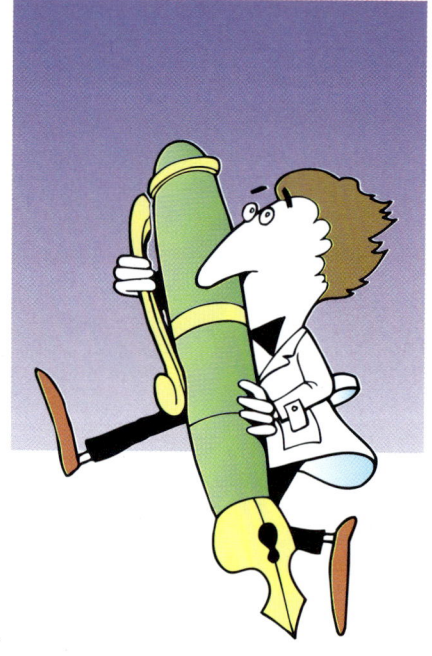

10 DESCRIBING A PROCESS

Study the diagrams below. Describe the process of mitosis in your own words. Use some of the words and expressions from exercise 7. The following words will also help you.

- ✔ network
- ✔ breaks up
- ✔ not apparent
- ✔ comes together
- ✔ two equal parts
- ✔ migrates
- ✔ opposite poles
- ✔ attracts
- ✔ duplicate
- ✔ arranged
- ✔ equator
- ✔ separate
- ✔ constricted
- ✔ dispersed

Notes

11 MOLECULAR BIOLOGY

Make as many words as you can with three or more letters from the words molecular biology. Each letter should be used only once per word, unless the letter appears more than once.

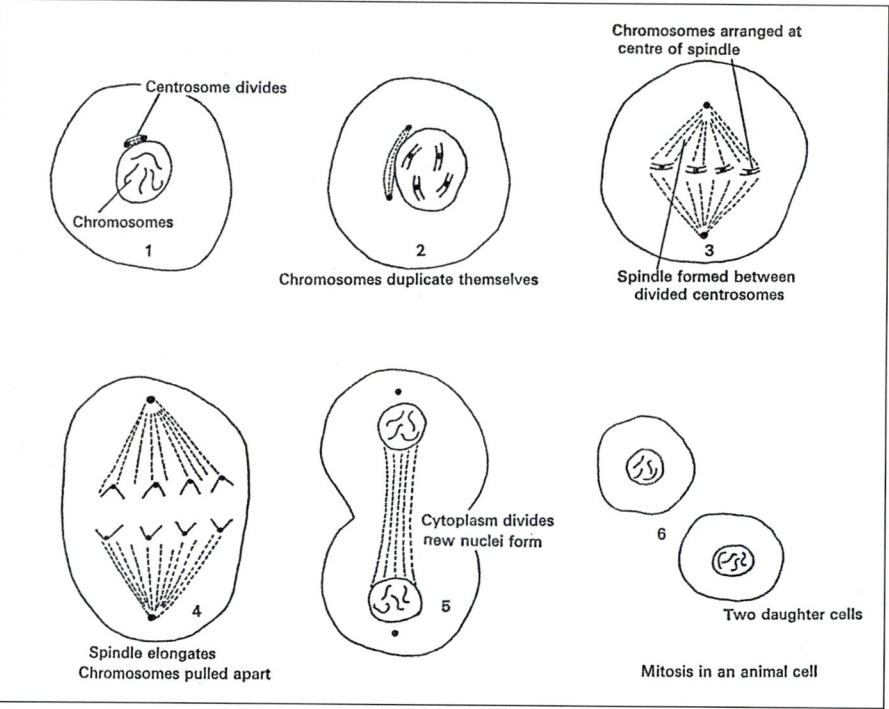

Centrosome divides

Chromosomes

1

Chromosomes duplicate themselves

2

Chromosomes arranged at centre of spindle

Spindle formed between divided centrosomes

3

Spindle elongates
Chromosomes pulled apart

4

Cytoplasm divides new nuclei form

5

Two daughter cells

6

Mitosis in an animal cell

SPEAKING

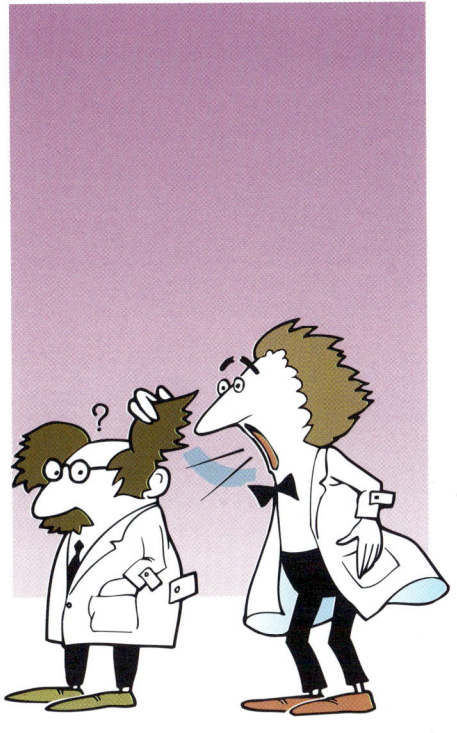

12 PRESENTATION

You are a T.V. presenter on the weekly programme "Science Today". Explain to the viewers the discovery made by Dr. Blackburn and her research group. Explain the importance of the discovery and the award she has just received. The words below will help you.

– discovery
– the way life works at the most basic level
– make copies of themselves before cell division
– chromosome ends
– difficult to study
– the National Academy of Sciences

13 INTERVIEW

Now interview Dr. Blackburn in person. Work with another student. One student takes the role of the interviewer and the other the doctor. The expressions below will help you.

– Can you tell me .... ?
– I wonder if you could explain .... ?
– Could you explain in detail .... ?
– How did you manage to .... ?
– What kind of difficulties .... ?

UNDERSTANDING IDIOMATIC ENGLISH

Explain the idiom.

I really put my foot in it

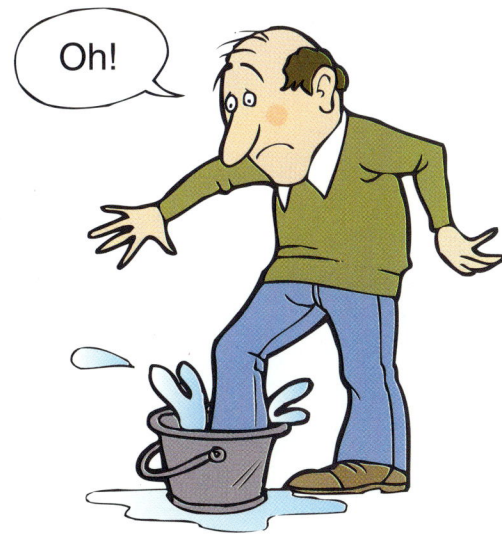

Oh!

UNIT 6

Deciphering the genetic code; gene therapy

The Gene Hunt

Scientists launch a $3 billion project to map the chromosomes and decipher the complete instructions for making a human being

Genome? The word evokes a blank stare from most Americans, whose taxes will largely support the project's estimated $3 billion cost. Explains biochemist Robert Sinsheimer of the University of California at Santa Barbara: "The human genome is the complete set of instructions for making a human being." Those instructions are tucked into the nucleus of each of the human body's 100 trillion cells* and written in the language of deoxyribonucleic acid, the fabled DNA molecule.

In the 35 years since James Watson and Francis Crick first discerned the complex structure of DNA, scientists have managed to decipher only a tiny fraction of the human genome. But they have high hopes that with new, automated techniques and a huge coordinated effort, the genome project can reach its goal in 15 years.

*Except red blood cells, which have no nucleus.

The goal: to map the human genome and spell out for the world the entire message hidden in its chemical code.

Mapping and sequencing the genes should accelerate progress in another highly touted and controversial discipline: gene therapy. Using this technique, scientists hope someday to cure genetic diseases by actually inserting good genes into their patients' cells. One proposed form of gene therapy would be used to fight beta-thalassemia major, a blood disease characterized by severe anemia and caused by the inability of hemoglobin to function properly.

University of Utah geneticist Mark Skolnick is convinced that mapping the genome will radically change the way medicine is practiced. "Right now," he says, "we wait for someone to get sick so we can cut them and drug them. It's pretty old stuff. Once you can make a profile of a person's genetic predisposition to disease, medicine will finally become predictive and preventive."

In a search coordinated by Wexler's foundation, geneticist James Gusella of Massachusetts General Hospital discovered a particular piece of DNA, called a genetic marker, that seemed to be present in people suffering from Huntington's disease. His evidence suggested that the marker must be near the Huntington's disease gene on the same chromosome, but he needed a larger sample to confirm his findings. This was provided by Wexler, who had previously traveled to Venezuela to chart the family tree of a clan of some 5,000 people, all of them descendants of a woman who died of Huntington's disease a century ago. Working with DNA samples from affected family members, Gusella and Wexler in 1983 concluded that they had indeed found a Huntington's marker, which was located near one end of chromosome 4.

Reading these genetic words and deciphering their meaning is apparently a snap for the clever machinery of a cell. But for mere scientists it is a formidable and time-consuming task.

Not only those with rare genetic disorders could benefit from the new technology. Says John Brunzell, a University of Washington medicine professor: "Ten years ago, it was thought that only 10% of premature coronary heart disease came from inherited abnormalities. Now that proportion is approaching 80% to 90%."

Harvard geneticist Philip Leder cites many common diseases—hypertension, allergies, diabetes, heart disease, mental illness and some (perhaps all) cancers—that have a genetic component. Unlike Huntington's and Tay-Sachs diseases, which are caused by a single defective gene, many of these disorders have their roots in several errant genes and would require genetic therapy far more sophisticated than any now even being contemplated. Still, says Leder, "in the end, genetic mapping is going to have its greatest impact on these major diseases."

VOCABULARY

Study the meaning of the following words and expressions as used in the text.

title a hunt
- a prolonged search
1 to launch
- to begin; to set in motion
1 to map
- to represent on a map
2 to decipher
- to translate from code
4 a stare
- a fixed look with eyes wide open
11 to tuck
- to fold
23 a goal
- the object of effort
28 to tout
- to make persistent attempts to sell
45 pretty
- very
45 stuff (fig.)
- a thing (often worthless)
73 a snap (coll.)
- an easy task
74 mere
- simple
74 formidable
- difficult; full of obstacles
75 a task
- hard or unpleasant work
87 to cite
- to refer to
97 far
- very much
99 still
- nevertheless

TEXT BASED EXERCISES

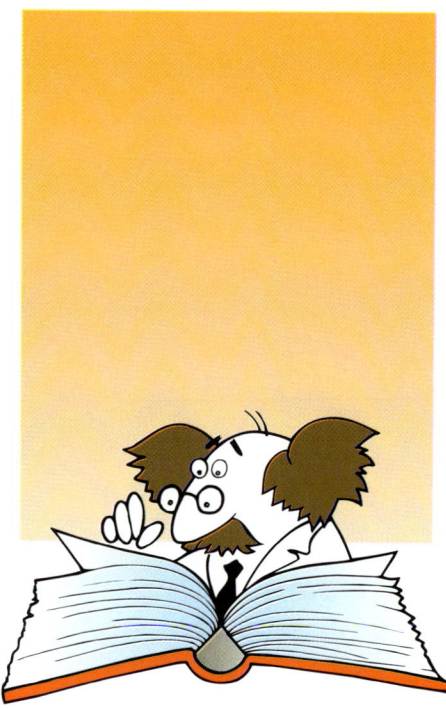

1

Say what the following words and expressions refer to in the text.

15 35 years
18 a tiny fraction
22 15 years
28 controversial discipline
35 a blood disease caused by the inability of hemoglobin to function properly
45 pretty old stuff
53 a particular piece of DNA
73 a snap
74 a formidable and time-consuming task
81 10%
84 80% to 90%
95 several errant genes

2 COMPREHENSION

Read the following statements. Say whether they are *TRUE* or *FALSE*. Correct the false statements.

1 Most Americans know what the Genome Project is.
2 Their taxes will completely support the project's cost.
3 The project will cost exactly $ 3 billion.
4 The structure of DNA is complicated.
5 Scientists have managed to decipher only a small part of the human genome.
6 It is difficult for a scientist to decipher and read these genetic words.
7 Geneticist Mark Skolnick believes that gene therapy will only slightly change the way medicine is carried out.
8 The 5,000 descendents of the woman who had died from Huntington's disease a century ago, had all been affected.
9 Huntington's disease is caused by a single defective gene.
10 It is unlikely that genetic mapping will have an impact on the major diseases.

3 ADJECTIVES

Fill in the blanks with the *adjectives* below as used in the text.

- ✔ complex
- ✔ formidable
- ✔ preventive
- ✔ affected
- ✔ estimated
- ✔ genetic
- ✔ high
- ✔ inherited
- ✔ complete
- ✔ controversal

a   an .... cost
b   a .... set
c   the .... structure
d   .... hopes
e   a .... task
f   a .... discipline
g   .... medicine
h   .... family members
i   .... disorders
j   .... abnormalities

4 MIXED VERBAL FORMS

Put the *verbs* in brackets into the verbal form used in the text.

1   In the 35 years since James Watson and Francis Crick first (discern) the complex structure of DNA, scientists (manage) to decipher only a tiny fraction of the human genome.

2   Mapping and (sequence) the genes (accelerate) progress in another highly touted and controversial discipline: gene therapy.

3   (use) this technique, scientists hope someday to cure genetic diseases by actually (insert) good genes into their patients' cells.

4   University of Utah geneticist Mark Skolnick (convince) that (map) the genome (change) radically the way medicine is practiced.

5   (Work) with DNA samples from affected family members, Gusella and Wexler in 1983 (conclude) that they (find) indeed a Huntington's marker, which (locate) near one end of chromosome 4.

6   Not only those with rare genetic disorders (benefit) from the new technology.

7   Unlike Huntington's and Tay-Sachs diseases, which (cause) by a single defective gene, many of these disorders have their roots in several errant genes and (require) genetic therapy far more sophisticated than any now (contemplate).

5 PREPOSITIONS

Fill in the blanks with a *preposition* as used in the text.

.... a search coordinated .... Wexler's foundation, geneticist James Gusella .... Massachusetts General Hospital discovered a particular piece .... DNA called a genetic marker, that seemed to be present .... people suffering .... Huntington's disease. His evidence suggested that the marker must be near the Huntington's disease gene .... the same chromosome, but he needed a larger sample to confirm his findings.
This was provided .... Wexler, who had previously traveled .... Venezuela to chart the family tree .... a clan .... some 5,000 people, all .... them descendants .... a woman who died .... Huntington's disease a century ago.
Working .... DNA samples .... affected family members, Gusella and Wexler .... 1983 concluded that they had indeed found a Huntington's marker, which was located near one end .... chromosome 4.

EXTENSION EXERCISES

6 WORD SUBSTITUTION

Substitute the following adverbs with another *word or phrase*.

a 5   largely.
b 28 highly.
c 31 actually.
d 37 properly.
e 40 radically.
f 48 finally.
g 61 previously.
h 72 apparently

7 NOUNS FROM VERBS

Complete the lists below with *a noun* related to each of the verbs.

e.g. to instruct → instruction

Verb	Noun	Verb	Noun
to map		to estimate	
to propose		to sample	
to project		to explain	
to cause		to confirm	
to predict		to conclude	
to convince		to progress	
to stare		to locate	
to prevent		to cure	
to support		to predispose	
to suggest		to accelerate	

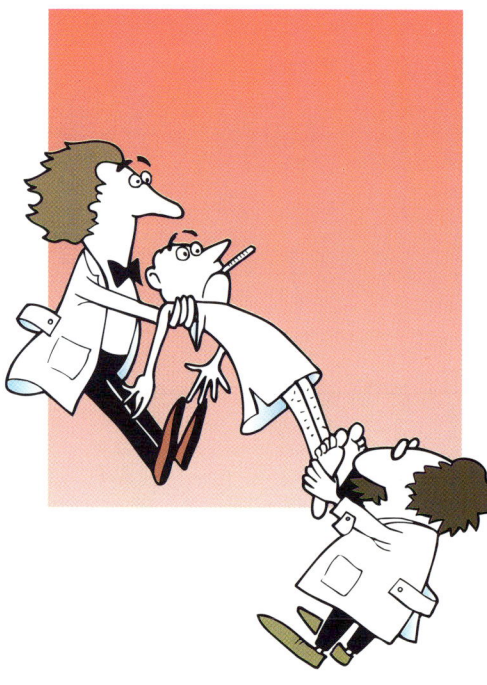

8

Fill in the blanks with the words below.

- ✓ tablets
- ✓ bandage
- ✓ plaster
- ✓ drops
- ✓ sticking plaster
- ✓ sling
- ✓ wheelchair
- ✓ stretcher
- ✓ syringe
- ✓ crutches

1 It's only a little cut on your finger. Put a .... on it.
2 Your ear-ache will soon heal. Put these .... in your ear morning and evening.
3 Jack had to go to hospital and have a .... put on his broken leg.
4 Use these .... They will take the weight off your legs until you can walk properly.
5 You can't walk to the ward. Sit down in this .... and I'll push it.
6 Take one of these .... three times a day. They will help your stomach-ache.
7 It isn't a serious wound. Put on a piece of gauze and a large ....
8 The patient was carried into the ambulance on a ....
9 It will help if you keep your arm bent. You should put it in a ....
10 When giving an injection, a hypodermic .... is used.

GRAMMAR POINT

SIMPLE PAST/ PRESENT PERFECT

Comparison of Simple Past and Present Perfect Tenses.

SIMPLE PAST	or	PRESENT PERFECT
I won		I have won.

THE SIMPLE PAST tells us *only about the past.*

> e.g. *He won* the prize.

THE PRESENT PERFECT tells us *about the present.*

> e.g. *He has won* the prize.

THE SIMPLE PAST
This is used for actions completed at *a definite time in the past.*
The time may be specified or understood.

> e.g. *I went* to London yesterday.
>
> The train *was* half an hour late.

THE PRESENT PERFECT
This is used for recent actions *when the time is not mentioned* or for actions further back in the past which *maintain a connection with the present.*

> e.g. *I have seen* Mr. Smith's report.

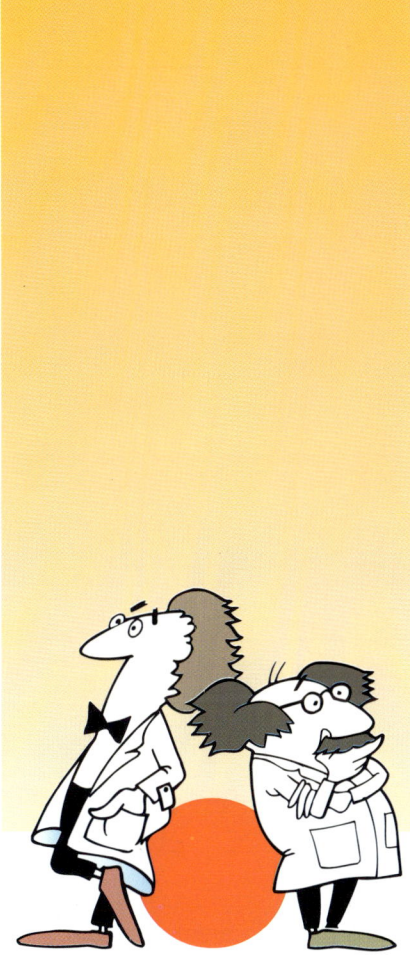

JUST + PRESENT PERFECT
Just is used for a recently completed action.

> e.g. He has *just* gone home.

N.B. Place just between the auxiliary and the main verb.

Put the verbs in brackets into the *Present Perfect* or the *Simple Past* as most appropriate.

1 When I (be) 19, I (start) my university course.
2 I (just hear) that Peter (be) admitted to hospital.
3 The doctor (leave) his house at 7.30 and (arrive) at the hospital at 8.15.
4 - How long (work) at the hospital?
   - I (work) there for six months, two years ago.
5 How long (be) in your present job?
6 - Would you like to check the results?
   - No, I (just check) them.
7 Dr. Black (be) ill yesterday. As he (have) to stay in bed, Dr. Brown (do) his rounds for him.
8 I (meet) Dr. Wilson last year at the International Conference in London.
9 Ten doctors (apply) for the job but so far nothing (be) decided.
10 Dr. Maxwell isn't in the hospital. I (just see) him leave.
11 I (look) for John everywhere but I (not find) him yet.
12 Carol (telephone) her sister this morning.
13 You (finish) yet?
14 They (be) in London on Friday?
15 Tony saw the film.
   - He (like) it?

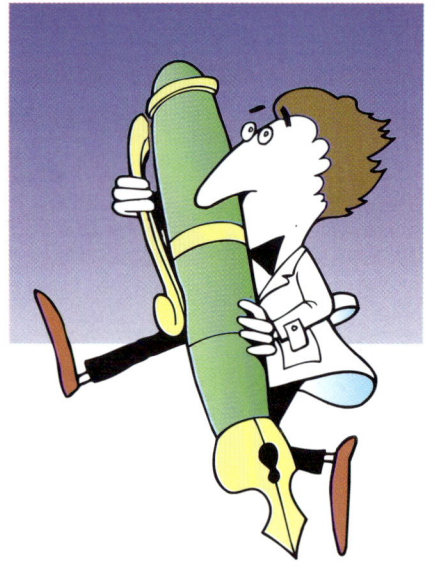

10 WRITING INFORMATION

Using your own words, fill in the spaces with information about each of the following:

The human genome

The goal of the scientists

Genetic predisposition

Gene therapy

Major diseases that have their roots in several errant genes.

SPEAKING

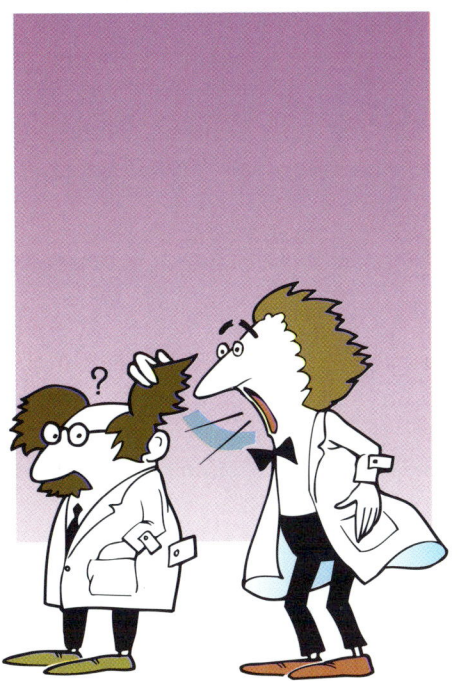

11 GROUP DISCUSSION

You are taking part in a public debate to discuss the pros and cons of gene therapy and the cost of the Genome Project. Each student should express the opinions of one of the following interested parties.

GROUP 1
Doctors and researchers working in the field of genetics. Use some of the expressions you have studied in presenting your case.

GROUP 2
Doctors and researchers working in other fields who fear that the government is spending too much money on this project and who fear, as a result, their research may receive less finance and less government support.

GROUP 3
Members of the public, worried about the possible problems that could arise from the misuse of genetic engineering.

UNDERSTANDING IDIOMATIC ENGLISH

Explain the idiom.

This will hurt me more than it hurts you

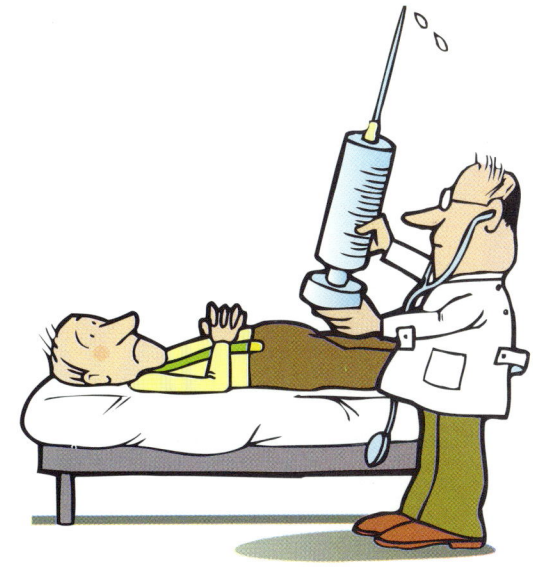

UNIT 7

Mapping chromosomes and sequencing genes

Treading on Heredity

MAPPING CHROMOSOMES

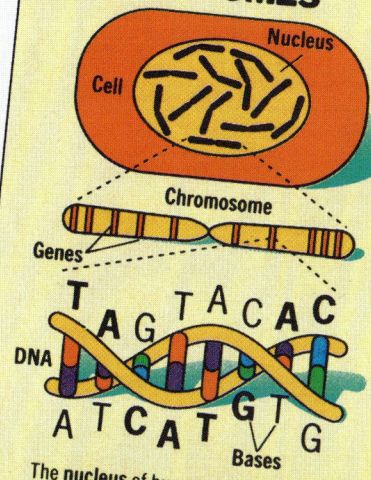

Cell — Nucleus

Chromosome

Genes

DNA — T A G T A C A C / A T C A T G T G

Bases

The **nucleus** of human cells contains a complete blueprint for a man or woman. That information resides on 46 **chromosomes** made primarily of long chains of **DNA**, the master chemical that controls the development and functioning of organisms. The crucial components of DNA are four nitrogenous **bases**: adenine, thymine, cytosine and guanine (A, T, C and G). The sequence of these bases determines the order in which amino acids are linked together to form proteins. A segment of the DNA chain that contains the instructions for a complete protein is called a **gene**.

During cell division, the DNA arranges itself into **23 pairs of complementary chromosomes**, each containing thousands of genes. The chromosomes in each pair have slight differences from each other that can be used as signposts or **markers** to help find genes. For every gene on a

chromosome, there is a corresponding gene on the other member of the chromosome pair.* One of the two genes came from the person's mother, and the other came from the father. The two genes may be the same or different, but they both affect the same characteristic.

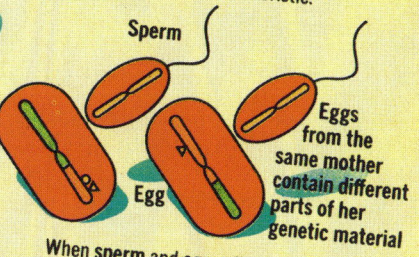

Sperm

Egg

Eggs from the same mother contain different parts of her genetic material

When **sperm** and **egg** cells are formed, they contain only one member of each chromosome pair. Before the chromosome pairs separate, they exchange pieces. In the process, some genes that were together on one chromosome wind up on different chromosomes and thus go into different sperm or egg cells. The closer two genes are to each other on a chromosome, the more likely they are to stay linked and be inherited together.

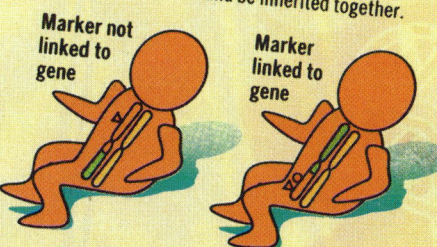

Marker not linked to gene

Marker linked to gene

That fact enables biologists to construct **maps of chromosomes**. To do so, the researchers must extract and analyze DNA from cells. They use a large set of chemicals known as restriction enzymes to chop up the DNA chain into much shorter pieces. Differences between these pieces are called restriction-fragment-length polymorphisms, or RFLPs (pronounced *rif*-lips). Gene mappers have identified a whole catalog of RFLPs, each with its own characteristic sequence of bases. By studying how frequently certain RFLPs are inherited

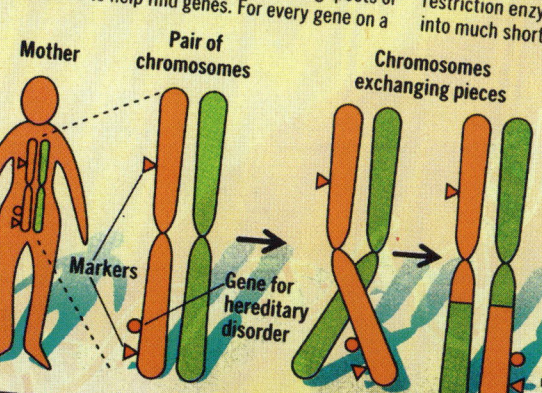

Mother

Pair of chromosomes

Chromosomes exchanging pieces

Markers

Gene for hereditary disorder

* An exception is a man's pair of sex chromosomes, which are called X and Y. A gene on the X chromosome does not necessarily have a complementary gene on the Y.

together in several generations of large families, and thus how close to one another the RFLPs are on the DNA chain, researchers can determine their approximate location on a chromosome.

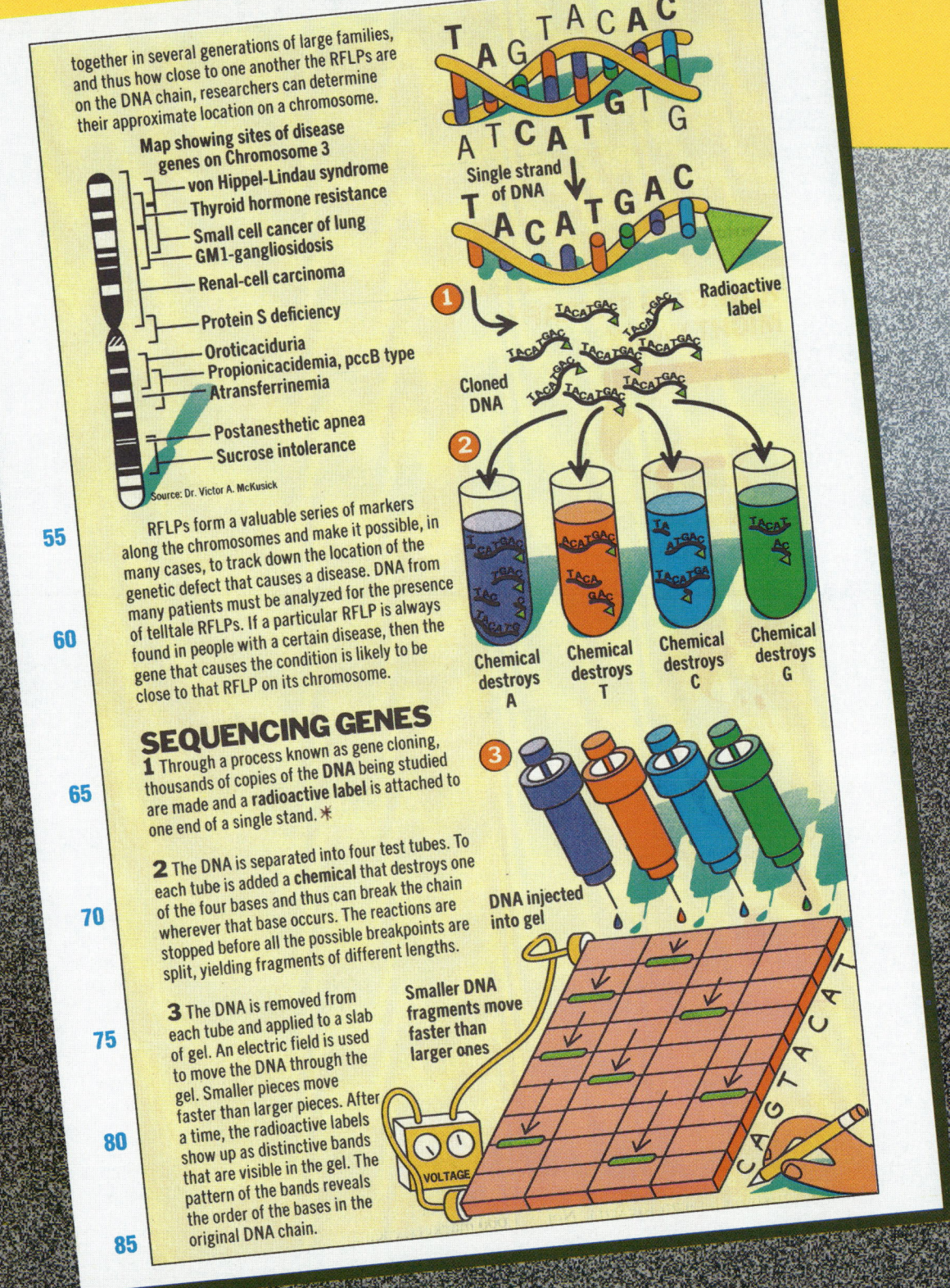

Map showing sites of disease genes on Chromosome 3

- von Hippel-Lindau syndrome
- Thyroid hormone resistance
- Small cell cancer of lung
- GM1-gangliosidosis
- Renal-cell carcinoma
- Protein S deficiency
- Oroticaciduria
- Propionicacidemia, pccB type
- Atransferrinemia
- Postanesthetic apnea
- Sucrose intolerance

Source: Dr. Victor A. McKusick

RFLPs form a valuable series of markers along the chromosomes and make it possible, in many cases, to track down the location of the genetic defect that causes a disease. DNA from many patients must be analyzed for the presence of telltale RFLPs. If a particular RFLP is always found in people with a certain disease, then the gene that causes the condition is likely to be close to that RFLP on its chromosome.

SEQUENCING GENES

1 Through a process known as gene cloning, thousands of copies of the **DNA** being studied are made and a **radioactive label** is attached to one end of a single stand. ✳

2 The DNA is separated into four test tubes. To each tube is added a **chemical** that destroys one of the four bases and thus can break the chain wherever that base occurs. The reactions are stopped before all the possible breakpoints are split, yielding fragments of different lengths.

3 The DNA is removed from each tube and applied to a slab of gel. An electric field is used to move the DNA through the gel. Smaller pieces move faster than larger pieces. After a time, the radioactive labels show up as distinctive bands that are visible in the gel. The pattern of the bands reveals the order of the bases in the original DNA chain.

Single strand of DNA

Radioactive label

Cloned DNA

Chemical destroys A

Chemical destroys T

Chemical destroys C

Chemical destroys G

DNA injected into gel

Smaller DNA fragments move faster than larger ones

VOLTAGE

55
60
65
70
75
80
85

TEXT BASED EXERCISES

VOCABULARY

Study the meaning of the following words and expressions as used in the text.

title to tread
- to walk on

2 a blueprint
- (fig.) a detailed plan

11 a segment
- a portion

14 to arrange
- to organize, to form

17 slight
- of small degree, extent or intensity

30 to wind up
- to finish up

33 likely
- probable

39 to chop up
- to cut into pieces

57 to track down
- to discover after a long search

60 telltale
- revealing a secret

67 a strand
- a single thread

73 to split
- to break; to become disunited

73 to yield
- to produce

75 a slab
- a large, flat piece

76 gel
- a solution which has set to a jelly

81 to show up
- to be clearly visible against a contrasting background

81 band
- a thin, narrow piece

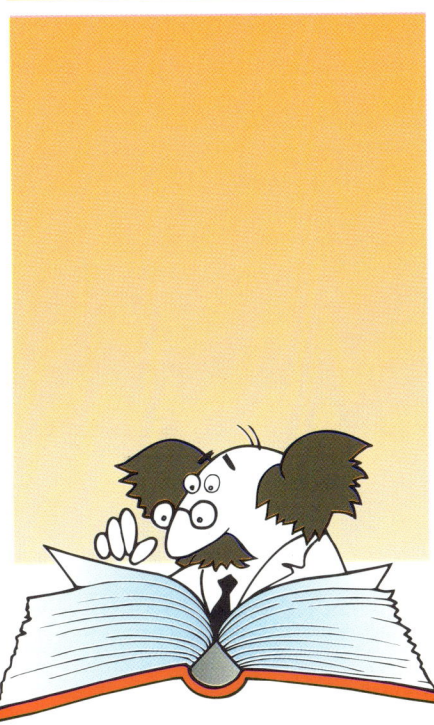

1 WORD CHECK

Explain what you understand by the following terms.

a A chromosome
b DNA
c Amino acids
d Maps of chromosomes
e Restriction-fragment-length-polymorphisms
f A genetic defect
g A test tube
h Gene cloning

2 COMPREHENSION

Answer the following questions.

1 Explain the following sentence: "The nucleus of human cells contains a complete blueprint for a man or a woman."

2 What do you understand by the use of the word *primarily* in line 4?

3 What factor determines the order in which amino acids are linked together to form proteins?

4 What fact enables biologists to construct maps of chromosomes?

5 What do researchers use to chop up the DNA chain into shorter pieces?

6 What factors have researchers studied that help them to determine the approximate location of RFLP's on a chromosome?

7 In what way has the determining of the position of RFLP's on a chromosome helped in finding the location of a genetic defect?

8 What is attached to the end of a single strand of cloned DNA when sequencing genes?

9 Why is a chemical that destroys one of the four bases added to each of the test tubes when sequencing genes?

10 Do the radioactive labels show up as distinctive bands immediately when passed through the gel?

3 NOUNS

Fill in the blanks with the *nouns* below as used in the text.

✓ copies	✓ order
✓ series	✓ chain
✓ sequence	✓ member
✓ pieces	✓ pair
✓ pairs	✓ instructions
✓ segment	✓ bases
✓ label	✓ pattern
✓ reactions	✓ strand
✓ set	✓ bands
✓ markers	✓ process

1 The .... of these .... determines the .... in which amino acids are linked together to form proteins.
2 A .... of the DNA .... that contains the .... for a complete protein is called a gene.
3 For every gene on a chromosome, there is a corresponding gene on the other .... of the chromosome ....
4 Before the chromosome .... separate, they exchange ....
5 They use a large .... of chemicals known as restriction enzymes to chop up the DNA chain.
6 RFLP's form a valuable .... of ....

7 Through a .... known as gene cloning, thousands of .... of the DNA being studied are made.
8 A radioactive .... is attached to one end of a single ....
9 The .... are stopped before all the possible breakpoints are split, yielding fragments of different lengths.
10 The .... of the .... reveals the order of the bases in the original DNA chain.

4

Some nouns and adjectives are formed by putting two words together.

e.g. *landmark* is made up of two words *land* and *mark*.

a Join one word from column 1 with one from column 2 in order to form a single word:

Column 1	Column 2
blue	tale
tell	points
sign	print
radio	posts
break	active

5

Fill in the blanks with one of the words below as used in the text.

✓ valuable	✓ complementary
✓ complete	✓ crucial
✓ large	✓ approximate
✓ electric	✓ shorter
✓ distinctive	✓ close

a The .... components of DNA.
b 23 pairs of .... chromosomes.
c They use a .... set of chemicals known as restriction enzymes to chop up the DNA chain into much .... pieces.
d By studying how frequently certain RELP's are inherited together in several generations of large families, and thus how .... to one another the RFLP's are on the DNA chain, researchers can determine their .... location on a chromosome.
e RFLP's form a .... series of markers along the chromosomes.
f An .... field is used to move the DNA through the gel.
g After a time, the radioactive labels show up as .... bands that are visible in the gel.
h A segment of the DNA chain that contains the instructions for a .... protein is called a gene.

6 ADJECTIVES

RENAL is the adjective used to describe the kidneys and their function. Some adjectives are similar to the part of the body they describe and others are different. Match the parts of the body with the corresponding adjective.

Part of the body	Adjective
1 the liver	a duodenal
2 the stomach	b oral
3 the duodenum	c epidermal
4 the lungs	d optic
5 the back	e hepatic
6 the skin	f gastric
7 the eyes	g dorsal
8 the mouth	h pulmonary

7

Study the use of the word *own* in the following sentence.
44 Gene mappers have identified a whole catalog of RFLP's, each with its *own* characteristic sequence of bases.

EXTENSION EXERCISES

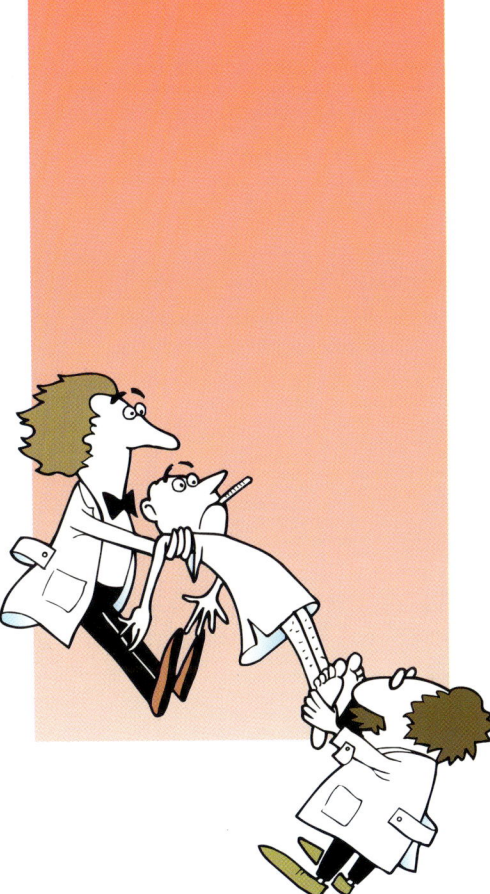

Own means exclusively possessed. My *own* room means that it is only mine and not shared with another person.

Read the following sentences . Change the sentences as in the example by using *own* and *a possessive adjective*.

e.g. He has a book.
He has *his own* book.

1 I have a business.
2 My wife has a car.
3 My son has a key.
4 She has ideas.
5 They have methods.
6 We have a house.
7 My grandmother has teeth.
8 Does he have a bank account?
9 They have rules.
10 The house has a garden.

8

I'm *on my own* means I'm alone. Fill in the blanks with a possessive adjective and the word *own*.

1 He's been travelling around Europe on ....
2 Jane's working on ....
3 I did the homework on ....
4 We're leaving the children with my mother and we're going on holiday on ....
5 They decided to set up a business on ....
6 You shouldn't do it on ....
7 Was he on .... when you saw him?
8 I went for a walk on ....

9 PHRASAL VERBS WITH COME

Study the meanings of the verbs below. They are all formed with the verb *TO COME*.

Complete the following sentences. Add the missing part of the phrasal verb.

1 As my father is a lawyer, he wanted me to join the family business. I told him I wanted to be a doctor. After a lot of persuading, he finally came ....

2 The team tried a new technique but it didn't come ....

3 Several specialists have applied for the post but Doctor Lincoln's application has come .... special consideration.

4 After a long anaesthetic, the patient still felt sick. He wasn't able to eat anything as it would have just come ....

5 Yesterday, I came .... an old photograph of my friends when we were medical students. I could hardly recognize some of them as they had changed a lot in ten years.

6 The surgeon thought that the operation would be straightforward. However, he came .... some unexpected problems when he began to operate.

7 "Isn't Doctor Fielding's wedding coming .... soon?"

8 The patient took several hours to come .... after the operation.

9 I'd like to apply for a job in Cardiology as soon as a vacancy comes ....

10 When it came .... that the hospital was going to be closed, the local residents formed a protest group.

Phrasal verb	Meaning
to come across	to find by chance
to come off (1)	to take place
to come off (2)	to succeed
to come out	to be revealed
to come round (1)	to finally accept a previously opposed suggestion
to come round (2)	to recover consciousness
to come up (1)	to be vomited
to come up (2)	to occur or arise (especially a vacancy or opportunity)
to come up against	to be faced with
to come up for	to be considered as an applicant or candidate

Notes

GRAMMAR POINT

THE PASSIVE

The passive is frequently used in medical writing.

a   *Construction.*
The OBJECT of the ACTIVE sentence becomes the SUBJECT of the PASSIVE sentence.

e.g. ACTIVE   Muscles *take* glucose out of the bloodstream.

PASSIVE   Glucose *is taken* out of the bloodstream by the muscles.

b   *The Agent.*
Often, the object (or agent) is *not* mentioned in the passive sentence.

e.g. ACTIVE   They found a cure.

PASSIVE   A cure was found.

When the agent is mentioned, it is preceded by the preposition BY and placed at the *end* of the clause.

e.g. ACTIVE   The pericardium protects the heart.

PASSIVE   The heart is protected *by* the pericardium.

c   The passive of an active tense is formed by putting the verb *to be* into the *same tense* as the active verb. The *past participle*

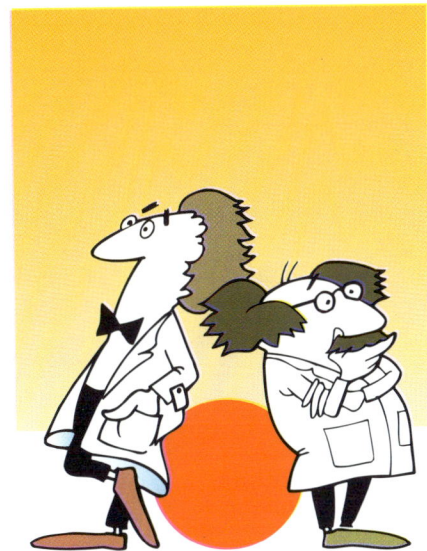

of the active verb is then added.

e.g. refers to   is referred to
ACTIVE   PASSIVE

d   *Some examples of passives.*

10 GRAMMAR CHECK

Turn the following active sentences into the *passive*.

1   Glands in the stomach wall secrete gastric juices.
2   The gall bladder stores bile.
3   The liver regulates the amount of sugar that passes into the general circulation.
4   The nervous system controls and co-ordinates the actions of the body.
5   Mineral salts provide many of the elements needed for growth.
6   The researcher separated the DNA into four test tubes.
7   They use a large set of chemicals to chop up the DNA chain into smaller pieces.
8   Researchers can determine their approximate location on a chromosome.
9   They add a chemical that destroys one of the four bases.

Tense and Verb Form	Active	Passive
Simple Present Tense	causes	is caused
Present Continuous	is causing	is being caused
Present Infinitive	to cause	to be caused
Perfect Infinitive	to have caused	to have been caused
Present Participle	causing	being caused
Perfect Participle	having caused	having been caused

WRITING

11 WRITING INSTRUCTIONS

Write instructions for sequencing genes. Make sentences with the words below. Use the *imperative* at the beginning of each sentence. The first two instructions are given as examples.

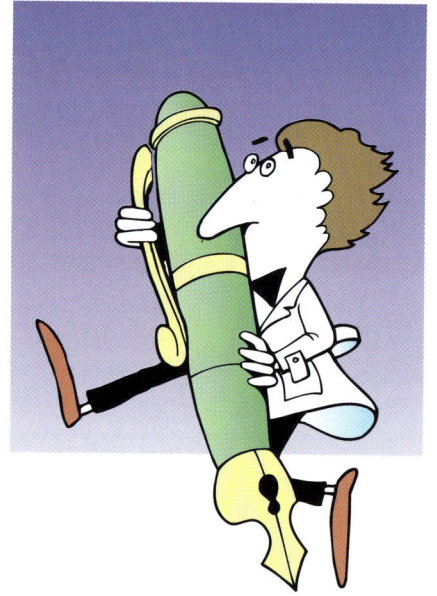

Notes

INSTRUCTIONS FOR SEQUENCING GENES	
copies	Make copies of the DNA.
a radioactive label	Attach a radioactive label to one end of a single strand.
test tubes	
a chemical	
the reactions	
each tube	
a slab	
an electric field	

SPEAKING

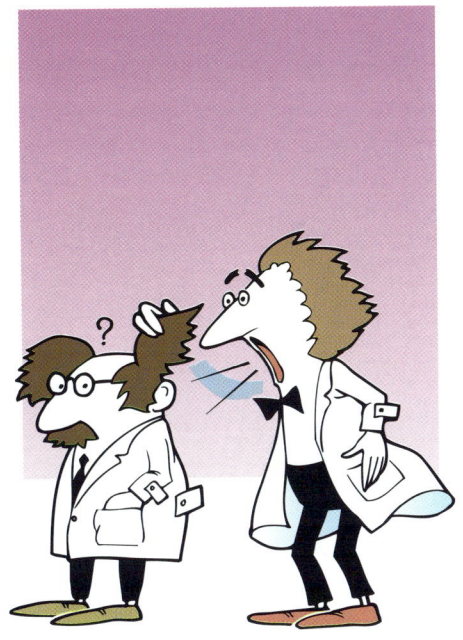

12 DESCRIBING

Describe the following in your own words:

— The structure of DNA
— Meiosis and its function
— Crossing-over

Notes

UNDERSTANDING IDIOMATIC ENGLISH

Explain the idiom.

He managed to
find his feet

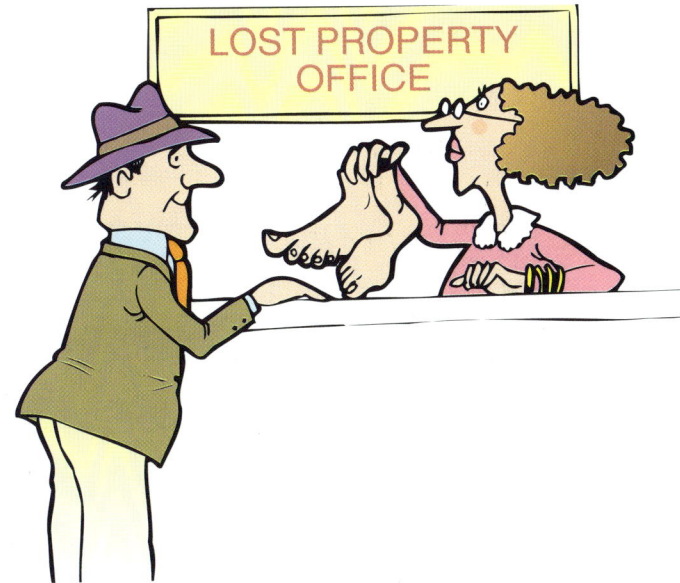

UNIT 8

Growth-hormone therapy

Can Hormones Stop the Clock?

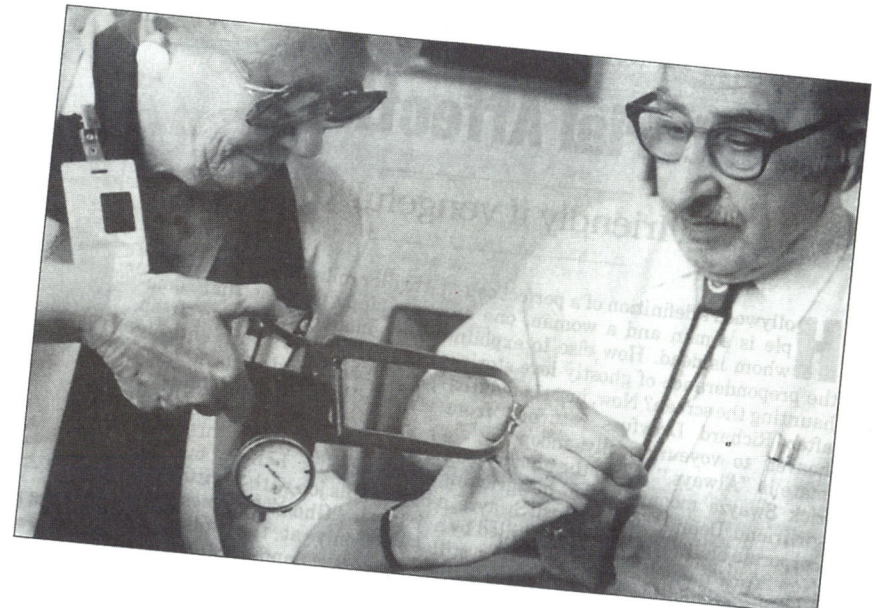

JAMES SCHNEPF

a gain in skin thickness.

Twelve seniors tone up

The American quest for the fountain of youth is never ending, and thanks to a study in last week's New England Journal of Medicine, old folks and Eli Lilly & Co. have a hot new prospect: human growth hormone. By injecting a synthetic version of the hormone into a handful of healthy, aging men for six months, researchers managed to reverse the process by which lean body mass gives way to fat. Indeed, the six-month regimen seemed to undo 10 to 20 years of skin, bone and muscle deterioration, prompting speculation that prolonged youth would one day be an option for anyone who could afford the treatment (it would cost about $14,000 a year at current prices). But don't hold your breath. As one expert puts it, "To think this is going to be an anti-aging panacea is a mistake."

The new study, funded in part by Lilly, was the first to test the effects of growth hormone on healthy oldsters, but the results were no great surprise. Previous trials have shown that growth-hormone therapy can slow muscle loss and fat buildup in young patients with endocrine deficiencies. Since advanced age brings similar changes in body composition—often accompanied by a decline in growth-hormone production—it stood to reason that aging patients might benefit from the treatment.

To find out, a team led by Dr. Daniel Rudman of the Medical College of Wisconsin and the Milwaukee VA Medical Center assembled 21 healthy men, 61 to 81, with low levels of growth hormone. For six months, 12 of the subjects received growth-hormone injections. The other nine didn't. The treated subjects enjoyed a 14 percent reduction in body fat and a 9 percent gain in lean body mass. They also showed slight gains in skin thickness and spinal density. By all these measures, they got younger.

So why not shout eureka? First, as Rudman and his colleagues duly note, the 12 men were by no means representative of the over-60 population. Though everyone slackens with age, only a third of the elderly experience the decline in growth hormone that this trial sought to counter. The treatment might do nothing for more typical aging males, or for women. A second reason for caution is that the observed effects don't necessarily represent improved health. The treatment may not enhance "muscle strength, mobility or the quality of life," Dr. Mary Lee Vance notes in an editorial accompanying the study. The treatment might even pose hazards. Potential side effects range from enlargement of the face and extremities to hypertension, arthritis and heart failure. There is also a possible cancer connection. People with acromegaly, a condition caused by excess growth hormone, are at increased risk of colon cancer. And one study of people taking human growth hormone for dwarfism found a rise in leukemia incidence.

As a medical field, hormone therapy holds rich possibilities. Last week alone, researchers reported in separate studies that the hormonal drug megestrol acetate could help emaciated cancer patients gain weight, and that treatment with a growth factor called TGF-beta might prevent some of the damage caused by heart attacks. Some statistical risks are justified when a treatment holds such promise. But until someone shows that the benefits of growth-hormone injections outweigh the risks to healthy adults, diet and exercise will be surer routes to good health.

GEOFFREY COWLEY *with* MARY HAGER *in Washington*

TEXT BASED EXERCISES

VOCABULARY

Study the meaning of the following words and expressions as used in the text.

1   a quest
    - a search
4   folks
    - people
10 lean
    - without fat
12 to undo
    - to cancel
15 to afford
    - to have enough money to pay for the treatment
19 a panacea
    - a remedy for all disorders
30 to stand to reason
    - to be of good sense
32 to lead
    - to act as chief (led-p.t.)
45 duly
    - appropriately
48 to slacken
    - to become less strong or solid
50 to counter
    - to neutralize the effects
55 to enhance
    - to increase or improve
59 a hazard
    - a risk
68 a dwarf
    - a person considerably below average size
75 to emaciate
    - to become excessively thin
76 to gain
    - to improve, increase, obtain
86 outweigh
    - are more than

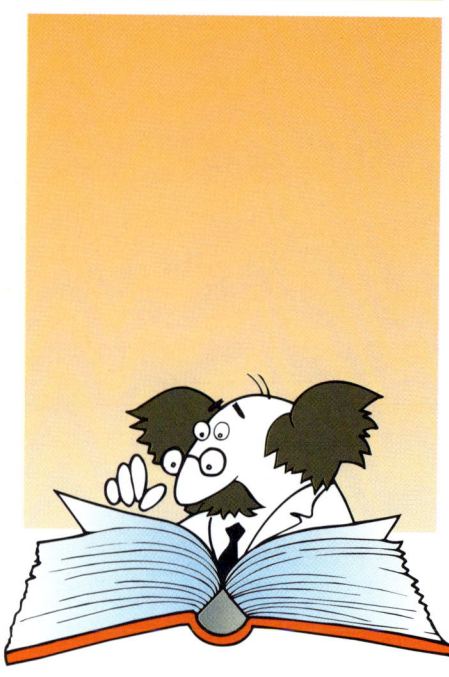

1 WORD CHECK

Explain the meaning of the following expressions as used in the text.

1   the fountain of youth
6   a synthetic version
11 a six-month regimen
19 an anti-aging panacea
22 healthy oldsters
24 growth-hormone therapy
26 endocrine deficiencies
60 potential side effects
69 leukemia incidence
88 surer routes to good health

2 COMPREHENSION

Read the following sentences. Say whether they are TRUE or FALSE.

1   The Americans have given up looking for a fountain of youth.
2   The results were a great surprise.
3   Previous trials have shown that growth-hormone therapy always slows muscle loss and fat buildup in young patients with endocrine deficiencies.
4   Only men with low levels of growth hormone took part in the trial.
5   All the 21 men who took part in the trial received growth-hormone injections.
6   Apart from a reduction in body fat and a gain in lean body mass, the treated subjects also showed a very small gain in skin thickness and spinal density.
7   The researchers shouted "Eureka!".
8   All elderly people experience a decline in growth hormone.
9   The treatment may not improve the quality of life.
10 There are no potential side effects connected with this treatment.
11 Working on hormone therapy could possibly make the researchers rich.
12 There is a possible cancer connection.

3

Join a word from column 1 with a word from column 2 in order to form an expression as used in the text.

Column 1	Column 2
body	buildup
endocrine	effects
body	cancer
heart	loss
colon	deficiencies
muscle	mass
fat	connection
side	composition
cancer	failure

Notes

4

Now use each of the expressions from exercise 3 to fill in the blanks below.

1 People with acromegaly are at increased risk of ....

2 Researchers managed to reverse the process by which lean .... gives way to fat.

3 Potential .... range from enlargement of the face and extremities to hypertension, arthritis and ....

4 Previous trials have shown that growth-hormone therapy can slow .... and .... in young patients with ....

5 Since advanced age brings similar changes in .... , it stood to reason that aging patients might benefit from the treatment.

6 There is also a possible ....

5 SENTENCE BUILDING

The sentences below all express possibility, doubt or uncertainty. Join a phrase from each of the three columns in order to form a sentence as used in the text.

Column 1	Column 2	Column 3
The six-month regimen	would	help emaciated cancer patients gain weight
It	possible	represent improved health
A second reason for caution is that the observed effects	seemed to	pose hazards
It stood to reason that aging patients	might even	cancer connection
The treatment	don't necessarily	undo 10 to 20 years of skin, bone and muscle deterioration
The treatment	might	enhance "muscle strength, mobility or the quality of life"
There is also a	could	cost about $ 14,000 a year at current prices
The hormonal drug megestrol acetate	may not	benefit from the treatment

6 IDIOMATIC EXPRESSIONS WITH COME

Study the following expressions. They are all formed with the verb *TO COME*.
Read the following sentences. Replace the part of the sentence *in italics* with one of the idioms below in the correct form.

1 The new hospital decided to adopt flexible visiting hours so that the visitors could *visit when they liked.*

2 Doctor Black to his colleague: "Jack, I'm giving a party tonight to celebrate my promotion. I hope you can come."
Doctor Fraser: "I'm sorry

EXTENSION EXERCISES

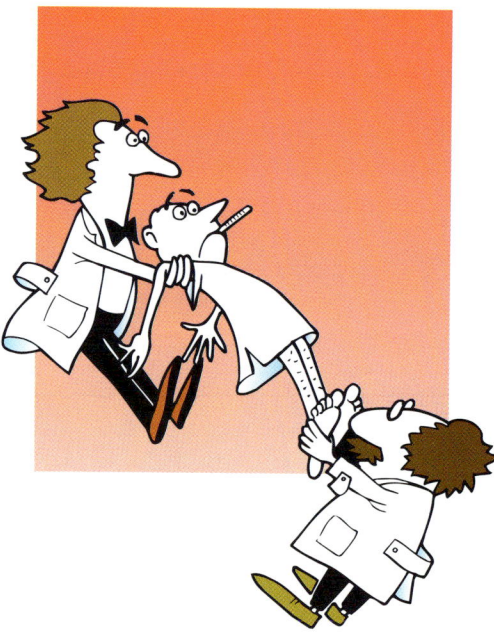

Mike. I won't finish work tonight until nine o'clock and I'll have to go home and change."
Doctor Black: "That's no problem Jack. You don't have to change. Come *in the clothes you are wearing.*"

3 Mr. Anderson was bored lying in bed all day long. When the nurse told him that he had a visitor, *his spirits lifted.*

4 Medical student to friend: "I'm going to study hard, pass all my exams with high marks, get a good job as a doctor, become a specialist before I'm 30, marry a beautiful wife, settle down and have two wonderful children."
Friend: "The best of luck. I hope you don't *meet with any problems that will cause you to modify your plans.*"
Medical student: "*Whatever happens,* I'll work hard at achieving my desires. I'll make them *happen just as I've dreamed.*"
Friend: "*Be reasonable.* Do you really think it's possible? Some problems are sure to occur. You can't always expect *to have the best possible results.*"
Medical student: "Well, now I *stop and think about it,* perhaps you're right. I've got my Pathology exam next week and there are a few things I'm not sure about. I could fail the exam. Perhaps I should try to be a specialist by the time I'm 32 instead of 30."

5 Tom liked studying medicine

Idiomatic expression	Meaning
to come alive	to come to life
to come as you are	to pay a visit or attend a function without dressing formally
to come out of one's shell	to overcome one's shyness
to come true	to actually happen as dreamed or hoped for
to come and go	to arrive and depart freely
now I come to think of it	now that the event etc. just mentioned has been thought of or recalled
come, come	expression used to urge someone to be sensible
come what may	whatever else may happen as a result of doing something
to come up roses	to happen in the best way possible
to come unstuck	to meet with a mishap or a reversal of a plan

but he had never managed to *overcome his shyness.* When he got his medical degree, he decided not to work with patients. He got a job in research and was successful and happy.

7

Study the following sentence.

48 Though everyone *slackens* with age, only a third of the elderly experience the decline in growth hormone that this trial sought to counter.

To slacken means to make or become slack.

Explain the meaning of each of the following verbs. Make a sentence in your own words with each of the verbs in any suitable form.

✓ to strengthen
✓ to weaken
✓ to lighten
✓ to loosen
✓ to flatten
✓ to quicken
✓ to widen
✓ to lengthen
✓ to shorten

Extract from a Medical Dictionary

hormone (hor'mōn) [Gr. *hormaein* to set in motion, spur on] a chemical substance, produced in the body by an organ or cells of an organ which has a specific regulatory effect on the activity of a certain organ; originally applied to substances secreted by various endocrine glands and transported in the blood stream to the target organ on which their effect was produced, the term was later applied to various substances not produced by special glands but having similar action. See also *endocrine system,* under *system.* **adaptive h.,** one, such as corticotropin or the corticoids, which is secreted during adaptation to unusual circumstances. **adenohypophyseal h.,** any hormone secreted by the adenohypophysis, including somatotropin (STH), thyrotropin (TSH), prolactin, follicle-stimulating hormone (FSH), luteinizing hormone (LH), melanocyte-stimulating hormone (MSH), and adrenocorticotropic hormone (ACTH). **adipokinetic h.,** 1. a hypothetical lipolytic hormone secreted by the pituitary gland. 2. lipolytic h. **adrenocortical h.,** any of the corticosteroids elaborated by the adrenal cortex, the major ones being the glucocorticoids and mineralcorticoids, and including some androgens, progesterone, and perhaps estrogens. See also *corticosteroid.* **adrenocorticotropic h.,** corticotropin. **adrenomedullary h's,** substances secreted by the adrenal medulla, including epinephrine and norepinephrine. **androgenic h's,** the masculinizing hormones, androsterone and testosterone. **anterior pituitary h.,** any of the several protein or polypeptide hormones secreted by the anterior lobe of the pituitary gland, including the corticotropic, growth, thyrotropic, and gonadotropic hormones. **antidiuretic h.,** a hormone secreted by the supraoptic nucleus of the hypothalamus, stored in the posterior pituitary and released on signal by osmoreceptors in the nucleus. It has a specific effect on the epithelial cells of the distal portion of the uriniferous tubule, stimulating reabsorption of water independently of solids, and resulting in concentration of urine. It also has vasopressor activity. Called also *vasopressin.* **Aschheim-Zondek h.,** luteinizing h. **chondrotropic h.,** growth h. **chromaffin h.,** epinephrine. **chromatophorotropic h.,** intermedin. **conjugated estrogen h's,** an amorphous preparation of naturally-occurring, water-soluble, conjugated forms of mixed estrogens. **corpus luteum h.,** progesterone. **cortical h.,** see *adrenocortical h.* **diabetogenic h.,** a substance in extracts of the anterior pituitary that tends to elevate the blood sugar by acting as an antagonist to insulin. It is probably not a distinct entity and its effects are probably related to those of known pituitary hormones, especially human growth hormone. **estrogenic h's,** substances capable of producing certain biological effects, the most characteristic of which are the changes which occur in mammals at estrus; the naturally occurring estrogenic hormones are b-estradiol, estrone, and estriol. **fat-mobilizing h's,** lipolytic h's. **follicle h.,** an estrogenic hormone produced by the graafian follicle. **follicle-stimulating h. (FSH),** one of the gonadotropic hormones of the anterior pituitary, which stimulates the growth and maturation of graafian follicles in the ovary, and stimulates spermatogenesis in the male. **follicle-stimulating hormone releasing h. (FSH-RH),** gonadotropin releasing h. **follicular h.,** one produced by the graafian follicle. **galactopoietic h.,** prolactin. **gastrointestinal h.,** hormones that originate in and regulate motor and secretory activity of the digestive organs, i.e., gastrin, secretin, and cholecystokinin. **gonadotropic h.,** any hormone that has an influence on the gonads. **gonadotropic h's, pituitary,** three hormones, including follicle-stimulating hormone and luteinizing hormone in mammals and prolactin in certain birds, secreted by the anterior pituitary gland which have an influence on the gonads. **gonadotropin releasing h. (Gn-RH)** a decapeptide hormone elaborated by the median eminence of the hypothalamus that stimulates the release of follicle-stimulating hormone and luteinizing hormone from the anterior lobe of the pituitary gland. **growth h. (GH),** any substance that stimulates growth, especially one secreted by the anterior pituitary, which exerts a direct effect on protein, carbohydrate, and lipid metabolism, and controls the rate of skeletal and visceral growth. Human growth hormone (HGH) is composed of a single chain of 188 amino acids without carbohydrate substituents. Called also *somatotropin.* **growth hormone release inhibiting h.,** somatostatin. **growth hormone releasing h. (GH-RH),** see under *factor.* **human (pituitary) growth h. (HGH),** see *growth h.* **hypophysiotropic h.,** any of the hormones of the hypothalamus that stimulate or inhibit the hypophysis, including the releasing factors. **inhibiting h's,** hormones elabnorated by one structure (as by the hypothalamus) that inhibit release of hormones from another structure (as from the anterior pituitary gland), e.g., *somatostatin* (growth hormone release inhibiting h.). The term is applied to substances of established clinical identity, whereas substances of unknown chemical structure are called *inhibiting factors* (see under *factor*). **inhibitory h.,** a substance that exerts a depressing influence on certain of its target organs, e.g., enterogastrone.

[From Dorland (adapted)]

UNDERSTANDING INCOMPLETE SENTENCES

Study the following sentence.

36 For six months, 12 of the subjects received growth-hormone injections. The other nine didn't.

Note the following points.

a It is *understood* that the second sentence means "didn't receive growth-hormone injections".
b This construction, using only the auxiliary, can be used when *the verb has already been stated* in the first sentence.
c The use of the auxiliary by itself thus *avoids a long second sentence* containing information already given.
d The auxiliary used, *must correspond* to the tense used in the first sentence.
e If the first sentence is affirmative, then the second is negative and viceversa.

   e.g.   These subjects *received* the treatment.
   AFFIRMATIVE

   The others *didn't*.
   NEGATIVE

   These subject *didn't receive* the treatment.
   NEGATIVE

   The others *did*.
   AFFIRMATIVE

GRAMMAR POINT

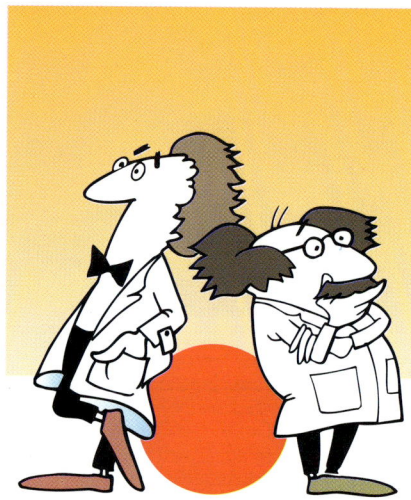

8 GRAMMAR CHECK

Complete the chart below by adding the corresponding negative short forms.

e.g. is ⟶ isn't
     are ⟶ aren't'

Affirmative	Negative	Affirmative	Negative
has		have	
do		does	
was		were	
did		had	
shall		will	
should		would	
can		could	
must		need	

9 GRAMMAR CHECK

Complete the following sentences using the words "the others" plus an appropriate auxiliary.

e.g. These tests were successful.
These tests were successful. The others weren't.

1 These treatments will have some side effects.
2 These patients couldn't afford the treatment.
3 These researchers want to repeat the test.
4 These men would take part in the trials if you asked them.
5 These tests were carried out for six months.
6 These women aren't at risk.
7 These old people don't like exercise.
8 These drugs could help cancer victims gain weight.
9 These subjects must follow a strict diet.
10 These trials haven't been tried on women.

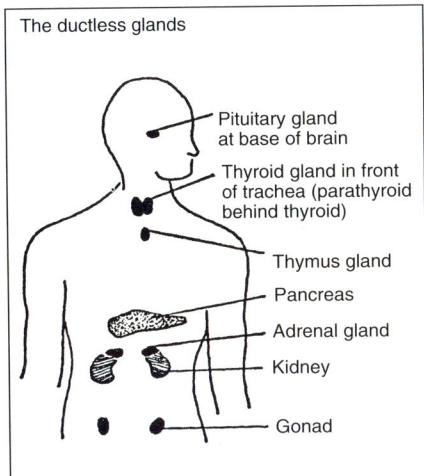

The ductless glands

- Pituitary gland at base of brain
- Thyroid gland in front of trachea (parathyroid behind thyroid)
- Thymus gland
- Pancreas
- Adrenal gland
- Kidney
- Gonad

VOCABULARY

15 pouchy
- loosely bulging
(a pouch
- a small bag)
40 to pour forth
- to pour out; to emerge in a stream
47 apt to be
- inclined, tend to be
50 to withstand
- to resist

Study the following passage.

ENDOCRINE GLANDS

In man's adaptations for life functions, there are glands which manufacture essential chemical substances. For example, gastric glands and the liver pour digestive juices through tubes called ducts into the stomach and intestine respectively to bring about digestion of food substances. Sweat glands in the skin and salivary glands in the mouth are other glands with ducts. The juices produced by these glands with ducts are called secretions. 5

During the 1920's scientists discovered that there are other glands in the body which have no ducts, and are therefore called ductless or **endocrine glands**. They produce or secrete chemicals called **hormones** (chemical messengers) directly into the blood stream. Hormones travel from the gland in which they are manufactured through the 10 blood stream to the organ or organs they affect.

Normal functioning of all the endocrine glands results in normal functioning of the cells of the body and general well-being.

The endocrine glands control our body activities. Some of their functions are generally familiar – e.g. the disorder in which the neck is much enlarged and pouchy- 15 looking and the eyes seem bulging. This swollen condition is known as goitre and is probably caused by an over-active **thyroid** gland in the neck region around the voice box. The thyroid secretes a hormone called **thyroxin** which controls the rate at which food is oxidized in the body (metabolism). The basal metabolism test determines this rate. Thyroxin contains iodine as part of its chemical make-up. 20

Abnormalities occur in the body where there is an insufficient production of thyroxin as well as where there is an overabundance of this hormone.

The **pituitary** gland, called the master gland, is located at the base of the brain. It merits its name because it seems to control other endocrine glands. Specifically, its functions are to control growth of the bony skeleton, to regulate metabolism of food, 25 to regulate the muscles of some internal organs, and to regulate the functioning of the kidneys.

Overactivity of the pituitary gland in childhood results in giantism – the famous giants of the circus. Underactivity of the master gland results in the opposite deformity, namely, dwarfism. 30

At the back of the thyroid gland and resting against the sides of the windpipe are two pairs of **parathyroid** glands. These glands regulate the use of calcium and phosphorus in bones and teeth. They also provide calcium to the skeletal muscles. Insufficient calcium causes great pain and lack of muscular control.

The **thymus gland** is located at the base of the trachea. Comparatively little is known 35 of its specific action, but it is thought that it plays a role in the build-up of antibodies.

The paired **adrenal** glands are located on top of each kidney. Extreme emotional disturbances – such as fright, fear, anger and joy, stimulate the **medulla** (centre of the gland) to produce the hormone **adrenalin**. This secretion activates the liver to pour forth more sugar into the blood for rapid oxidation in the muscles and in the 40 brain cells – this results in more rapid, sometimes immediate, thinking and muscular responses. Thus it works in antagonism to insulin.

Adrenalin also aids in blood clotting by constricting blood vessels, decreasing shock and stimulating heart action. It helps relieve asthmatic conditions due to constriction of the trachea and bronchial tubes. 45

Adrenalin may be synthesised from animal secretions and is sometimes injected into the body during operations where there is apt to be excessive bleeding, and directly into the heart muscles in cases of heart failure.

The adrenal **cortex** (outer layer) secretes several hormones affecting salt retention, blood sugar concentration and the ability to withstand stress. 50

WRITING

10 HORMONES

Explain what you understand by the expression "hormones are chemical messengers".

Notes

11 ENDOCRINE GLANDS

Write a few sentences about each of the following.

the thyroid gland
the pituitary gland
the parathyroid glands
the thymus gland
the adrenal glands

Notes

SPEAKING

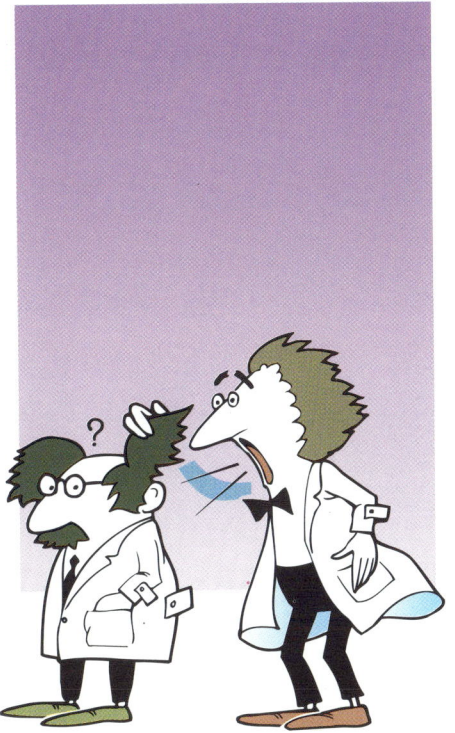

12 ASKING QUESTIONS

Group work.
One student takes the part of Dr. Daniel Rudman of the Medical College of Wisconsin who led the team working on the growth-hormone study. Another student should take the part of Dr. Mary Lee Vance who wrote an editorial accompanying the study. The other students should ask questions about the details of the study, the results, the potential side effects and the future possibilities connected with hormone therapy.

13 DOCTOR/PATIENT DIALOGUE

Work in pairs.
Conduct the following doctor/patient dialogue.

An elderly male patient wants to stay as young and healthy as possible.
He has read about the benefits of hormone therapy and has come to ask his doctor for advice.

The doctor should briefly explain the advantages and disadvantages of the treatment. He should also give advice on other ways of maintaining good health.

UNDERSTANDING IDIOMATIC ENGLISH

Explain the idiom.

He got a dose
of his own medicine

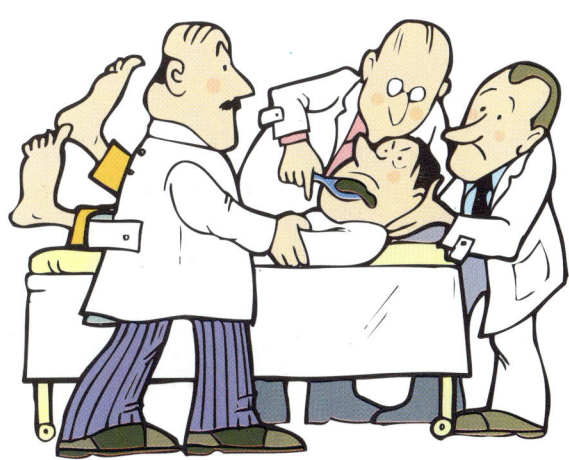

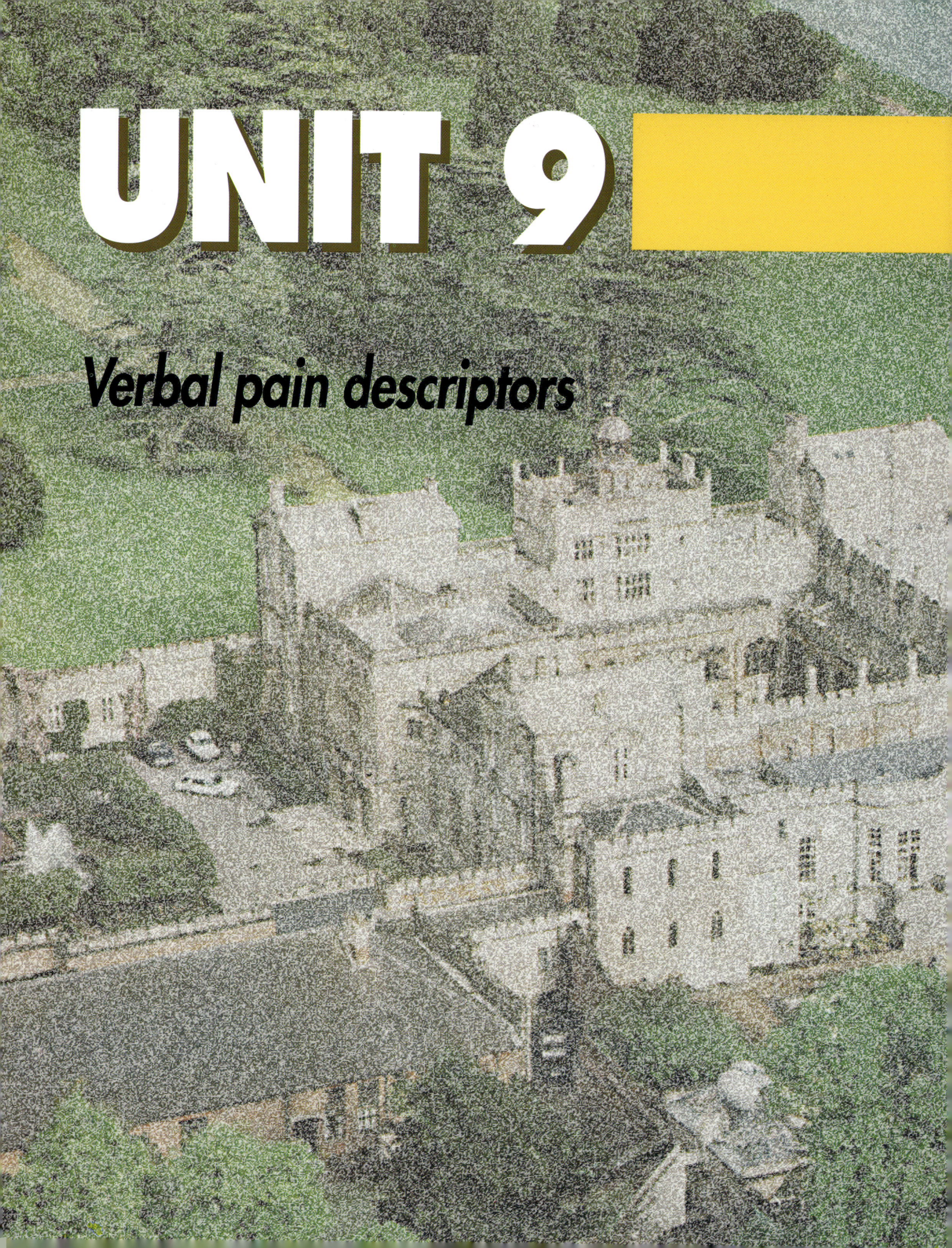

UNIT 9

Verbal pain descriptors

Measuring pain quality: validity and reliability of children's and adolescents' pain language

Summary Although considerable research has been conducted to identify children's and adolescents' language of pain, research is lacking regarding a method to quantify the pain quality described by this language. Three descriptive studies involving 1223 children, aged 8–17 years, were conducted in school and hospital settings. The aims were to develop and examine the validity and reliability of a word list for measuring pain quality that was free of age, gender, and ethnic biases. A word list with 43 words was developed and resulted in sensory, affective, evaluative, and total scores that correlated with pain location and pain intensity scores ($r = 0.19$–0.44; $P \leqslant 0.01$). Pain quality scores decreased over time in a postoperative pain model. Test–retest reliability of the word list scores was high ($r = 0.78$–0.95; $P < 0.001$). This word list was revised and resulted in a word list with 56 words relatively free of gender, ethnic, and developmental biases. Additional research is needed to assess the psychometric properties of this word list in pediatric populations experiencing different pain syndromes.

Key words: Pain; Quality; Descriptors; Assessment; (Children); (Adolescents)

Introduction

In clinical practice, pain quality has been operationalized by words that individuals use to describe their pain. These verbal pain descriptors are recognized as an important assessment parameter, especially when they are theoretically organized in a tool, such as in the McGill Pain Questionnaire [13], the Tursky Pain Perception Profile [25], or verbal descriptor scales of painfulness [7]. These scales have been used to differentiate pain syndromes [3,27] and to determine the effectiveness of pain therapy in adult populations [8]. However, children's pain descriptors, which have been found to be both similar and different from adult pain words, have not been organized in a tool that provides a method of quantifying pain quality [11]. Development of a measure of pain quality is important to help characterize pediatric pain syndromes and to determine the influence of different analgesic therapies on pediatric pain quality.

Study 1

Purpose and sample. Study 1 was designed to construct a developmentally appropriate list of words known and used by multiethnic samples of children and adolescents to describe pain. Three samples of children, 8–17 years of age, were included: (1) 433 students in school classroom settings, 44% male, 27% white, 34% Chinese, and 39% from other ethnic groups; (2) 525 students in school classroom settings, 49% male, 56% white, 9% black, 10% Hispanic and 25% from other ethnic groups; and (3) 35 hospitalized children experiencing pain, 80% less than 14 years of age, 66% male, and 63% white. English was *not* the first language for 25% of the 993 children. Most students (64%) had been hospitalized at least once.

Instruments and procedures. The available domain of children's pain descriptors was reviewed, i.e., research conducted or reported before 1985 [1,2,14,15,17,21,22,24]. One hundred and twenty-nine words were identified as used by children for pain description. Each of the 129 words was printed on a 2.5×3.5 inch card. Individually, the children were asked to sort the 129 cards into 3 stacks representing (1) words they knew and used to describe pain, (2) words they knew but would not use to describe pain, and (3) words not known to them. Two weeks after this sorting procedure, 64 students from the first school sample and 44 students from the second school sample repeated the procedure. Because some of the hospitalized children had greater difficulty completing the procedures than did the students, the test–retest component was not included with the third hospital sample.

Results. To include a word on a pain quality word list, a criterion was set of at least 50% of the sample knowing and using a particular word. Forty-three of the 129 words met this criterion for the first student sample, 72 words for the second student sample, and 36 words for the hospitalized sample. When the data from the 2 student samples were combined (n = 958), 67 words met the 50% criterion. All but 8 of the 36 words from the hospitalized sample met the 50% criterion for the student samples (i.e., angry, always there, exhausting, frustrating, nervous, sad, scary, and tiring did not).

As found in previous research [10], in the combined student sample, an age-related trend was observed in the number of words not known which supports the general assumption that vocabulary influences children's description of pain. All of the 129 words were known by at least 50% of the

TABLE 1

SECOND-GENERATION WORD LIST CATEGORIZED BY SENSORY, AFFECTIVE, AND EVALUATIVE DIMENSIONS

Dimension [a]	Word	Dimension	Word	Dimension	Word	Dimension	Word
E	Annoying [b]	S	Biting [c]	S	Itching [b,c]	A	Crying [c]
	Bad [c]		Cutting [b,c]		Like a scratch		Frightening [b,c]
	Horrible [c]		Like a pin [c]		Like a sting		Screaming
	Miserable [b,c]		Like a sharp knife		Scratching [c]		Terrifying [b,c]
	Terrible [c]		Pinlike		Stinging [b,c]		
	Uncomfortable [c]		Sharp [b,c]			A	Dizzy
			Stabbing [c]	S	Shocking [c]		Sickening [b,c]
S	Aching [b,c]				Shooting [c]		Suffocating [b,c]
	Hurting [b,c]	S	Blistering [c]		Splitting		
	Like an ache		Burning [b,c]			E	Never goes away [c]
	Like a hurt		Hot [b,c]	S	Numb [b,c]		Uncontrollable
	Sore [b,c]				Stiff		
		S	Cramping [b,c]		Swollen [c]		
			Crushing [b,c]		Tight [b]		
S	Beating [b,c]		Like a pinch				
	Hitting		Pinching [b,c]	A	Awful [c]		
	Pounding [b,c]		Pressure [b,c]		Deadly [c]		
	Punching [c]				Dying [c]		
	Throbbing [b]				Killing [c]		

[a] S = sensory; A = affective; E = evaluative.
[b] Words grouped similarly to the McGill Pain Questionnaire (like a bullet was not included on the second word list).
[c] One of the 42 words included on the first word list.

adolescents aged 14–17 years, but 13 words were not known by 50% or more of the children, aged 8–9 years.

A first-generation word list was constructed with the 43 words identified from the first student sample. These 43 words were organized theoretically by 5 clinical nurse specialists independently categorizing the words into groups that described similar qualities of pain. The clinical specialists were instructed to use the McGill Pain Questionnaire as a model [13]. Twelve word groups resulted which included sensory, affective, evaluative, and miscellaneous words. This list was used subsequently in study 2 and study 3.

Eleven of the 67 words identified from the combined student samples were selected as a pain descriptor by less than 50% of the subjects from at least 2 of the 5 2-year age groups. These 11 words were judged by the investigators to be ineligible for a word list intended to be free of developmental bias. Therefore, 56 words were included in a second-generation word list and are listed in Table I. All but 1 of the 43 first-generation words were on the second-generation word list (like-a-bullet was not eligible).

Age (grouped by 2-year intervals), gender, or ethnic differences in words selected as known and used to describe pain were tested. Each of the 56 words was examined with a pairwise comparison of proportion for each level of the 3 variables of interest. A significance criterion of 0.001 was used for each comparison. Findings indicated that: (1) 3 words were selected in different proportions by 3 or more of the 2-year age groups (pounding, cramping, numb); (2) 4 words were selected more frequently by girls (crying, frightening, miserable, sickening); and (3) none of the words was selected

differently by the 6 ethnic groups (n ≥ 73 for each group). Therefore, 49 words exhibited no selection bias by age, gender, or ethnicity of the children. The investigators elected to not remove the 7 possibly biased words at this stage of instrument development but to examine children's use of the word list with other samples experiencing pain.

The 56 words with limited age, gender, and ethnic biases were organized theoretically by the 5 clinical nurse specialists who had organized the first-generation word list. They independently categorized the words into groups that they believed described similar sensory, affective, or evaluative qualities of pain using the McGill Pain Questionnaire and the first word list as models [13]. Their majority assignment determined the categorization and produced a revised, 13-group word list (Table I). Twenty-four words were assigned to a group similar to their classification in the McGill Pain Questionnaire; 3 words were assigned differently than in the McGill Pain Questionnaire (stabbing, shooting, splitting). The remaining 29 words do not appear in the McGill Pain Questionnaire.

In the first student sample, the test–retest procedure using the McNemar test indicated moderate to high consistency in the children's sorting of the 43 words. The percentage of the 64 children who sorted the words the same each time, i.e., as used or not used/not known, ranged from 63% to 89%. For 34 of the words, the percentage of consistent classification was at least 70%. Low test–retest reliabilities were noted for 9 words; these 9 words (pounding, scratching, terrifying, dying, frightening, deadly, horrible, terrible, uncomfortable) were reclassified consistently by less than 70% of the children.

TEXT BASED EXERCISES

VOCABULARY

Study the meaning of the following words and expressions as used in the text.

3 settings
- surroundings

5 a score
- number of points gained by a competitor in a game or test

45 to review
- to revise; to re-examine

51 to sort
- to separate into classes

52 a stack
- a mass of things lying on top of one another

74 scary
- frightening

115 to pound
- to beat heavily

116 cramp
- involuntary, violent and painful contraction of muscles

116 numb
- without feeling; stiff through cold

118 to sicken
- to make one feel sick

140 to stab
- to pierce or wound with a pointed weapon

141 shooting
- moving with great speed.

From table 1

to ache
- to feel continuous pain

to hurt
- to cause injury or pain

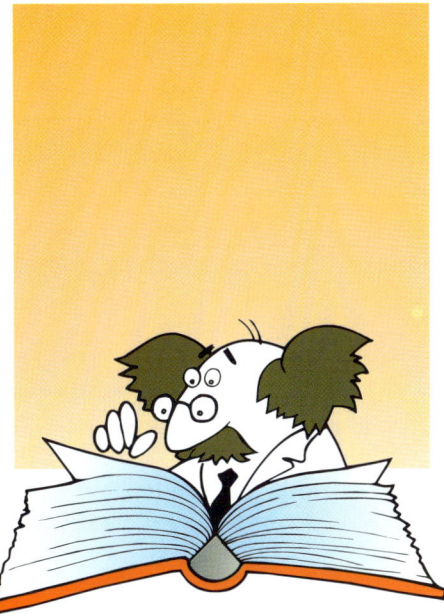

sore (adj.)
- painful when touched

an itch
- a sensation of irritation on skin causing desire to scratch

to sting
- to pierce with a sting (a sting - an organ used as a weapon by an animal esp. if containing poisonous or inflammatory liquid)

dizzy
- suffering from vertigo

to throb
- to pulsate

a blister
- a small swelling on the skin filled with serum

1 COMPREHENSION

Ask questions to which the following are the answers.

1 They were conducted in school and hospital settings.

2 They have been found to be both similar and different.

3 In order to help characterize pediatric pain syndromes and to determine the influences of different analgesic therapies on pediatric pain quality.

4 Children between the ages of 8 and 17.

5 Group 1 represented words they knew well and used to describe pain.
Group 2 represented words they knew but would not use to describe pain.
Group 3 represented words not known to them.

6 At least 50% of the sample had to know and use a particular word.

7 67 words.

8 An age-related trend was observed in the number of words not known.

9 It supports the general assumption that vocabulary influences children's description of pain.

10 Crying, frightening, miserable and sickening.

11 49 words exhibited no selection bias by age, gender or ethnicity of the children.

12 Pounding, scratching, terrifying, dying, frightening, deadly, horrible, terrible and uncomfortable.

2

Fill in the blanks below with the following adjectives and nouns. Try to complete the exercise without referring to the text.

> ✓ clinical specialists
> ✓ additional research
> ✓ general assumption
> ✓ pediatric pain syndromes
> ✓ important assessment parameter
> ✓ analgesic therapies
> ✓ hospitalized children
> ✓ sorting procedure
> ✓ age-related trend

1 These verbal pain descriptors are recognized as an ....

2 The .... were instructed to use the McGill Pain Questionnaire as a model.

3 Two weeks after this .... , 64 students from the first school sample and 44 students from the second school sample repeated the procedure.

4 .... is needed to assess the psychometric properties of this word list in pediatric populations

experiencing different pain syndromes.

5 As found in previous research, in the combined student sample, an .... was observed in the number of words not known which supports the .... that vocabulary influences children's description of pain.

6 Because some of the .... had greater difficulty completing the procedures than did the students, the test-retest component was not included with the third hospital sample.

7 Development of a measure of pain quality is important to help characterize .... and to determine the influence of different .... on pediatric pain quality.

3

Find a word in table I that *best describes* the following expressions.

a Like an ache.
b Like a hurt.
c Like a pin.
d Like a sharp knife.
e Like a pinch.
f Like a scratch.
g Like a sting.

4

Choose *one* of the three words given below that *best describes* the word in capitals.

1 ANNOYING
   (a) uncomfortable
   (b) pinlike
   (c) uncontrollable

2 ACHING
   (a) sore
   (b) burning
   (c) itching

3 THROBBING
   (a) swollen
   (b) pounding
   (c) shooting

4 STABBING
   (a) stiff
   (b) blistering
   (c) sharp

5 CRAMPING
   (a) stinging
   (b) numb
   (c) tight

6 ITCHING
   (a) scratching
   (b) blistering
   (c) stabbing

7 KILLING
   (a) dizzy
   (b) sickening
   (c) uncontrollable

8 AWFUL
   (a) shooting
   (b) terrible
   (c) suffocating

5 MIXED VERBAL FORMS

Put the verbs in brackets into *the verbal form as used in the text*.

a These verbal pain descriptors (recognize) as an important assessment parameter, especially when they (organize) theoretically in a tool, such as in the McGill Pain Questionnaire, the Tursky Pain Perception Profile, or verbal descriptor scales of painfulness. These scales (use) to differentiate pain syndromes and to determine the effectiveness of pain therapy in adult populations. However, children's pain descriptors, which (find) to be both similar and different from adult pain words (not organize) in a tool that provides a method of quantifying pain quality.

b The available domain of children's pain descriptors (review). One hundred and twenty nine words (identify) as used by children for pain description. Each of the 129 words (print) on a 2.5 x 3.5 inch card. Individually, the children (ask) to sort the 129 cards into three stacks representing (1) words they (know) and (use) to describe pain, (2) words they (know) but (not use) to describe pain and (3) words (not know) to them. Two weeks after this sorting procedure, 64 students from the first school sample and 44 students from the second school sample (repeat) the procedure. Because some of the hospitalized children (have) greater difficulty completing the procedures than did the students, the test-retest component (not include) with the third hospital sample.

c The 56 words with limited age, gender and ethnic biases (organize) theoretically by the five clinical nurse specialists who (organize) the first-generation word list. They independently (categorize) the words into groups that they (believe) described similar sensory, affective, or evaluative qualities of pain using the McGill Pain Questionnaire and the first word list as models. Their majority assignment (determine) the categorization and (produce) a revised 13-group word list with each group representing a single dimension.

Notes

EXTENSION EXERCISES

6 SYNONYMS

Give suitable *synonyms* for the following words.

   8 additional
   8 needed
  30 construct
  50 individually
  64 set
  74 sad
114 selected

7

Study the use of the words ending in *ing* in the following sentence.

63 To include a word on a pain quality word list, a criterion was set of at least 50% of the sample *knowing* and *using* a particular word.

Now change the following *infinitives as in the example below*.

e.g.: To know and to use - *knowing and using.*

a To see and to believe.
b To test and to retest.
c To include and to exclude.
d To report and to review.
e To seek and to find.
f To construct and to identify.
g To organize and to categorize.
h To select and to reject.
i To examine and to compare.
j To determine and to produce.

8 NOUNS FROM VERBS

a Give *nouns* from the following verbs.

e.g. to locate → location

Verb	Noun
to assess	
to organize	
to practise	
to develop	
to review	
to assume	
to combine	
to observe	
to research	
to describe	

b Write sentences *in your own words* which contain each of the nouns.

Notes

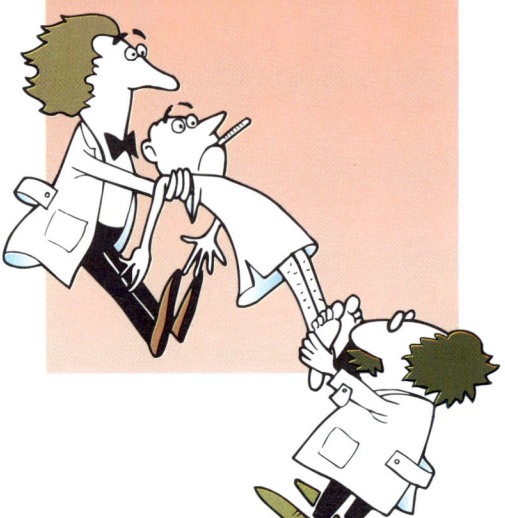

PAST PERFECT TENSE

This tense is formed with *HAD* and the *past participle*.

affirmative	He had arrived
negative	He hadn't arrived
interrogative	Had he arrived?

a The Past Perfect is the past equivalent of the Present Perfect. However, it differs from the Present Perfect in that *the time of the action can be mentioned.*

e.g. He had been in London only yesterday.

b The Past Perfect is also the past equivalent of the Simple Past. Although the Simple Past is used to talk about what happened in the past, *the Past Perfect looks even further back into the past.*

e.g. I arrived at the hospital.
SIMPLE PAST

When I arrived at the hospital, I realized that *I had left* my brief-case on the train.
PAST PERFECT

c When *just* is used it is placed between had and the past participle.

e.g. Dick had *just* gone out when I phoned him.

GRAMMAR POINT

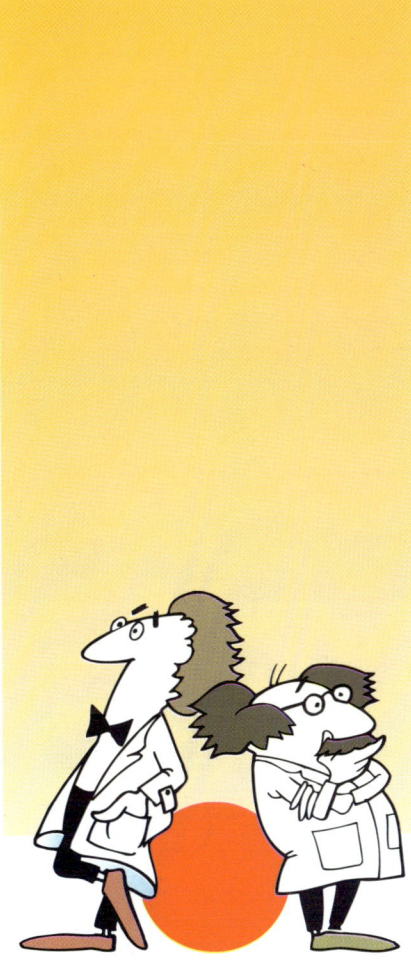

d Note the use of *till* and *until* in the following examples.
He didn't go home *till* he had finished writing the report.
He waited *until* he had received confirmation of his new appointment before telling his friends.

9 GRAMMAR CHECK

Read the sentences below. Add a second sentence to each that gives further information about events in the past. Use the *Past Perfect*.

e.g. The patient was very surprised when the doctors told him that he had a heart condition.

He hadn't suspected anything.

1 Barbara had a plaster on her leg.
2 Dr. Blake was very happy.
3 I saw water coming from under the bathroom door.
4 The surgeon was very tired.
5 Jack was disappointed.
6 Dr. Lawson didn't read the report.
7 The letter was still in her pocket.
8 Dr. Fielding was late for work.

10 GRAMMAR CHECK

Read the following sentences. Give an explanation in your own words using *just* and the *Past Perfect*.

e.g. He wasn't hungry.
He had just eaten.

a She wasn't tired.
b They weren't thirsty.
c John wasn't in when I called.
d His father was very angry.
e We arrived at the meeting late.
f He had to take a taxi home.

11 NERVE CELLS

Read the following passage:

NERVE CELLS

The smallest unit of the nervous system is a neuron or nerve cell. These cells are very specialized. A nerve cell is made up of three parts, each of which has a special function:

Cell body – irregular in shape, with branches leading from it. Its function is to regulate the activities of the entire cell.

Axon – one long insulated fibre leading from the cell body and branching at its end. Its function is to relay a stimulus to the next nearest neuron.

Dendrites – small branches from many sides of the cell body. Their function is to receive stimuli. There are three kinds of neurons, each adapted for a particular function:

Afferent or sensory neuron – These receive stimuli and send an impulse to the central nervous system.

Associative neuron – in the central nervous system, where the stimulus message is interpreted and action is taken.

Efferent or *Motor neuron* – carries impulse from CNS for action to a muscle or gland.

Nerve – fibres which run parallel and bound in a common coat.

WRITING

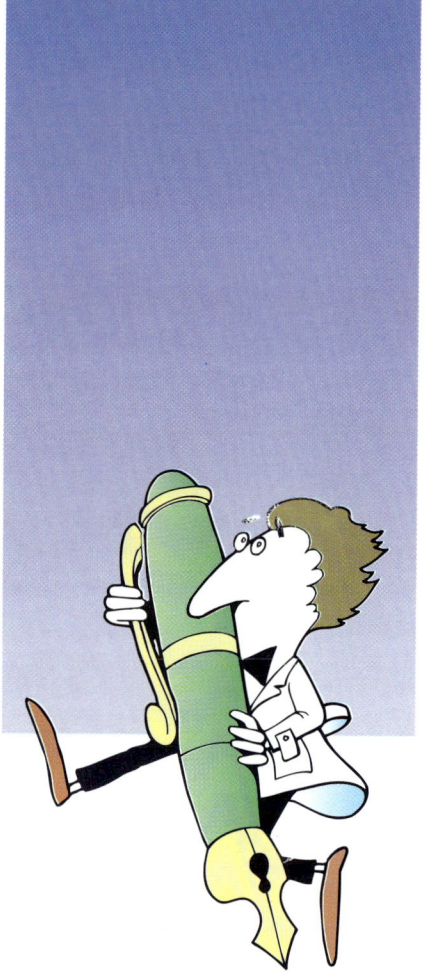

Neurons do not actually connect one with the other by touching. A *synapse* is formed, over which an impulse jumps very much like electricity will jump over a small space between open ends of wires that almost touch. A synapse is the very small space between the terminal ends of the axon of an afferent nerve and the dendrites of an efferent nerve.

In order to have control over the body and to adapt it to the environment, nerve pathways have been established within man's nervous system. Some responses made to stimuli are voluntary; others are involuntary.

Briefly decribe, in your own words, the difference between voluntary and involuntary responses.

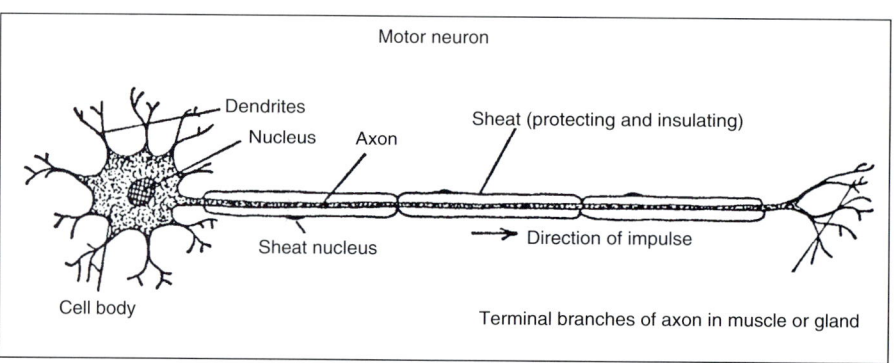

Motor neuron

Dendrites
Nucleus
Axon
Sheat (protecting and insulating)
Sheath nucleus
→ Direction of impulse
Cell body
Terminal branches of axon in muscle or gland

SPEAKING

12 DOCTOR/PATIENT DIALOGUE

Work in pairs.
Conduct the following doctor/patient dialogue.

The patient is describing his pain to the doctor. Try to use some of the words in table I. The doctor should try to ask accurate questions to obtain as much exact information as possible.

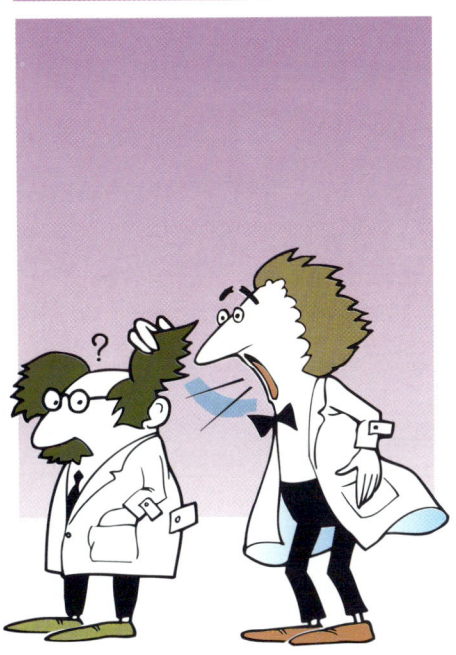

13 DESCRIBING NEURONS

Read the sentences below.
Continue the descriptions. Use the terms you have studied in exercise 11.

a A nerve cell is made up of three parts, each of which has a special function.

b There are three kinds of neurons, each adapted for a particular function.

UNDERSTANDING IDIOMATIC ENGLISH

Explain the idiom.

After his speech, doctor Spencer was given a big hand

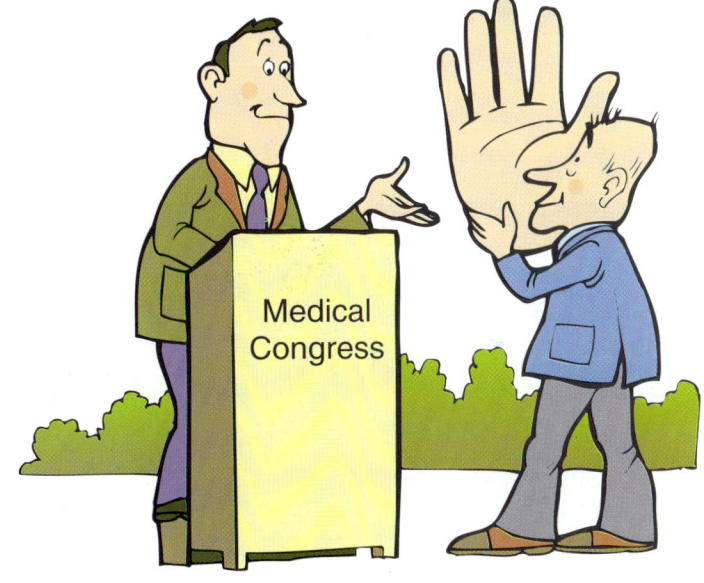

UNIT 10

Purifying peptides

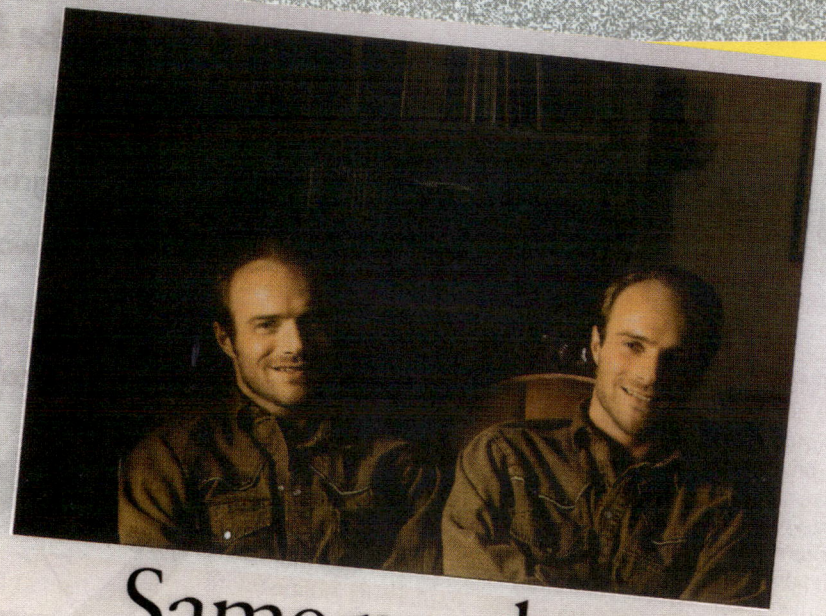

VOCABULARY

Study the meaning of the following words and expressions as used in the text.

3 right away
   - immediately
8 trouble
   - difficulty
13 a lot
   - a large quantity
21 a pore
   - a very small opening
24 to pack
   - to put into a container for travel or storage
29 scale-up
   - increase according to a specific ratio
34 maybe
   - perhaps, possibly
35 a triplet
   - each of three children born at one birth

TEXT BASED EXERCISES

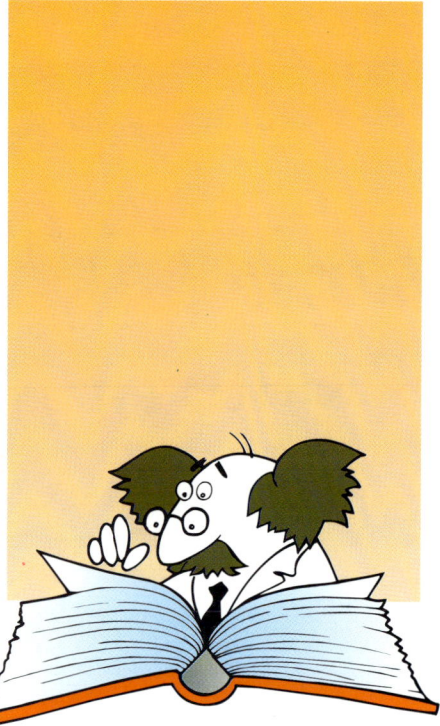

1 WORD CHECK

Explain the following words and expressions.

4 a helping hand
6 a challenge
12 over 3 decades
15 insight
21 pore size
26 available

2

Explain the idea the writer conveys by the choice of the following words.

5 typical
19 new
22 high
30 simple
15 unique
21 selective
24 popular
31 difficult

3 NOUNS

Fill in the blanks with one of the *nouns* below.

> purification
> resolution
> dimensions
> capabilities
> experience
> analysis
> system
> phase
> size
> work

We've put some of this .... to work in a new reversed-............ HPLC medium, Super Pac Pep-S. With its highly selective, IOOA pore ...., this medium is ideal for high .... peptide .... and .... Packed in the popular SuperPac cartridge ...., this medium is available in 3 different cartridge .... There are columns for analitical ...., and for preparative work with direct scale-up ....

4 VERBS

Fill in the blanks with the *verbs* below in the form used in the text.

e.g. (be) But they .... not twins.
But they *are* not twins.

- ✓ learn
- ✓ put
- ✓ reverse
- ✓ be
- ✓ synthesize
- ✓ offer
- ✓ gain
- ✓ purify
- ✓ separate
- ✓ associate
- ✓ relate
- ✓ work
- ✓ prepare
- ✓ select
- ✓ pack

1 How .... this possible?
2 You've .... a peptide.
3 Pharmacia can .... a helping hand.
4 We've been .... peptides for over 3 decades.
5 Over the years, we've not only .... a lot about what makes peptides so special, but also .... insight into some of the unique problems .... with peptide purification.
6 We've .... some of this experience .... in a new .... - phase HPLC medium SuperPac Pep-S.
7 With its highly ...., 100A pore size, this medium is ideal for high resolution peptide purification and analysis.
8 .... in the popular SuperPac cartridge system, the medium is available in 3 different cartridge dimensions.
9 There are columns for analytical work and for .... work with direct scale-up capabilities.
10 Not only can it help you .... two closely .... peptides, but maybe even to see the unpredictable triplet.

5 PREPOSITIONS

Fill in the blanks with a suitable *preposition*.

1 You've synthesised a peptide, but are having trouble separating it .... a closely related analogue.
2 We've gained insight .... some .... the problems associated .... peptide purification.
3 We've put some .... this experience to work .... a new reversed-phase HPLC medium, SuperPac Pep-S.
4 .... its highly selective, 100A pore size, this medium is ideal .... high resolution peptide purification and analysis.
5 The medium is available .... 3 different cartridge dimensions.
6 There are columns .... analytical work and .... preparative work .... direct scale-up capabilities.
7 It is packed .... the popular SuperPac cartridge system.
8 They have the same mother and father and the same date .... birth.
9 Few people see it right away- at least not .... a helping hand.
10 .... the years we've learned a lot .... what makes peptides so special.

Notes

EXTENSION EXERCISES

6 PREFIXES

Give the opposite of the words below by adding *prefixes*. Make your own sentences using each of the newly-formed words.

e.g. known → *un*known

Although a lot of research is being carried out, the cause of the disease is still *unknown*.

a Popular.
b Available.
c Direct.
d Predictable.
e Possible.
f Related.
g To pack.
h To associate.

7 NOT ONLY ... BUT ALSO

Note the use of the conjunctions *not only... but also* on line 13. Join the following sentences inserting *not only... but also* in the most appropriate position. Make any changes necessary.

e.g. We've learned a lot about what makes peptides so special. We've gained insight into some of the unique

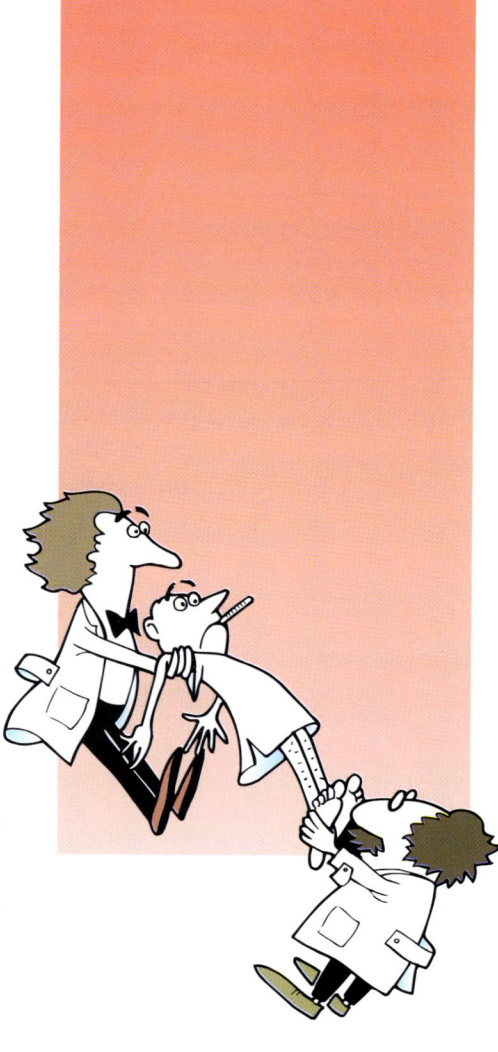

problems associated with peptide purification.
We've *not only* learned a lot about what makes peptides so special, *but also* gained insight into some of the unique

problems associated with peptide purification.

1 There are columns for analytical work.
There are columns for preparative work.

2 I have studied many new expressions.
I have learned some phrasal verbs and idiomatic expressions.

3 I have passed the Biology exam.
I have passed the Anatomy exam.

4 It can help you to separate two closely related peptides.
It can help you to see the unpredictable triplet.

5 This medium is ideal for high resolution peptide purification.
This medium is ideal for analysis.

6 They have the same mother and father.
They have the same date of birth.

7 The research group has studied chromosome ends.
The research group has identified a key enzyme.

8 Those with rare genetic disorders could benefit.
Those who suffer from diabetes could benefit.

9 The treatment is very long.
The treatment is very expensive.

10 The new procedure takes less than an hour.
The new procedure requires no stitches.

GRAMMAR POINT

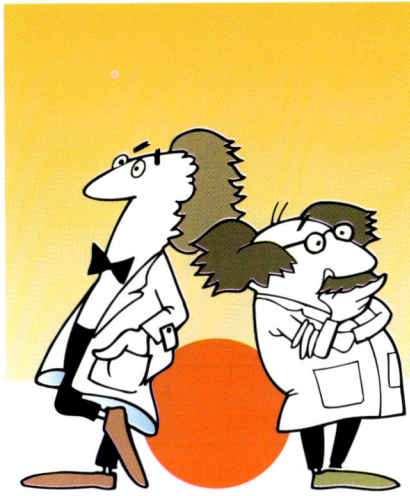

PRESENT PERFECT CONTINUOUS TENSE

a   This tense is formed by using the Present Perfect of the verb to be (e.g. I have been) + the present participle.

e.g.   *We've been purifying peptides for over three decades.*

negative:
We haven't been purifying peptides.

interrogative:
Have we been purifying peptides?

b   This tense is used to say *how long* something has been happening.

e.g.   I've been studying English for eight years.

c   Some verbs are *not* normally used in the continuous form.

e.g.   to prefer
          to like
          to see
          to hear
          to know
          to believe
          to seem
          to remember

d   When asked how long you have been doing something, *DO NOT ANSWER WITH THE PRESENT TENSE.*

e.g.   How long have you been studying medicine?

right   *I've been studying medicine for six years.*

wrong   (I study medicine for six years.)

e   It is *also* possible to use the *Present Perfect* for actions repeated over a long period.

e.g.   *Present Perfect Continuous*
       I've been studying English for three months.

       Present Perfect
       I've studied English for three months.

8   FOR/SINCE

BOTH WORDS begin phrases which indicate how long something has been happening. Use SINCE when you say when the action began i.e. *A SPECIFIC TIME.*

e.g.

since 10 o'clock

since Sunday

since Easter

since September

since he left

Use FOR when you don't say when the action began i.e. *NOT SPECIFIC*

e.g.

for an hour

for two days

for a year

for a month

for a long time

e.g.   He's been working here *since* January.

       He's been working here *for* two months.

9 GRAMMAR CHECK

Fill in the blanks with *FOR* or *SINCE*.

1 I have known him .... six years.
2 I have known him .... I was a child.
3 Have you been studying English .... a long time?
4 I've lived in Manchester .... 1989.
5 She's been in hospital .... a week.
6 He's been going for tests every six weeks .... October.
7 The nurses' strike lasted .... five days.
8 Doctor Gibson has been waiting .... six o'clock.

10 GRAMMAR CHECK

Work in pairs.
Student 1: Ask questions using the construction "How long...?"
Student 2: Answer the questions *in your own words* using the Present Perfect Continuous tense.

e.g. (you) wait to see the doctor?

Student 1: How long have *you* been waiting to see the doctor?

Student 2: I've been waiting to see the doctor *for* half an hour.

1 (He) try to give up smoking?
2 (Jack) look for a parking space?
3 (They) work at the hospital?
4 (You) wait for them to telephone?
5 (She) try to find a job?
6 (Dr. Fielding) talk to the patient?
7 (The patient) take these tablets?
8 (Linda) put off going to see her doctor?
9 (We) stand in the queue?
10 (Mrs. Oliver) learn to drive?

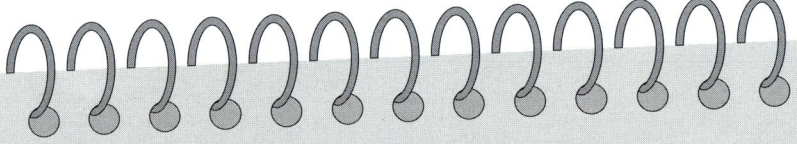

Notes

WRITING

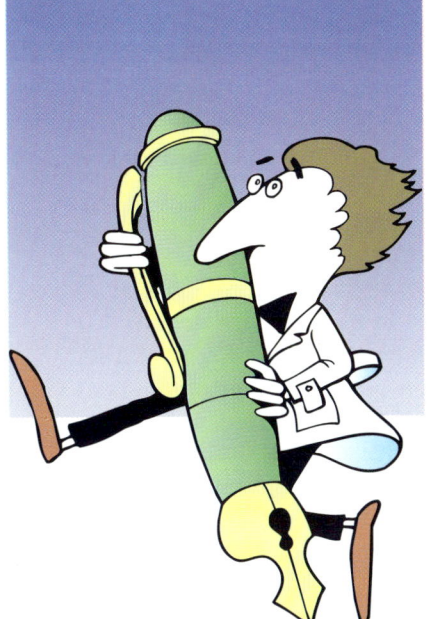

11 FORM FILLING

A *date of birth* is usually written in numbers i.e. 20.3.65.
You are going to attend a medical conference in Greece.
You will arrive on 16th May and stay at the hotel Splendid for 3 days.
Fill in the booking form below.

12 LETTER WRITING

Write *a short letter* to Pharmacia. Explain that you have read their advertisement for the SuperPac Pep-S and that you would like further information about their products and if possible, a sample. Add any other information you consider necessary.

Notes

SURNAME	....
CHRISTIAN NAME(S)	....
DATE OF BIRTH	....
PLACE OF BIRTH	....
NATIONALITY	....
ADDRESS	....
PROFESSION	....
DATE OF ARRIVAL	....
NUMBER OF NIGHTS	....
SIGNATURE	.... DATE ....

Read the following passage.

A peptide is a compound in which amino acids are covalently linked together through secondary amide or peptide bonds (–CO.NH–). The term protein, derived from the Greek word *proteios* ("primary"), was coined before anything was known about the chemical structures of these natural macromolecules. It is conventional to retain this term for large molecules and to use the term peptide for molecules which are built up from only a small number of amino acid residues. Nature, however, is not influenced by terminological conventions and the molecular sizes of natural peptides and proteins cover a fairly continuous spectrum. It is debatable, therefore, whether adrenocorticotropic hormone, which is built up from thirty-nine amino acid residues, is a large peptide or a small protein. Use of the terms oligopeptide and polypeptide are similarly vague; in addition, the latter term has been reserved by some authors for artificial macromolecules built up from only one type of amino acid residue. It is probably too late to hope for universal acceptance of a more systematic nomenclature. Fortunately, the meanings of the various terms are usually quite clear from the context in which they occur. In particular cases, the size of a molecule may be specified by a prefix, e.g. undecapeptide. In sport, an analogous situation exists with the word team. This term applies to any group who play together against another team or teams and might range from two (e.g. tennis) to a very large number (e.g. a national team in an athletics or swimming fixture).

5

10

15

20

2	a bond - that which binds; a link holding atoms together
4	to coin - (fig.) to invent a new word or phrase
6	to retain - to keep
10	fairly - rather
11	debatable - open to discussion
14	latter - second; the more recently mentioned of two
17	systematic - methodical; based on a system
17	nomenclature - system of naming, esp. for classification
23	to range - to extend
24	a fixture - a sporting event to be held on a date fixed in advance

Secondary bands of a protein

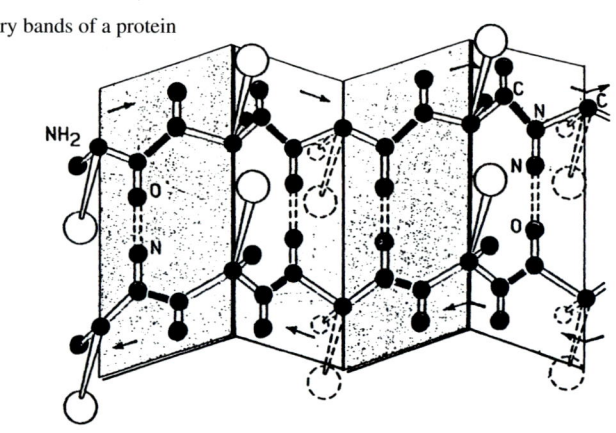

Notes

SPEAKING

13 SUMMARIZING

Summarize the passage you have just read in your own words. The words below will help you.

- peptide - compound - amino acids - covalently linked - secondary amide or peptide bonds
- protein - conventional - this term
- large molecules
- term peptide - molecules - built up - small number of amino acid residues
- adrenocorticotropic hormone - thirty-nine amino acid residues - large peptide or a small protein
- oligopeptide - polypeptide - similarly vague
- probably too late - universal acceptance - more systematic nomenclature

- fortunately - meanings of the terms - clear from the context - they occur
- particular cases - size of a molecule - specified - prefix

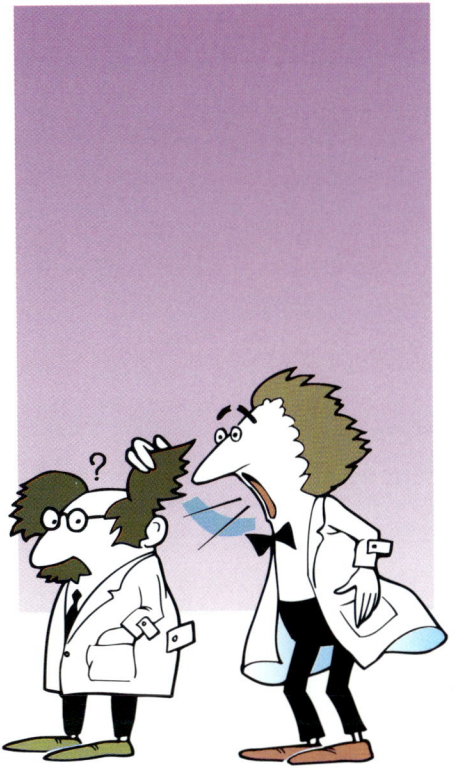

14 DOCTOR/PATIENT DIALOGUE

Work in pairs.
Conduct the following doctor/patient dialogue.

A patient comes to you for advice. Her teenage daughter has decided to become a vegetarian. Her mother wants to know what foods she should eat and if she will lack necessary proteins following this type of diet.

UNDERSTANDING IDIOMATIC ENGLISH

Explain the idiom.

Take this medicine
it will do the trick

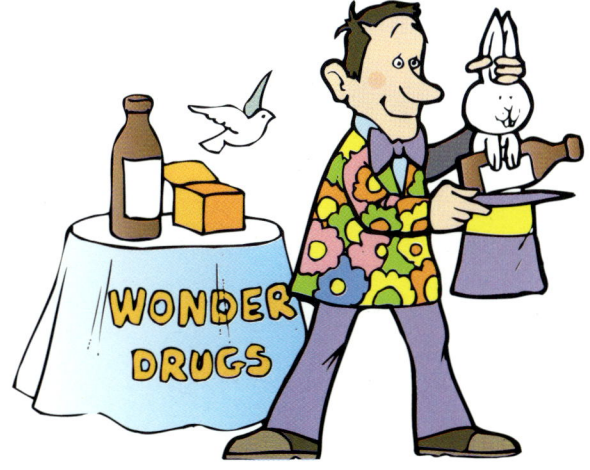

WONDER DRUGS

UNIT 11

Major surgery on a fetus

The Tiniest Patients

Doctors perform the first major surgery on a fetus, opening the door to more lifesaving therapies

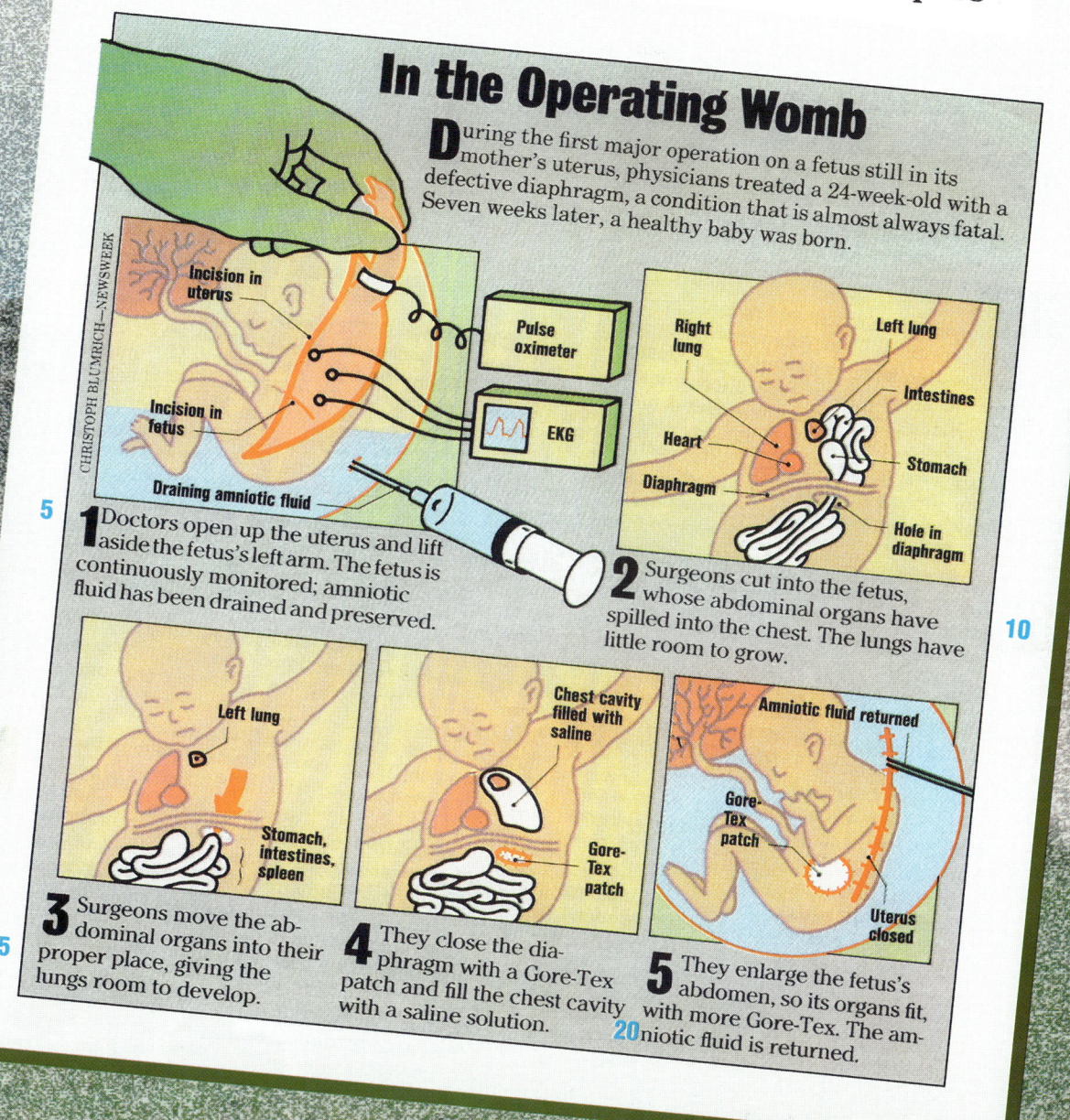

In the Operating Womb

During the first major operation on a fetus still in its mother's uterus, physicians treated a 24-week-old with a defective diaphragm, a condition that is almost always fatal. Seven weeks later, a healthy baby was born.

CHRISTOPH BLUMRICH—NEWSWEEK

Incision in uterus

Incision in fetus

Draining amniotic fluid

Pulse oximeter

EKG

1 Doctors open up the uterus and lift aside the fetus's left arm. The fetus is continuously monitored; amniotic fluid has been drained and preserved.

Right lung

Left lung

Intestines

Heart

Stomach

Diaphragm

Hole in diaphragm

2 Surgeons cut into the fetus, whose abdominal organs have spilled into the chest. The lungs have little room to grow.

Left lung

Stomach, intestines, spleen

3 Surgeons move the abdominal organs into their proper place, giving the lungs room to develop.

Chest cavity filled with saline

Gore-Tex patch

4 They close the diaphragm with a Gore-Tex patch and fill the chest cavity with a saline solution.

Amniotic fluid returned

Gore-Tex patch

Uterus closed

5 They enlarge the fetus's abdomen, so its organs fit, with more Gore-Tex. The amniotic fluid is returned.

Scores of obstacles confront a fetus struggling to grow from a mere fertilized egg into a sentient, conscious human being. There are fingers to mold from featureless blobs, brains to craft from undifferentiated protoplasm. One of the higher hurdles looms at the eighth week. That's when the diaphragm, separating the abdomen and chest, should close. But for unknown reasons, in about one of 2,500 fetuses in the United States it remains open. As a result the stomach, intestines, spleen and part of the liver can spill into the chest,

leaving the lungs with no room to grow. About 75 percent of such babies die—often right in the delivery room—unable to gasp even the tiniest breath. Now, at least for those fetuses in which the hernia has been detected by ultrasound, there is hope. Last week in The New England Journal of Medicine, a team of physicians led by Dr. Michael Harrison of the University of California, San Francisco, reported that in two life-threatening cases, they had reached into the womb itself to repair the defect.

These triumphs represent the first successful major surgery on a fetus. With other such operations in the offing, says UCSF's N. Scott Adzick, "fetal therapy is here to stay." It has been slow in coming. For years obstetricians have given transfusions to anemic fetuses, steroids to those with underdeveloped lungs and other medications to those with abnormal metabolisms. But doctors wanted to do more, and none more badly than Harrison.

In 1982 Harrison for the first time operated on a fetus directly, rather than through its mother. The surgery, to unblock a urinary tract, worked again. But the baby's lungs and kidneys were so damaged that he died within hours of birth. Since then, Harrison and his team have reported four more such operations. All were technical successes, but in half the cases the fetus had suffered so much damage from the blockage that it could not live. That showed how crucial it is to identify fetuses whom surgery has a chance of helping.

By the mid-1980s the UCSF team was ready to try repairing hernias of the diaphragm. None of their first six patients lived. Then, last year, Harrison and his team operated on a 24-week fetus with the defect. The surgeons made a small incision in the womb of his mother, Beth Schultz of Michigan, and lifted aside the fetus's left arm (diagram). They opened the baby's chest and pushed the abdominal organs into their proper place. The surgeons then closed the diaphragm with a patch of Gore-Tex, waterproof material commonly used in parkas. They also made an incision in the abdomen, to enlarge it enough to accommodate the returned organs, and patched it with more Gore-Tex. The operation took 54 minutes. Seven weeks later, Blake was born. He spent three weeks on a respirator, but at eight months, he is home and thriving. A girl who had the same defect was operated on this March; now six weeks old, she is also developing normally.

'The mom': Technical difficulties aside, fetal surgery is plagued by a perceived conflict between maternal and fetal rights. Some physicians and ethicists argue that it is wrong to endanger a woman—through general anesthesia and major surgery—in order to benefit a fetus, especially if the benefits are far from assured. As Harrison says, to save the baby, "We have to put at risk an innocent bystander—the mom." And bioethicists worry that courts may *require* women to submit to such surgery. Partly for that reason, the UCSF team emphasizes that the mothers understand the risks, consent to them, and are not harmed by the procedure. In the six cases where the fetus with the defective diaphragm died, all four of the mothers who tried to conceive again delivered healthy babies.

Although heroic medicine usually carries a stiff price tag, this operation may not. At $15,721, it costs less than the intensive care given babies born with a herniated diaphragm—most of whom die anyway. Insurance companies, however, view the procedure as "experimental" and will not pay for it. This isn't a cure-all. In some babies, the damage is so great that even if the defect is corrected, the newborn doesn't stand a chance at life. In others, the hernia is so mild that, says Adzick, "it should be treated after birth, with the operation reserved for worse cases." Still, while the procedure will never be routine (only the UCSF team knows how to perform it), it may pave the way for other in utero surgery. The UCSF surgeons are already eying the possibility of operating on fetal lung tumors, for instance. Medicine cannot reduce the hurdles to a healthy birth, but it can help at least some fetuses over them.

VOCABULARY

Study the meaning of the following words and expressions as used in the text.

title womb
- uterus

6 aside
- to one side

8 to drain
- to extract liquid

19 a patch
- a piece of material used to repair a hole

31 a hurdle (fig.)
- an obstacle

31 to loom (fig.)
- to appear important and menacing

58 in the offing (fig.)
- likely to come or happen

102 to thrive
- to develop healthily

107 plagued
- persistently troubled

110 to endanger
- to expose to danger

115 a bystander
- a spectator or onlooker

126 stiff (coll.)
- excessive

141 to pave the way for
- to facilitate the coming of

142 to eye
- to look at

TEXT BASED EXERCISES

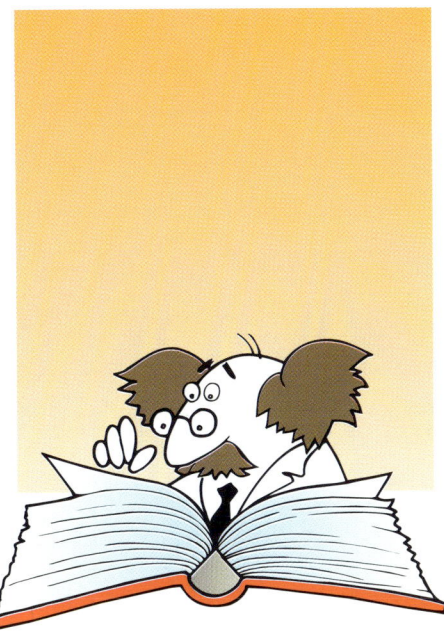

1 WORD CHECK

Explain what you understand by the following expressions.

3 a defective diaphragm
8 amniotic fluid
10 the abdominal organs
45 ultrasound
59 fetal therapy
62 obstetricians
64 steroids
64 underdeveloped lungs
67 abnormal metabolisms
101 a respirator

2 SENTENCE RECONSTRUCTION

Make *complete sentences* from the following. Add the missing words.

1 Doctors - the uterus - lift aside - fetus's left arm.

2 Surgeons - the fetus - abdominal organs - spilled - the chest.

3 Surgeons - abdominal organs - their proper place - the lungs - room - develop.

4 They - diaphragm - a Gore-Tex patch - the chest cavity - a saline solution.

5 They - the fetus's abdomen - organs - fit - more Gore-Tex.

6 The stomach, intestines - spleen - part - liver can spill - the chest - the lungs - no room - grow.

7 For years obstetricians - transfusions - anemic fetuses, steroids - those - underdeveloped lungs - other medications - those - abnormal metabolisms.

8 Last year, Harrison - team, operated - 24-week fetus - the defect.

9 He - three weeks - a respirator.

10 Only - the UCSF team - how - perform - it.

3 USING COMMAS TO SEPARATE CLAUSES

Join the following sentences. Make one complete sentence as in the example. *Use commas to separate the clauses*. Make any necessary changes.

e.g. The surgery worked again. The surgery was to unblock a urinary tract.

The surgery, to unblock a urinary tract, worked again.

1   Bile emulsifies fats. Bile is produced in the liver.
2   Villi extend inward from the intestinal wall. Villi are finger-like projections.
3   That's when the diaphragm should close. The diaphragm separates the abdomen and chest.
4   Now there is hope. At least there is hope for those fetuses in which the hernia has been detected by ultrasound.
5   People with acromegaly are at increased risk of colon cancer. Acromegaly is a condition caused by excess growth hormone.
6   The pituitary gland is located at the base of the brain. The pituitary gland is called the master gland.
7   Geneticist James Gusella discovered a particular piece of DNA that seemed to be present in people suffering

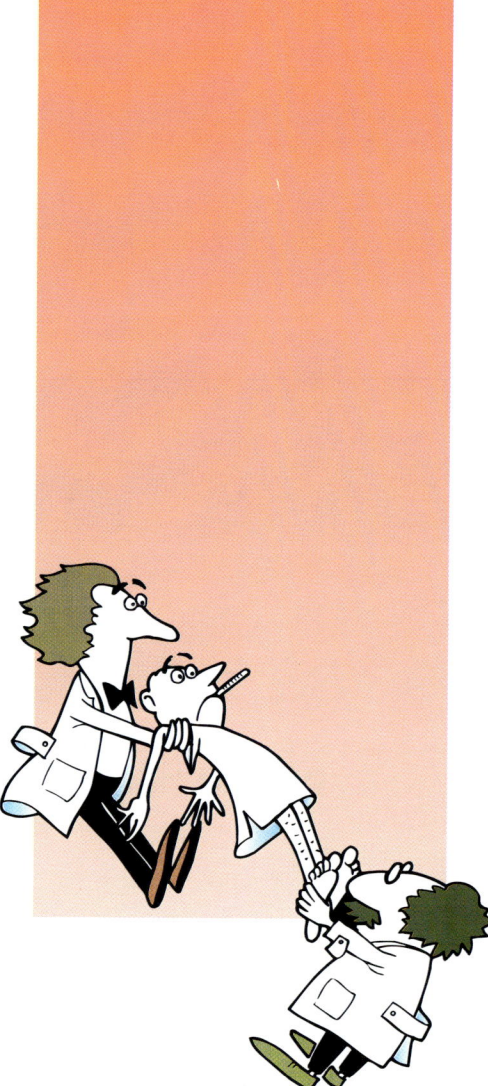

from Huntington's disease. The piece of DNA is called a genetic marker.

8   Lower back pain is the price human beings pay for walking upright. Lower back pain is as prevalent as the common cold.

4 ADJECTIVES WITH "LESS"

Study these sentences.

28 There are fingers to mould from *featureless* blobs, brains to craft from undifferentiated protoplasm.
55 These triumphs represent the first *successful* major surgery on a fetus.

Success*ful* means having success.

Feature*less* means without features.

Give the *opposite* of the following adjectives by adding the suffix *less*. Make a complete sentence *in your own words* for each of the opposites.

✓ careful
✓ harmful
✓ helpful
✓ painful
✓ powerful
✓ thoughtful
✓ useful
✓ colourful

5

A fetus of 24 weeks is a *24-week fetus*.

N.B. In the hyphenated expression, *the word week is singular*.

Now change the following into *hyphenated expressions*.

a An incision of two inches.
b A contract of three months.
c An operation of fifty minutes.
d A search of twenty years.
e A regimen of six months.
f A waiting list of five years.
g A reaction of sixty seconds.
h A therapy of ten days.

6

The surgeon *made* a small incision. *Made* is the Simple Past of *make*.

Put the verbs in brackets into the *Simple Past*.

1 The operation (take) 54 minutes.
2 In 1982 Harrison for the first time (operate) on a fetus directly, rather than through its mother.
3 The baby's lungs and kidneys were so damaged that he (die) within hours of birth.
4 They (open) the baby's chest and (push) the abdominal organs into their proper place.
5 Doctor Harrison (lead) the team of physicians.
6 Seven weeks later, Blake (be) born.
7 They (close) the diaphragm with a Gore-Tex patch and (fill) the chest cavity with a saline solution.
8 The UCSF team (emphasize) that the mothers (understand) the risks.
9 Obstetricians (give) transfusions to anemic fetuses.
10 He (spend) three weeks on a respirator.

7 PHRASAL VERBS WITH DO

Study the meanings of the verbs below. They are all formed with the verb *TO DO*.
Read the following sentences.

Replace the part of the sentence *in italics* with one of the phrasal verbs in the correct form. Make any changes necessary.

a Doctor Crawford: "Thanks for helping with the operation Andrew. We didn't expect the emergency and we couldn't have *managed if you hadn't helped*."
b Doctor Benson to colleague: "The next time I perform an operation, I don't want you anywhere near the operating theatre. All you do is criticize my every move. I *do not require* that kind of help."
c Doctor Edwards: "Let me sit down. I've listened to patients' problems all day long. I've made several house calls and put in many hours at the hospital. I'm *dog tired*."
d One of the surgical wards is closed at the moment. It's being *renovated*.

Phrasal verb	Meaning
to do for	to manage to obtain
to do well	to achieve success
to do badly	not to do well
to do up	to renovate or modernize
to do with	to need or want
what to do with oneself	how to occupy one's time
to do without (1)	to manage without
to do without (2)	not to require or to resent having
done in	exhausted

e Nurse Peters: "I've got a lot of work at the moment. I could *use* a helping hand."

f Robert worked very hard at school. He *was first in his class* and went on to be a doctor. Unlike his brother who never studied and *failed all his exams*. When he left school, he didn't know *how to spend his time* or what he was going to do *about* money. Then he married a rich woman twice his age and invested her money. His risks turned out to be successful. Now he earns more than his brother and lives in a beautiful villa in the south of France.

Notes

GRAMMAR POINT

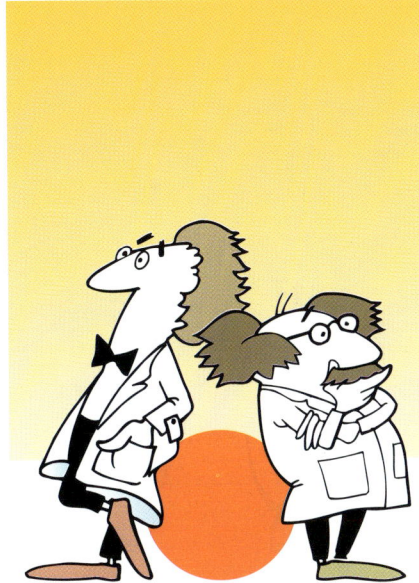

SO/SUCH

a The use of *SO* and *SUCH* make the meaning stronger.

b *SO* is *an adverb* used in front of adjectives *not followed* by their nouns or in front of adverbs.

e.g. In some babies, the damage is *so great*.

He always operates *so carefully*.

c *SUCH* is an adjective used in front of an adjective + a noun.

e.g. It was *such a difficult case*.

d *SUCH* is *never* used in front of much and many.

SO is used even when much and many are followed by nouns.

e.g. The fetus had suffered *so much damage* from the blockage that it could not live.

e *SUCH* can also mean "*of that kind*"

e.g. About 70% of *SUCH* babies die.

SO is *not* used in this construction.

8 GRAMMAR CHECK

Fill in the blanks with *SO* or *SUCH*.

1 There are .... many benefits to be gained from the new treatment.
2 The operation was .... successful that they wrote about it in the Lancet.
3 .... cases always require surgery.
4 There is .... a shortage of nurses at the hospital that the situation is becoming serious.
5 In some babies, the damage is .... great that even if the defect is corrected, the newborn doesn't stand a chance at life.
6 Harrison and his team have reported four more .... operations.

9 GRAMMAR CHECK

Change the structure of the following sentences. Use *such* in each sentence. Begin with the word given in brackets. *Make any changes necessary.*

e.g. His cold was *so* bad that he had to stay in bed. (He)
He had *such* a bad cold that he had to stay in bed.

1 The investigation took so long that I thought they wouldn't find a solution. (It)
2 The man looked so healthy that nobody believed be was ill. (He)
3 The medicine was so horrible that the patient stopped taking it. (It)
4 The treatment was so expensive that few patients could afford it. (It)
5 The procedure is so painless that patients are soon able to return home. (It)
6 The incision was so small that it didn't leave a scar. (It)

WRITING

10 DESCRIBING FETAL SURGERY

Following the diagrams below, describe the operation on the 24 - week - old fetus with a defective diaphragm. Describe the operation in your own words.

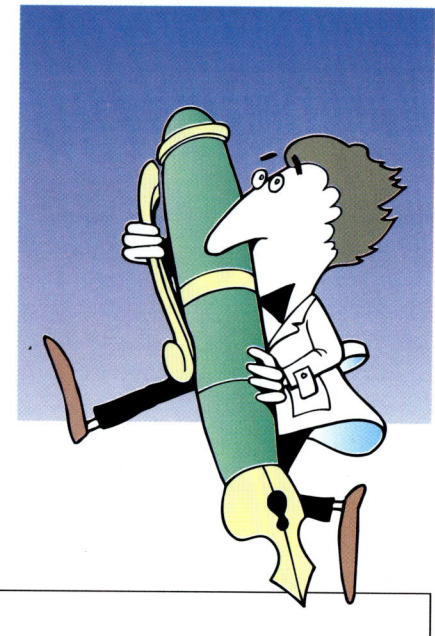

Notes

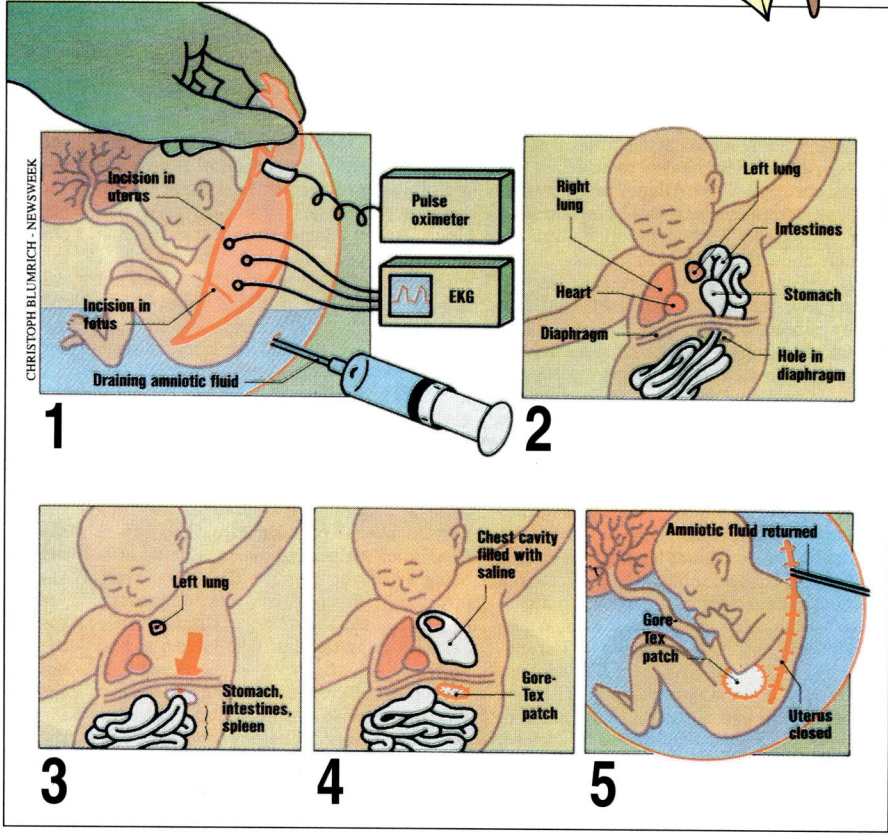

CHRISTOPH BLUMRICH - NEWSWEEK

1
- Incision in uterus
- Incision in fetus
- Draining amniotic fluid
- Pulse oximeter
- EKG

2
- Right lung
- Left lung
- Intestines
- Heart
- Stomach
- Diaphragm
- Hole in diaphragm

3
- Left lung
- Stomach, intestines, spleen

4
- Chest cavity filled with saline
- Gore-Tex patch

5
- Amniotic fluid returned
- Gore-Tex patch
- Uterus closed

SPEAKING

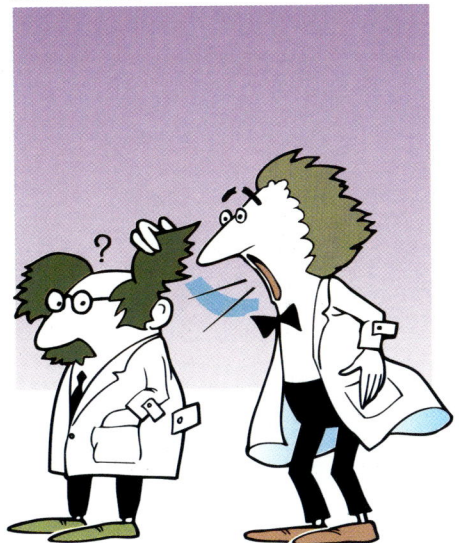

11 DISCUSSING FETAL THERAPY

Group work.
A public debate has been called to discuss fetal therapy. The chairman should propose the motion that "Medicine cannot reduce the hurdles to a healthy birth, but it can help at least some fetuses over them".

The speakers should include:
A surgeon from the UCSF team who believes that fetal therapy "is here to stay".

A mother who had a successful operation.

A bioethicist who is worried that courts may require women to submit to such surgery.

A representative from an insurance company who views the procedures as "experimental" and will not pay for it.

The public should ask questions after each person has briefly given their point of view.

UNDERSTANDING IDIOMATIC ENGLISH

Explain the idiom.

Her new car cost her an arm and a leg

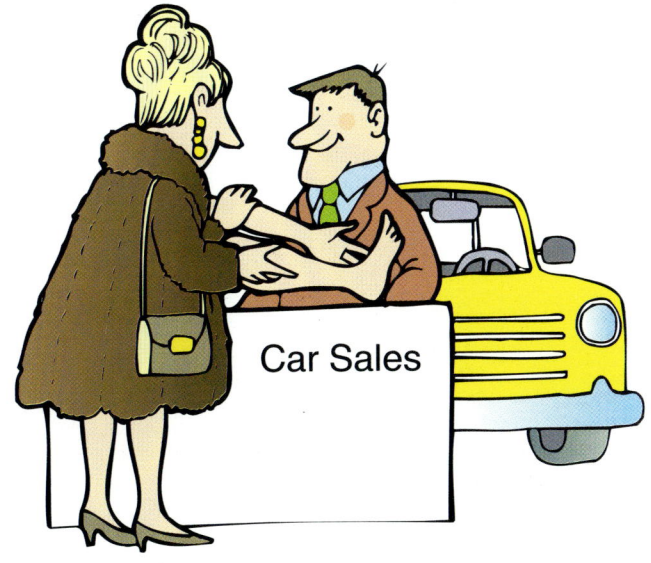

UNIT 12

An "uncommon"
neurological disorder

A nommocnu impairment

Stuart Sutherland

A CURIOUS neurological disorder, called unilateral neglect, was first noticed towards the beginning of this century: in 1941 the syndrome was more fully delineated by an English neurologist, aptly named R. Brain. People suffering from unilateral neglect have difficulty in responding to stimuli on the opposite side to their brain lesion and may fail to manipulate objects on that side of the body, for example by pulling on only one trouser leg.

In this issue (*Nature* **346**, 267–269; 1990), Alfonso Caramazza and Argye Hillis report a new impairment that is unexpected and potentially informative. They investigated a patient with unilateral neglect caused by a lesion in the left parietal lobe; they found that she could read the left sides of words well but made gross errors with right halves. This is a not uncommon defect in such patients. With considerable ingenuity, however, Caramazza and Hillis presented her with words in other forms, in particular with words spelled backwards and with words in which the letters were arranged in a vertical string. In both cases she had problems with the second half of the words as normally written. For example, if shown 'common' spelt backwards as 'nommoc' she would read out 'com' but would make errors on 'mon' even though as far as the eye is concerned the 'mon' (transformed into 'nom') was physically presented on the side (her left) that should not have been subject to neglect. Similarly, when words were shown vertically she still had difficulty with their second halves although there was no difference in the position of any of the letters along the horizontal axis.

In a further series of tests, using among other tasks forward and backward spelling, the authors obtained exactly the same results. The patient performed almost perfectly on the first half of each word but made a large number of errors on the second half (over 50 per cent on the final letter). They concluded that the centre of a word must somehow occupy a fixed point in the recognition and production systems for written words and conducted a further very clever test of this hypothesis. If it is correct, the subject should perform better at recognizing 'contrast' in the word 'contrastiveness' than when presented simply with 'contrast'. Amazingly, this is exactly what happened (it would incidentally be nice to know what would happen if the additional letters were a random string so that no word is completed).

Caramazza and Hillis rightly insist that their results show that unilateral neglect can operate at a central level far removed from the topographical layout of the scene on the retina and in the early visual centres. To recognize a word, one must access its representation in memory: the results suggest that this representation preserves the left-to-right ordering of the letters in words, as indeed it must. What is puzzling is that they also suggest that words are positioned in this representation by their centre point. It is well known that words are accessed by their initial letter. When asked, most people say that more words begin with 'r' than have 'r' as the third letter but they are wrong: because we address words by their initial letter, it is difficult to retrieve words, such as 'street' that have an 'r' as their third letter. Moreover, in reading, words are usually fixated just to the right of their beginning. These facts might explain why the left-hand side of a word is easier to recognize than the right, but they do not begin to explain why a given letter string is easier to recognize if it has extra letters tacked onto the end.

Some earlier work, not mentioned by the authors, is however relevant. In their chapter in *Neuropsychology of Visual Perception* (Lawrence Erlbaum, 1989), G. Gainotti *et al.* described how they asked unilateral-neglect patients to copy a drawing of a series of objects, such as trees and houses, arranged in a horizontal row. Some of the patients copied all the objects, not just those on the same side as the lesion. But they tended to miss out those parts of each object that lay on the opposite side to the lesion (see figure). Only patients with right-sided lesions did this. It would be interesting to test Gainotti's patients with upside-down objects to see whether they would neglect the half presented contralateral to the lesion or the half of the object if the object be contralateral to the lesion if the object

were in its normal orientation (as Caramazza and Hillis's patients did with words).

One possibility is that just as the left hemisphere is dominant for words, the right is dominant for the representation of objects, and that attention to the side of the representation of a word or object that is contralateral to the dominant hemisphere is impaired if input from the non-dominant hemisphere is faulty as a result of a lesion. Even this explanation, like most of those put forward by neuropsychologists, remains vague.

Nevertheless neuropsychology is coming of age: whereas in the past it concerned itself with *where* a function is carried out, it is now investigating *how* it is carried out. Its findings must be taken into account by those trying to explain how the mind works, but unfortunately many results, such as those discussed here, remain baffling. □

Stuart Sutherland is at the Centre for Research on Perception and Cognition, University of Sussex, Brighton BN1 9QG, UK.

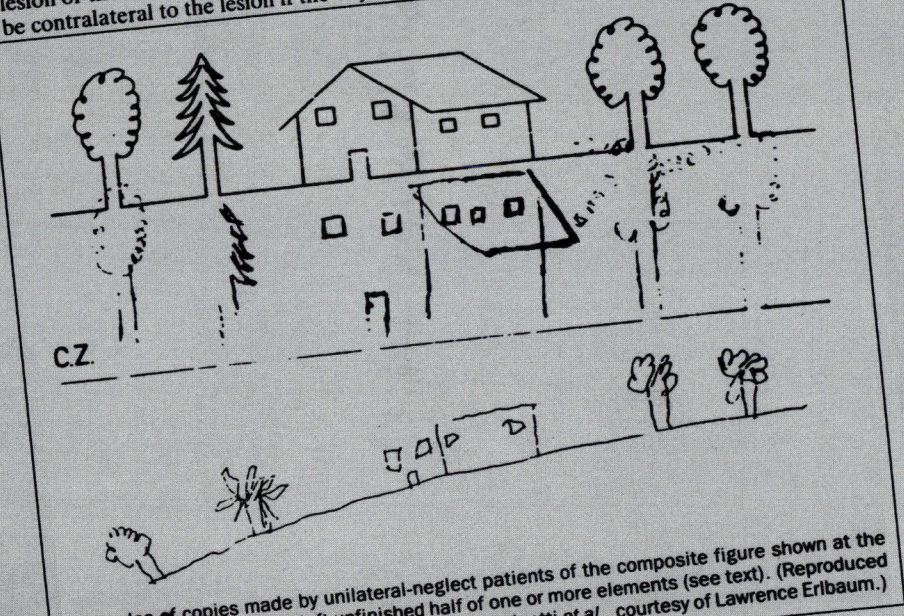

C.Z.

Examples of copies made by unilateral-neglect patients of the composite figure shown at the top. In each case patients left unfinished half of one or more elements (see text). (Reproduced from *Neuropsychology of Visual Perception* by G. Gainotti *et al.*, courtesy of Lawrence Erlbaum.)

VOCABULARY

Study the meaning of the following words and expressions as used in the text.

title to impair
  - to injure or weaken
2 to neglect
  - to leave out; not to notice
5 to delineate
  - to describe
6 aptly
  - suitably
23 ingenuity
  - skill
26 to spell
  - to say or write the letters that form a word in the correct order
28 a string
  - a series of things in close succession
51 somehow
  - in a way unknown or unspecified
61 random
  - made or done without method; left to chance
66 layout
  - plan
73 to puzzle
  - to confuse
90 to tack
  - to fix; to fasten with tacks
99 a row
  - a line
120 faulty
  - defective; with faults
124 to come of age
  - to reach maturity
132 to baffle
  - to puzzle

TEXT BASED EXERCISES

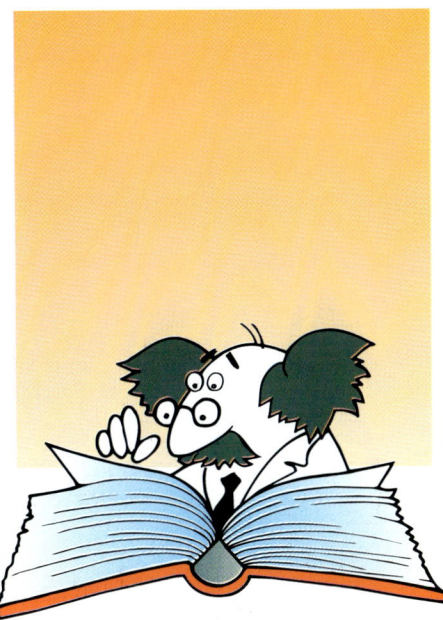

1 WORD CHECK

Explain the meaning of the following words and expressions as used in the text.

  1 curious
  3 towards
  6 aptly named
  43 further
  51 somehow
  54 clever
  92 relevant
  97 such as
  122 put forward
  128 taken into account

2 COMPREHENSION

Answer the following questions.

1 What is unilateral neglect syndrome?

2 When was this syndrome first noticed?

3 What had caused the syndrome in the patient investigated by Caramazza and Hillis?

4 What common defect did Caramazza and Hillis's patient have when reading?

5 In what other forms were words presented to the patient?

6 How did the patient respond when the words were shown vertically?

7 What did they conclude about the centre of a word in the recognition and production systems for written words?

8 Why would most people say that more words begin with "r" than have "r" as the third letter?

9 What were the results when patients were asked to copy a drawing of a series of objects arranged in a horizontal row?

10 In the writer's opinion, why is neuropsychology coming of age?

3

Fill in the blanks with the words below as used in the text.

- ✔ suffering
- ✔ puzzling
- ✔ noticed
- ✔ earlier
- ✔ side
- ✔ explanation
- ✔ suggest
- ✔ difficulty
- ✔ disorder
- ✔ positioned
- ✔ mentioned
- ✔ forward
- ✔ well-known
- ✔ stimuli
- ✔ however
- ✔ fail

a A curious neurological (1) .... , called unilateral neglect, was first (2) .... towards the beginning of this century.

b People (3) .... from unilateral neglect have (4) .... in responding to (5) .... on the opposite (6) .... of their brain lesion and may (7) .... to manipulate objects on that side of the body.

c What is (8) .... is that they also (9) ....

that words are (10) .... in this representation by their centre point.

d Some (11) .... work, not (12) .... by the authors, is (13) .... relevant.

e Even this (14) .... , like most of those put (15) .... by neuropsychologists, remains vague.

f It is (16) .... that words are accessed by their initial letter.

4 OPPOSITES

Give the opposite of the following words and expressions which are *all to be found in the text.*

e.g. right → left

a forwards
b horizontal
c the opposite
d the end
e right-hand side
f common
g without fault
h dominant

5 VERBS

Fill in the blanks with the following *verbs* in the form used in the text.

- ✔ show
- ✔ tend
- ✔ find
- ✔ make
- ✔ cause
- ✔ spell
- ✔ read
- ✔ lie
- ✔ be
- ✔ arrange
- ✔ read
- ✔ have

a They investigated a patient with unilateral neglect (1) .... by a lesion in the left parietal lobe; they (2) .... that she (3) .... the left sides of words well but (4) .... gross errors with right halves.

b If shown "common" spelt backwards as "nommoc", she (5) .... out "com" but would make errors on "mon" even though as far as the eye is concerned the "mon" was physically presented on the side that (6) .... subject to neglect.

c Similarly, when words (7) .... vertically, she still (8) .... difficulty with their second halves although there was no difference in the position of any of the letters along the horizontal axis.

d They (9) .... to miss out those parts of each object that (10) .... on the opposite side to the lesion.

e Caramazza and Hillis presented her with words in other forms, in particular with words (11) .... backwards and with words in which the letters (12) .... in a vertical string.

6 PREPOSITIONS

Fill in the blanks with a suitable *preposition*.

1 People suffering .... unilateral neglect have difficulty .... responding to stimuli .... the opposite side to their brain lesion and may fail to manipulate objects .... that side .... the body, for example .... pulling .... only one trouser leg.

2 Gainotti described how they asked unilateral neglect patients to copy a drawing .... a series .... objects, such as trees and houses, arranged .... a horizontal row.

3 They tended to miss .... those parts .... each object that lay .... the opposite side to the lesion.

4 Caramazza and Hillis rightly insist that their results show that unilateral neglect can operate .... a central

level far removed .... the topographical layout .... the scene .... the retina and .... the early visual centres.

5 .... a further series .... tests, using among other tasks forward and backward spelling, the authors obtained exactly the same results.

6 .... 1941 the syndrome was more fully delineated .... an English neurologist, aptly named R. Brain.

7 This is a not uncommon defect .... such patients.

8 .... both cases she had problems .... the second half .... the words as normally written.

7 ADVERBS

Fill in the blanks with the *adverbs* below as used in the text.

✔ potentially   ✔ vertically
✔ perfectly   ✔ amazingly
✔ usually   ✔ similarly
✔ fully   ✔ exactly
✔ incidentally

a In 1941 the syndrome was more .... delineated by an English neurologist.

b In this issue, Alfonso Caramazza and Argye Hillis report a new impairment that is unexpected and .... informative.

c ...., when words were shown .... she still had difficulty with their second halves although there was no difference in the position of any of the letters along the horizontal axis.

d The patient performed almost .... on the first half of each word but made a large number of errors on the second half.

e ...., this is .... what happened (it would .... be nice to know what would happen if the additional letters were a random string so that no word is completed).

f Moreover, in reading, words are .... fixated just to the right of their beginning.

Notes

EXTENSION EXERCISES

8 PHRASAL VERBS WITH PUT

Study this sentence.
121 Even this explanation, like most of those *put forward* by neuropsychologists, remains vague.

In this sentence put forward means to suggest or propose.

Study the meanings of the verbs below. They are all formed with the verb TO PUT.

Read the following sentences. Fill in the blanks with one of the phrasal verbs in the correct form.

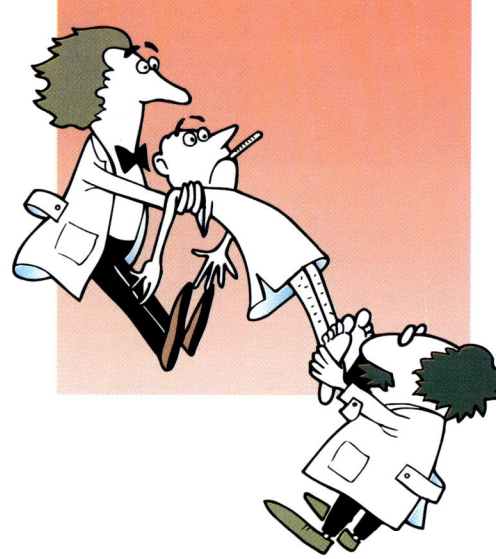

Phrasal verb	Meaning
to put across	to communicate
to put away (1)	to put something in a box or drawer etc.
to put away (2)	to save
to put forward (1)	to suggest or propose
to put forward (2)	to recommend
to put forward (3)	to move the hands of a clock forward
to put in	to insert; to include
to put in for	to apply for a job
to put off	to postpone
to put a person off	to tell him to postpone his visit to you

1 He tried to ....
.... a suggestion but it wasn't accepted.
2 Professor Baker always gives an interesting lecture. He is very good at .... his subject ....
3 The football match was .... because of bad weather.
4 I have decided to ....
.... the job I told you about yesterday.
5 My sister was due to spend the weekend with us. When the doctor said the children had measles, I immediately
....
....
6 Jack's desk is always untidy. He never .... his papers ....
7 Paul's chief was very pleased with his work. He .... him .... for promotion.
8 Read the sentence and .... the missing word.
9 If you want to go to the Bahamas on holiday, you should start to ....
some money ....
10 Clocks are ....
.... one hour at the beginning of official Summer Time.

9* VERBS FROM NOUNS

Give the *verbs* from the nouns below. Make sentences in your own words using the verb in any form.

e.g. memory

The teacher asked the class *to memorize* the new words.

a	8	stimuli
b	44	spelling
c	52	recognition
d	52	production
e	68	centre
f	69	representation
g	97	a drawing
h	128	findings

GRAMMAR POINT

FUTURE PERFECT

a   The *FUTURE PERFECT* is formed by using WILL+HAVE+THE PAST PARTICIPLE.

e.g. We'll go on holiday in September. George *will have taken* his exams by then and he'll be able to come with us.

Study the construction of the above sentence.

George will have taken his exams
subject + auxiliary will + have + past participle + object

b   *The Future Perfect is used for an action which at a precise future time will already be in the past. It is normally used with a time expression beginning with by.*

e.g. By the end of the month, *I'll have worked* at Sussex General Hospital for ten years.

FUTURE PERFECT CONTINUOUS

a   This tense is formed with WILL+HAVE+BEEN+THE PRESENT PARTICIPLE.

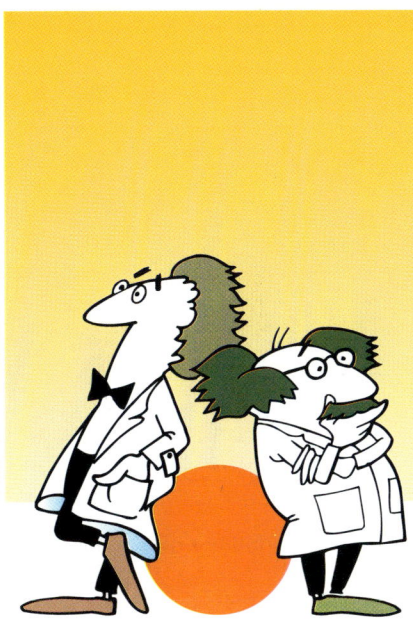

b   Like the Future Perfect, it is normally used with a time expression beginning with *by*.

c   *The Future Perfect Continuous can be used when the action is continuous or when expressed as a continuous action.*

e.g. By the end of this week, *we'll have been testing* the drug for two years.

Study the construction of the above sentence.

We'll have been testing
subject + will + have + been + present participle

10 GRAMMAR CHECK

Now change the following sentences from the *Future Simple* to the *Future Perfect* as in the example. Complete the sentences with the time expression *by* and the words in brackets.

e.g. I'll finish this work. (tomorrow)
I'll have finished this work *by* tomorrow.

1 She'll read the report. (tomorrow morning)
2 They'll spend the money on the project. (next year)
3 Will John leave? (six o'clock)
4 The laboratory will complete the tests. (tonight)
5 The doctor won't finish his rounds. (midday)
6 They'll announce the results of the competition. (June)
7 He'll return the book he borrowed. (Wednesday)

11 GRAMMAR CHECK

Now form *complete* sentences from the words below. Put the verbs in brackets into the *Future Perfect Continuous*.

e.g. By August, I (live) - this house - for six years
By August, *I'll have been living* in this house for six years.

1 By the end of this week, they (work) on the research project for four months.
2 By six o'clock, I (type) for two hours.
3 By the end of this term, we (study) English for eight years.
4 By the time he retires, he (operate) for 30 years.
5 By the end of the month, Carol (live) in Manchester for six weeks.
6 By Christmas, I (follow) the exercise programme for two months.
7 By the time they buy a house, they (save up) for five years.

Notes

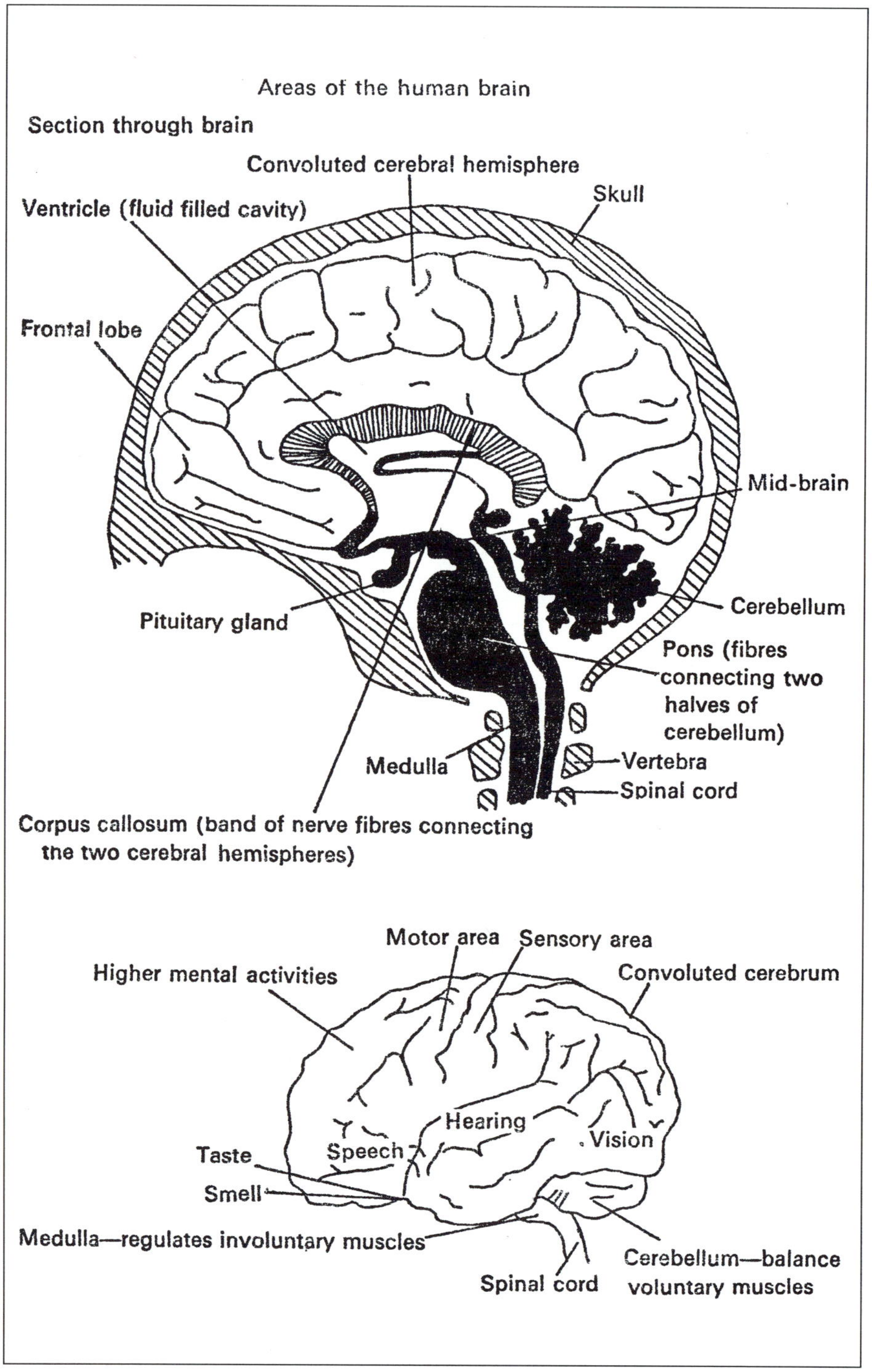

Areas of the human brain

Section through brain

Convoluted cerebral hemisphere

Ventricle (fluid filled cavity)

Skull

Frontal lobe

Mid-brain

Pituitary gland

Cerebellum

Pons (fibres connecting two halves of cerebellum)

Medulla

Vertebra

Spinal cord

Corpus callosum (band of nerve fibres connecting the two cerebral hemispheres)

Higher mental activities

Motor area   Sensory area

Convoluted cerebrum

Taste

Speech

Hearing

Vision

Smell

Medulla—regulates involuntary muscles

Spinal cord

Cerebellum—balance voluntary muscles

Study the following terminology.

PATHOLOGY

Pathology is the scientific study of disease, its causes and its effects; disease in any disturbance of normal body structure or function.

5 Pathological changes are neither constant nor static as there is always continual interaction between the causative agent or agents and the body's natural responses; nevertheless, fairly consistent patterns emerge, and these are the foundations of pathological practice.

BASIC TERMINOLOGY IN PATHOLOGY

10 *Aetiology* is the actual cause or causes of the disease.
Pathogenesis is the sequence of events in disease development from outset to termination, and includes any influencing factors; thus, it is the means whereby the aetiological agent brings about disease. Although not synonymous, aetiology and pathogenesis
15 are usually considered together.
Predisposing factors are pre-existing pathological or physiological states which increase the likelihood of developing the disease.
Natural history is the 'normal' course of any disease,
20 unmodified and unaffected by treatment, from beginning to end.
Symptoms are abnormalities or subjective complaints noticed by the patient.
Physical signs are abnormalities found or elicited on clinical examination. Some disease may be well established or even
25 fairly advanced before symptoms and/or physical signs appear.
Lesions are the pathological structural abnormalities. They may be *macroscopical* (i.e. visible on naked eye examination) or *microscopical* (i.e. detectable only by appropriate microscopy).
Diagnosis is an opinion, based on all available evidence, of the
30 disease process or processes present. Anyone can attempt to make a diagnosis; often, it is relatively easy, but sometimes considerable experience and numerous different investigational techniques are necessary; rarely, only a list of possible diseases can be provided (i.e. *differential diagnoses*), with further tests
35 required before an accurate *definitive diagnosis* can be made.
Prognosis is a prediction of the likely outcome of any disease, and is obviously influenced by treatment given.
Morbidity reflects ill-health, incapacity or sickness associated with non-fatal disease.
40 *Mortality* related to deaths from disease.

USEFUL APPROACH TO PATHOLOGY

It is always very useful (and in examinations, important) to have a logical and systematic approach to pathological conditions and diseases and it is well worth while developing such an approach at the outset. Below is the outline of a series of questions worth
45 applying to any pathological entity.
Definition. A clear, concise and accurate definition of the appropriate condition is an essential starting point.
Incidence. How common is it? A knowledge of the approximate incidence of different conditions enables anyone to put them
50 into perspective and into order of frequency. The old adage that common things are common will always be applicable to pathology, and it is important to begin by discussing the most likely possibilities.
Aetiology. What is the cause? Is more than one cause known? Is
55 it idiopathic? Are any predisposing factors recognised?
Pathogenesis. What is the natural sequence of events in its evolution? Are any influencing factors known?
Age. When does it usually develop-infancy, childhood, old age, etc.? Can it appear at any age?
60 *Sex.* Is it obviously more common in males or females, or is the sex incidence approximately equal?
Geographical distribution. Is it more common in particular areas or countries? Is this related to affluence, poverty, climatic conditions or certain socio-economic groups?
65 *Lesions.* What does it look like macroscopically? What are the microscopic appearances? Are these features specific for the disease concerned? What is required for definitive clinical or pathological diagnosis? Is a differential diagnosis appropriate?
Clinical features. What are the usual presenting symptoms?
70 What physical signs are found? How specific are these features? Are they diagnostic? Are any other investigations (radiology, biochemistry, microbiology, etc.) diagnostic?
Spread. Does it spread locally? Does distant spread occur? How does it spread? What effects does spread produce?
75 *Treatment.* Does any treatment exist? How specific and how effective is treatment? Are there significant side effects?
Prognosis. What is the natural history? What is the likely outcome? What factors influence prognosis? What complications may develop? Does it predispose to any other
80 disease?

VOCABULARY

12	outset - start	13	to bring about - to cause	36	outcome - result
13	whereby - by means of which	17	likelihood - probability	51	an adage - a saying

WRITING

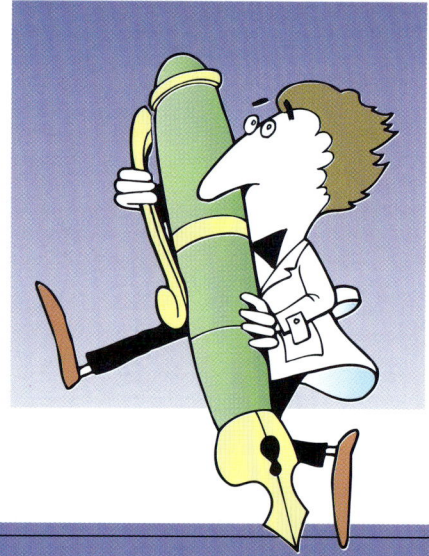

12

Write a short explanation of the following statement in your own words.

4   "Pathological changes are neither constant nor static."

13

Fill in the chart below. Write about a disease of your choice.

Definition	
Incidence	
Aetiology	
Pathogenesis	
Age	
Sex	
Geographical distribution	
Lesions	
Clinical features	
Spread	
Treatment	
Prognosis	

SPEAKING

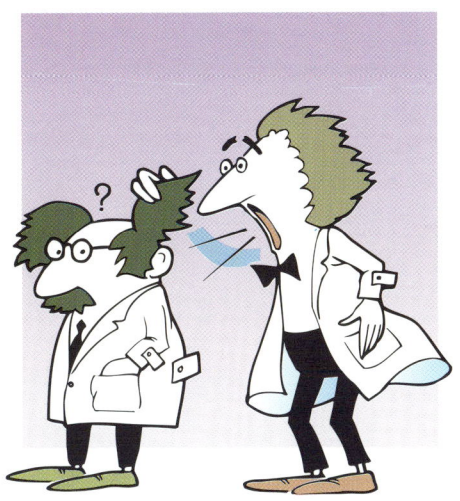

14 SPELLING

Spell the words below.

NEUROLOGICAL
CURIOUS
UNILATERAL
IMPAIRMENT
INGENUITY
SYNDROME

VERTICAL
AXIS
HORIZONTAL
BACKWARDS
TOPOGRAPHICAL
PHYSICALLY
FAULTY
VAGUE
NEUROPSYCHOLOGY
HYPOTHESIS
ORIENTATION
HEMISPHERE

15 TERMINOLOGY

Explain the following terminology
in your own words.

Predisposing factors
Natural history
Symptoms
Physical signs

Differential diagnoses
Prognosis
Morbidity
Mortality

UNDERSTANDING IDIOMATIC ENGLISH

Explain the idiom.

He's got two left feet

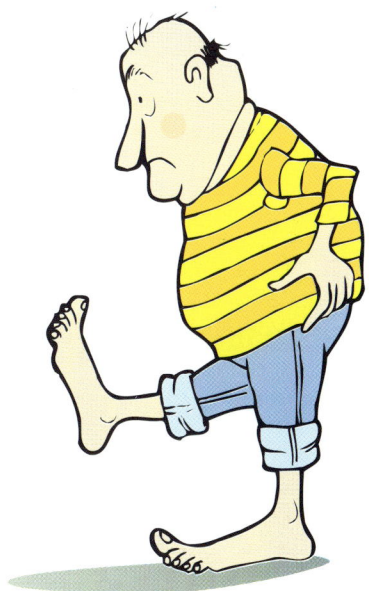

UNIT 13

Atherosclerosis:
reversing the damage

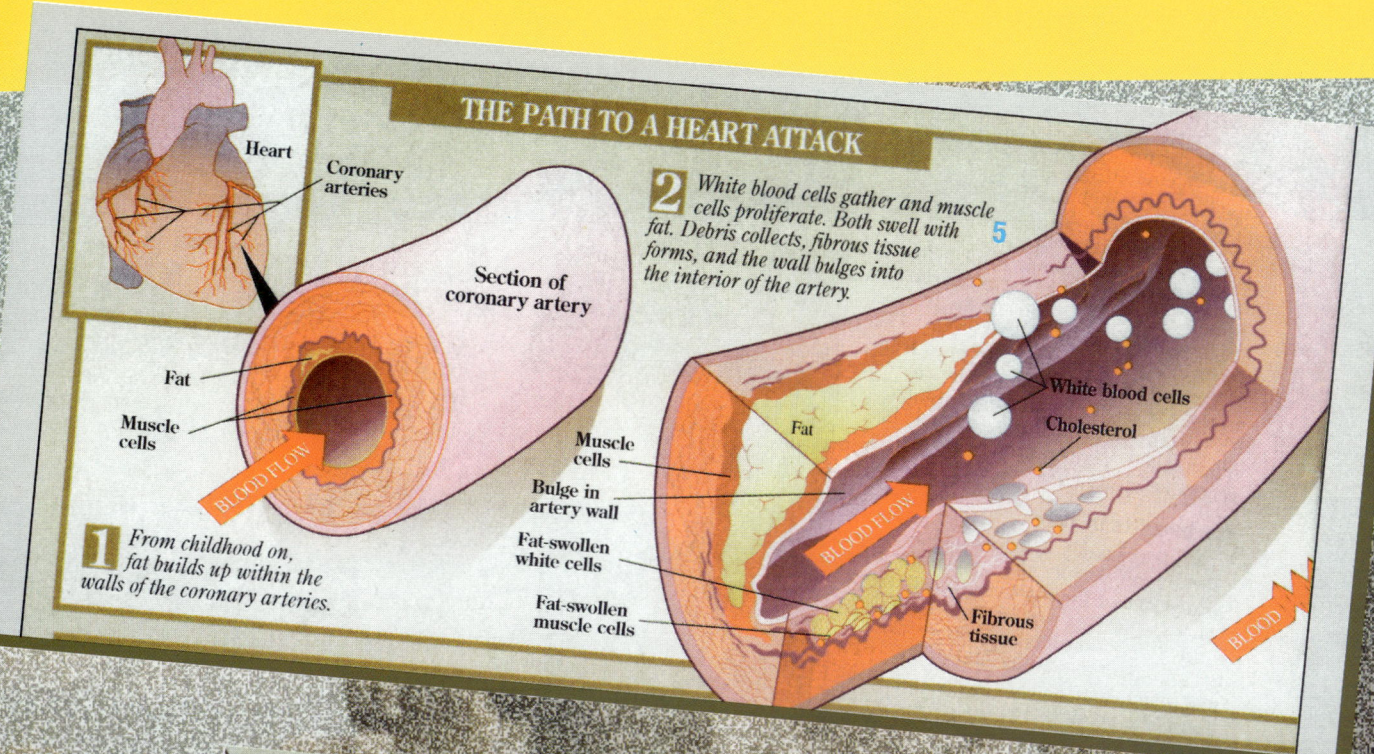

THE PATH TO A HEART ATTACK

Heart

Coronary arteries

Section of coronary artery

Fat

Muscle cells

1 From childhood on, fat builds up within the walls of the coronary arteries.

2 White blood cells gather and muscle cells proliferate. Both swell with fat. Debris collects, fibrous tissue forms, and the wall bulges into the interior of the artery.

5

White blood cells

Cholesterol

Muscle cells

Bulge in artery wall

Fat-swollen white cells

Fat-swollen muscle cells

Fat

Fibrous tissue

BLOOD FLOW

BLOOD

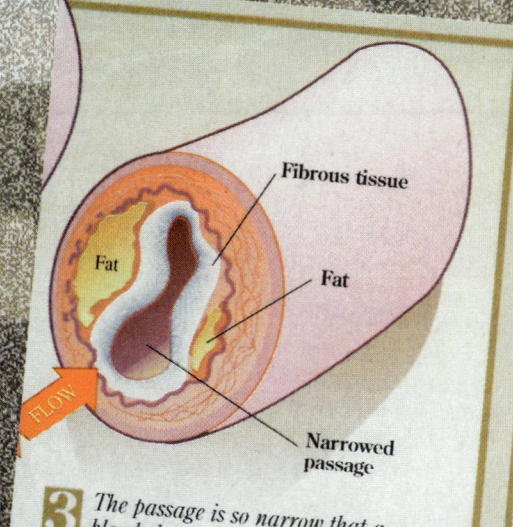

Fibrous tissue

Fat

Fat

FLOW

Narrowed passage

3 The passage is so narrow that a blood clot or a spasm of the artery can shut off blood flow, resulting in a heart attack.

10

REVERSING THE DAMAGE

Reduced bulge

What happens during reversal is unknown. One possibility: The extra cells and much of the fat simply break down. Although cleaner, the artery walls may still be scarred.

15

Imagine a man en route to a heart attack. The blood nourishing his heart fights its way through coronary arteries that have slowly narrowed over time. The heart attack strikes: A clot or spasm clamps a stretch of narrowed artery completely shut, depriving part of the heart muscle of its lifeblood. The muscle dies— and so does the man, if his remaining heart muscle cannot compensate.

How the coronary arteries narrow is well understood. The process, called atherosclerosis, is not a matter of globs of fat and cholesterol building up like hardened deposits inside decrepit plumbing. Rather, it happens within the artery walls themselves. The muscle cells that line the arteries divide and swell with fat. White blood cells congregate, scooping up more fat. Fibrous tissue forms, cholesterol and other debris pile up and the wall bulges into the interior of the artery, impeding blood flow.

Just what triggers the narrowing is less clear. In the early 1970s, Russell Ross and John Glomset of the University of Washington proposed that the artery is responding to a perceived injury. Their hypothesis, since refined, is that high levels of cholesterol in the blood irritate the artery lining, which lets white blood cells enter. Those cells, and the muscle cells in the wall, divide; both types of cells accumulate fat. High blood pressure, diabetes and smoking also set off the process. Less fat builds up, but the artery still narrows.

In some people, says biochemist David Hajjar of Cornell University, the on-signal may come from the herpes virus responsible for cold sores. In the laboratory, the virus both impairs the muscle cells' ability to produce an enzyme that normally breaks down cholesterol and forces infected cells to turn out a molecule that makes other cells divide.

Or it may be a matter of oxidation, the chemical reaction that rusts iron and steel. In the body, the same reaction alters low-density lipoproteins (LDL's), molecules that carry cholesterol from the blood into the artery wall, where it can get picked up by the white cells and muscle cells. Dr. Daniel Steinberg of the University of California at San Diego has shown that it is primarily oxidized LDL that collects in cells. In lab tests, antioxidants like vitamin E have kept cells from swallowing oxidized LDL.

VOCABULARY

Study the meaning of the following words and expressions as used in the text.

4   to gather
- to assemble or collect

7   to bulge
- to swell outwards

17   to scar
- to mark with a scar

22   a clot
- part of blood which thickens and separates from the serum

23   to clamp
- to press firmly; to hold together with a clamp (*a clamp* - a metal or wood fastening for holding things firmly together)

30   a glob
- a drop; a globule

36   to scoop up
- to lift by using a scoop (*a scoop* - a shovel for lifting and moving liquids or loose substances)

38   to pile up
- to accumulate

41   to trigger
- to initiate a violent or destructive process by a comparatively small act

62   to turn out
- to produce

TEXT BASED EXERCISES

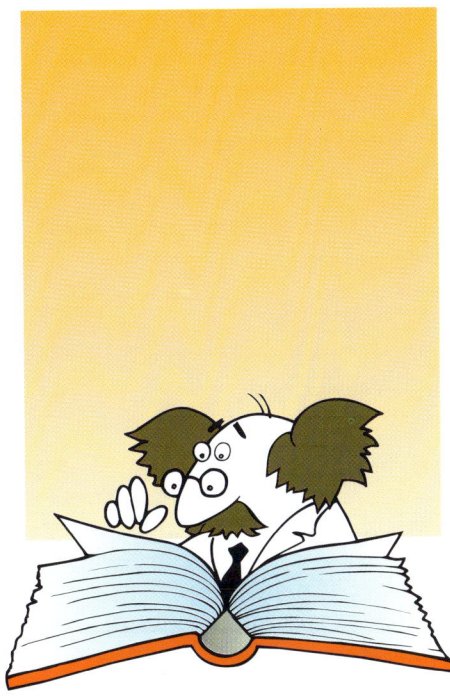

1 WORD CHECK

Explain the following expressions in your own words.

title   The Path To A Heart Attack

11   shut off blood flow
20   fights its way through
20   coronary arteries
21   slowly narrowed over time
32   decrepit plumbing
52   set off the process
diagram   reduced bulge

2 ASKING QUESTIONS

Write questions to which the following are the answers.

1   It happens from childhood on.
2   It deprives part of the heart of its lifeblood.
3   Atherosclerosis.
4   No, it happens within the artery walls themselves.
5   The artery wall eventually bulges into the interior of the artery.
6   The high levels of cholesterol in the blood.
7   High blood pressure, diabetes and smoking.
8   It both impairs the muscle cells' ability to produce an enzyme that normally breaks down cholesterol and forces infected cells to turn out a molecule that makes other cells divide.
9   Dr. Daniel Steinberg of the University of California at San Diego.
10   Antioxidants like vitamin E.

3 PREPOSITIONS

Fill in the blanks with prepositions.

1   The blood nourishing his heart fights its way

.... coronary arteries that have slowly narrowed over time.

2 White blood cells congregate, scooping .... more fat.

3 Fibrous tissue forms, cholesterol and other debris pile .... and the wall bulges .... the interior .... the artery, impeding blood flow.

4 High blood pressure, diabetes and smoking also set .... the process.

5 Less fat builds .... but the artery still narrows.

6 .... the laboratory, the virus both impairs the muscle cells' ability to produce an enzyme that normally breaks .... cholesterol and forces infected cells to turn .... a molecule that makes other cells divide.

7 .... the body, the same reaction alters low-density lipoproteins, molecules that carry cholesterol .... the blood .... the artery wall, where it can get picked .... by the white cells and muscle cells.

8 Dr. Daniel Steinberg .... the University .... California .... San Diego has shown that it is primarily oxidized LDL that collects .... cells.

4 VERBS

Fill in the blanks with the *verbs* below in the form used in the text.

✓ understand
✓ build up
✓ line
✓ form
✓ congregate
✓ happen
✓ impede
✓ swell
✓ bulge
✓ call

How the coronary arteries narrow is well .... The process, ... atherosclerosis, is not a matter of globs of fat and cholesterol .... like hardened deposits inside decrepit plumbing. Rather, it .... within the artery walls themselves. The muscle cells that .... the arteries divide and .... with fat. White blood cells ...., scooping up more fat. Fibrous tissue ...., cholesterol and other debris pile up and the wall .... into the interior of the artery, ... blood flow.

5 NOUNS

Fill in the blanks with the following *nouns* as used in the text.

✓ narrowing
✓ lining
✓ blood
✓ process
✓ enzyme
✓ blood pressure
✓ virus
✓ molecule
✓ levels
✓ wall
✓ sores
✓ injury

Just what triggers the .... is less clear. In the early 1970's, Russell Ross and John Glomset of the University of Washington proposed that the artery is responding to a perceived .... Their hypothesis, since refined, is that high .... of cholesterol in the .... irritate the artery ...., which lets white blood cells enter. Those cells, and the muscle cells in the ...., divide; both types of cells accumulate fat. High ...., diabetes and smoking also set off the .... Less fat builds up, but the artery still narrows.

In some people, says biochemist David Hajjar of Cornell University, the on-signal may come from the herpes .... responsible for cold .... In the laboratory, the virus both impairs the muscle cells' ability to produce an .... that normally breaks down cholesterol and forces infected cells to turn out a .... that makes other cells divide.

EXTENSION EXERCISES

6 NOUNS FROM VERBS

Give *nouns* related to the verbs below.

e.g. to *proliferate* → *proliferation*

Verb	Noun
to gather	
to bulge	
to fight	
to strike	
to clamp	
to deposit	
to divide	
to irritate	
to infect	
to alter	
to swell	
to form	
to narrow	
to collect	
to compensate	
to impair	
to pile up	
to perceive	
to oxidize	
to accumulate	

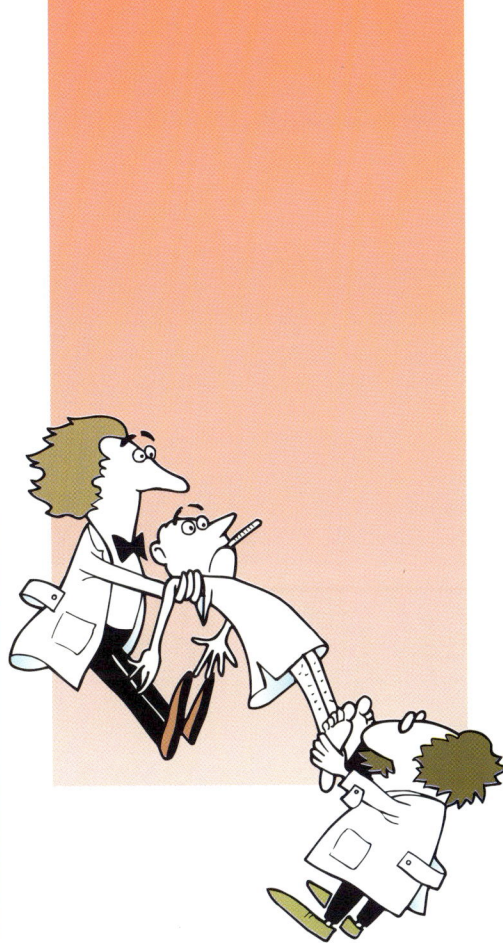

7 INTERROGATIVE SENTENCES

Ask questions as in the example. Begin each question with an auxiliary.

e.g. The artery narrows.
Does the artery narrow?

1 Fibrous tissue forms.
2 A heart attack is life-threatening.
3 Both types of cells accumulate fat.
4 Jack will have to stop smoking in order to reduce his risk of having a heart attack.
5 Mike could take more exercise, if he really wanted to.
6 Mr. Collins has had two heart attacks this year.
7 They would lose a lot of weight if they went on a strict diet.
8 Antioxidants like vitamin E have kept cells from swallowing oxidized LDL.
9 White blood cells can congregate, scooping up more fat.
10 Fat builds up within the walls of the coronary arteries.

8 NEGATIVE SENTENCES

Make the following sentences negative.

1 The blood fights its way through coronary arteries.
2 They have narrowed over time.
3 It happens within the artery.
4 White blood cells congregate.
5 It may be a matter of oxidation.
6 It can get picked up by the white cells.
7 The cells will swell with fat.
8 The researchers would like to do further lab tests.
9 He could have avoided a heart attack.
10 He was told he had high blood pressure.

9 IDIOMATIC EXPRESSIONS WITH DO

Study these idioms formed with the verb *TO DO*. Read the idioms in column 1 and try to join them to their corresponding meaning in column 2.

Column 1	Column 2
1 to do one's best	a to visit patients at home or in the hospital
2 to do the donkey work	b to do something to oblige someone else
3 to do someone a favour	c to do practical jobs like house-painting etc. instead of getting them done by tradesmen
4 to do more harm than good	d to do something completely and thoroughly
5 to do the rounds	e to be very beneficial
6 to do-it-yourself	f to do something as well as one can
7 to do a world of good	g to achieve an effect which is more dangerous than beneficial
8 to do nothing by halves	h to do the hard or unpleasant part of the work as contrasted with the parts that require skill

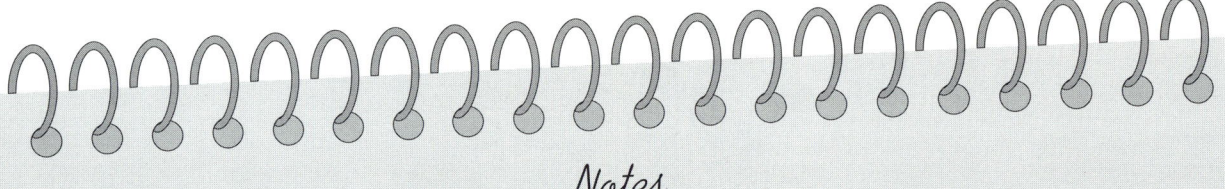

Notes

PAST CONTINUOUS TENSE

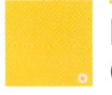

a   The Past Continuous Tense is formed by using the past tense of the verb *to be* + the present participle.

  e.g. *He was talking* while *I was trying* to study.

b   The Past Continuous is mainly used for past actions which continued for some time.

  e.g. *They were having difficulty in finding the cause of the illness.*

c   As we have already seen, the Present Continuous can be used to express a definite future arrangement.

  e.g. I'm taking my exam tomorrow.

  In the same way, the Past Continuous can express this type of future in the past.

  e.g. He was ready to go to hospital as *he was having* an operation the next day.

d   *Always* can be used to convey *a habitual past continuous action.*

GRAMMAR POINT

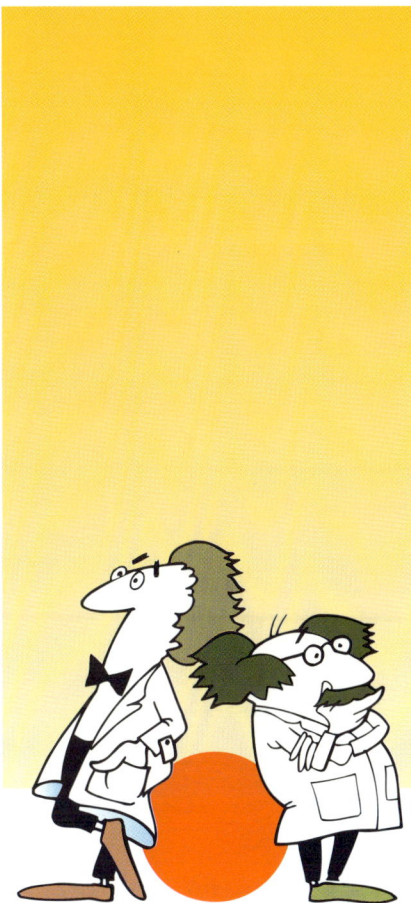

  e.g. When I was at school, my teachers *were always telling* me to study hard.

e   The *Past Continuous* and the *Simple Past* are often used together to say that something happened in the middle of something else.

  e.g. While *I was watching* television, *the phone rang.*

10 GRAMMAR CHECK

Use the verbs in brackets to form *the Simple Past or the Past Continuous.*

1   Doctor Baxter (have) his lunch when he (receive) an emergency call.
2   As she (drive) into the hospital car park she (see) someone take her parking space.
3   Since he (want) to specialize in heart surgery, he (think) about going to America to study some new techniques.
4   While the teacher (give) the lecture, most of the students (sleep).
5   Is your leg sore? I (see) you yesterday and you (limp).
6   When the doctor (arrive) at his surgery, his patients (wait) for him.
7   He (not like) school. His teachers always (tell) him that he (be) hopeless.
8   The cardiologist (tell) his patient to take up a sport as he (not get) enough exercise.

WRITING

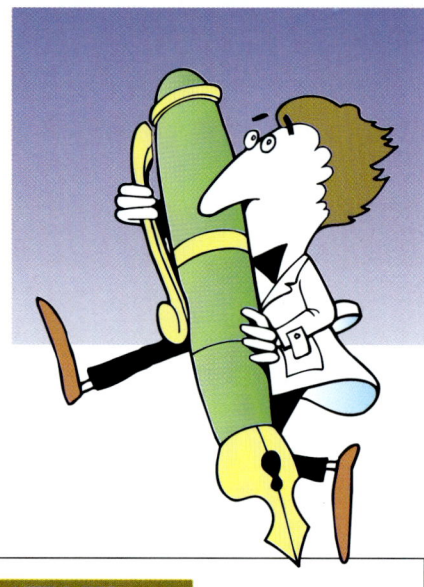

11 HEART ATTACK

Study the diagram below. Write an explanation of the path to a heart attack based on the text. Begin with the words "From childhood on ..."

Notes

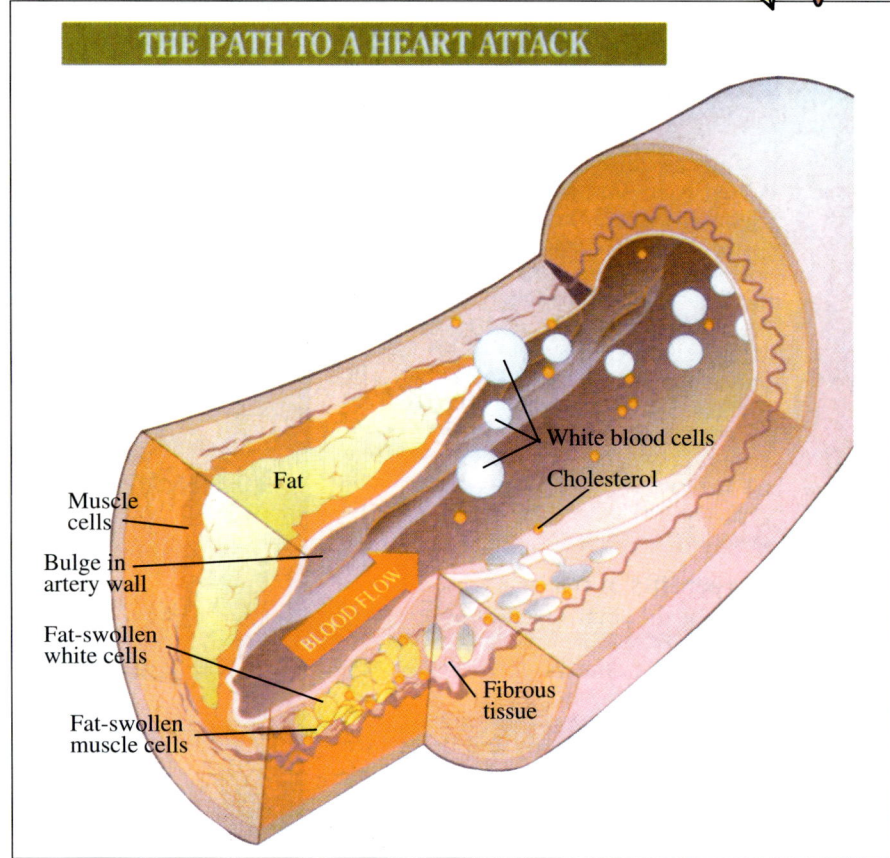

THE PATH TO A HEART ATTACK

Muscle cells

Fat

White blood cells

Cholesterol

Bulge in artery wall

BLOOD FLOW

Fat-swollen white cells

Fibrous tissue

Fat-swollen muscle cells

Read the following passage.

BLOOD VESSELS

The blood vessels are well adapted for their special jobs in the body. There are three types of blood vessels, namely, arteries, capillaries and veins. An artery is a blood vessel which carries blood away from the heart to all parts of the body. The aorta is the largest artery in the body. It leads directly from the left ventricle of the heart with a large supply of oxygenated blood. 5

Arterial blood generally appears bright red due to its supply of oxygen.

The term 'blood pressure' refers to the force of the blood within artery walls.

The doctor uses an instrument called a sphygmomanometer to measure this force. A rough standard for normal blood pressure has been established depending upon the sex and age of the individual. Any deviation above the norm is called high blood 10 pressure or hypertension. Continuous physical and mental strain, calling for over-activity on the part of the heart, may result in hypertension.

As an individual grows older all the muscles of the body become less elastic.

The muscular walls of the arteries, as well, lose their elasticity and gradually become hardened. As they become less flexible, the passageways in the arteries be- 15 come smaller, the pressure of the blood against these walls increases and the heart has to work harder to pump blood through them.

In order to reach all cells of the body, the vessels carrying the blood must necessarily branch from larger into smaller tubes. Thus large arteries branch into smaller arteries and finally into very tiny branches called capillaries. 20

These are vessels with walls of one-celled thickness, allowing digested food and oxygen to pass directly into the cells which they surround by the process of diffusion.

Gas and liquid wastes from the cells enter the bloodstream in these capillaries and are carried by veins into which they branch. Tiny veins join up to form larger veins until they become main veins, the superior and inferior venae cavae, which enter the 25 heart.

Veins are blood vessels which carry blood back to the heart from all organs of the body. These are relatively thin-walled and inelastic. Within them are small valves that prevent backflow of blood, especially where the blood has to flow against the pull of gravity (that is, from the lower trunk, legs and arms). Blood in the veins is 30 generally purplish because it contains less oxygen. It is generally on its way back to the heart to be sent to the lungs for oxygenation.

Let us trace the blood through the circulatory system.

Blood, with fresh oxygen, returns to the left auricle of the heart through the pulmonary veins. It passes through valves into the left ventricle. From here it is pumped 35 with great force into the largest artery, the aorta, which branches into smaller arteries and finally into capillaries. Oxygen and digested food enter the cells of the body; waste gases (carbon dioxide) and liquids leave the cells and diffuse into the thin-walled capillaries. Blood, carrying these substances, enters small veins which branch into larger veins. Blood from the lower part of the body returns to the right 40 auricle of the heart through the large, vein, the inferior vena cava. Blood from the upper part of the body returns through the superior vena cava into the right auricle; the blood passes through valves into the right ventricle. From here it is pumped directly through the pulmonary artery into the lungs where the waste gas carbon dioxide is given off together with water vapour and fresh oxygen is taken in. 45 Oxygenated blood then returns to the left ventricle of the heart via pulmonary veins and the cycle is repeated rhythmically.

Liquid wastes are extracted from the blood as it passes through the kidneys in its circuit round the body. Note that all the deoxygenated blood from the stomach and intestines passes to the liver in the hepatic portal vein before passing to the interior 50 vena cava in the hepatic vein. In the liver the blood sugar level is controlled.

Notes

VOCABULARY

9 norm
 - recognized standard

15 to harden
 - to become hard

23 waste
 - refuse

31 purplish
 - like purple

12 BLOOD VESSELS

Write a short summary, in your own words, of the passage you have just read.
The words below will help you.

BLOOD VESSELS:
3 types.

ARTERY:
away from the heart - the aorta - oxygenated blood.

BLOOD PRESSURE:
force - a sphygmomanometer - hypertension - physical and mental strain - overactivity.

CAPILLARIES:
one-celled thickness - diffusion - gas and liquid wastes - enter the bloodstream.

VEINS:
thin-walled - inelastic - valves - backflow - join up to form - superior and inferior venae cavae.

THE CIRCULATORY SYSTEM:
left auricle - pulmonary veins - valves - left ventricle - the aorta - oxygen and digested food - carbon dioxide and liquids - right auricle - right ventricle - pulmonary artery - the lungs.

Notes

SPEAKING

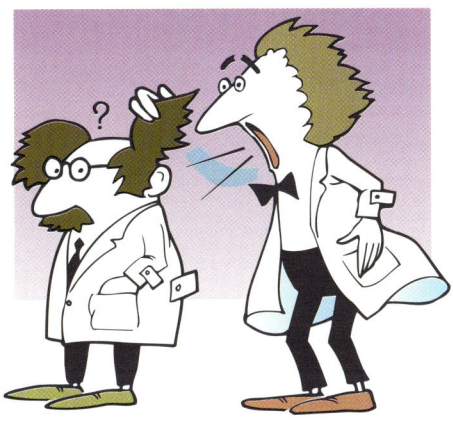

NordicTrack
A CML Company

Free Brochure & Video
Call Toll Free in U.S. and Canada
1-800-328-5888

❑ Please send me a free brochure.
❑ Also a free video tape ❑ VHS ❑ BETA

Name _____

Street _____

City_____ State_____ Zip_____

Phone (   ) _____
141C Jonathan Blvd. N. • Chaska, MN 55318
385H0

VOCABULARY

jarring	- hard
upkeep	- maintenance

Take a walk on NordicTrack and discover why it's 8 ways better than a treadmill.

1. **Better exercise.**
   NordicTrack simulates cross-country skiing, the world's best total-body exercise.

2. **Non-jarring.**
   NordicTrack eliminates unsafe jarring motions which can damage joints & ligaments.

3. **Safer.**
   NordicTrack uses no electric motors or high-speed belts that can throw off a user.

4. **You are in control.**
   No panic starts and stops as with motorized devices.

5. **Quieter.**
   NordicTrack eliminates the pounding foot step noise associated with treadmills.

6. **No electric cord or outlet required.**
   With NordicTrack you are not constrained by outlet locations.

7. **Costs far less for equal quality.**
   NordicTrack needs no expensive electric motors and speed controls. And little upkeep is required.

8. **Non-boring.**
   7 out of 10 owners are still using their machines more than 3 times a week, 5 years after purchasing one.

The world's best aerobic exerciser.

NordicTrack
A CML Company

---

13 THE BENEFITS OF A NORDICTRACT

Read the advertisement for the NordicTrack. You are a doctor working with a group of patients who have all had heart attacks and are being monitored on an exercise programme taking place at your hospital. You would like the hospital to buy an aerobic exerciser. You have read the advertisement for the NordicTrack.

Explain its benefits to your colleagues. They will ask you some questions. Explain the details in your own words. Use the following headings as a guideline.

1 Better exercise.
2 Non-jarring.
3 Safer.
4 You are in control.
5 Quieter.
6 No electric cord or outlet required.
7 Costs far less for equal quality.
8 Non-boring.

UNDERSTANDING IDIOMATIC ENGLISH

Explain the idiom.

He's pulling your leg

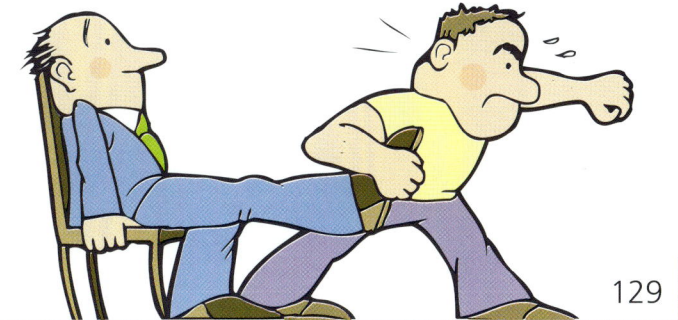

UNIT 14

Heart Tests

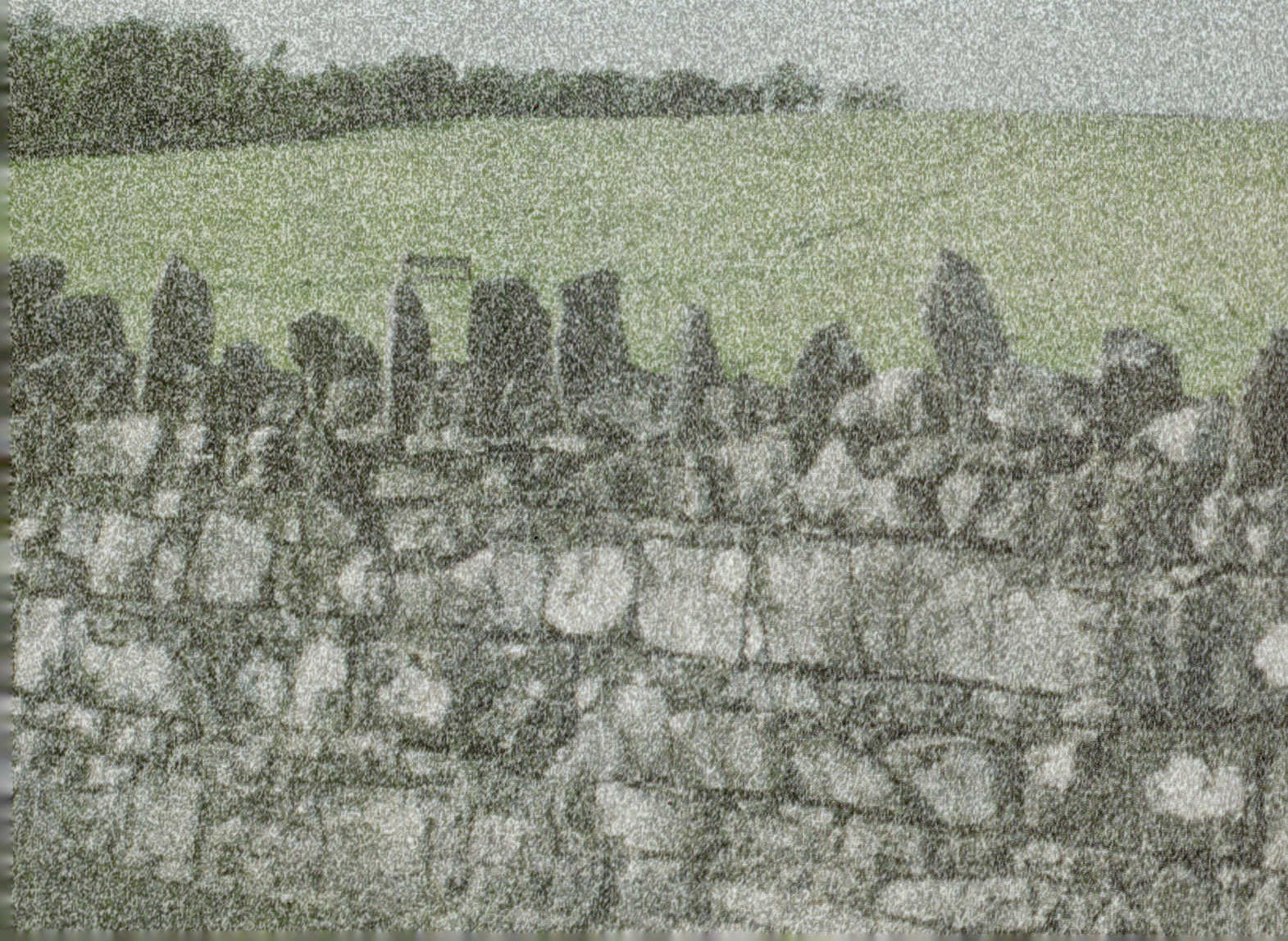

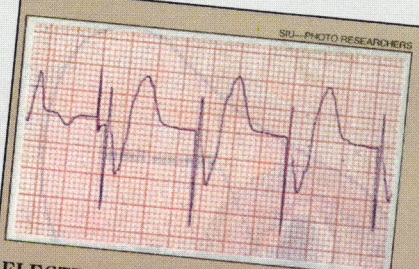

SRU—PHOTO RESEARCHERS

ELECTROCARDIOGRAM (EKG)

Designed as a first rough screening, the EKG provides tracings of the heart's electrical activity. Abnormal patterns suggest disorders of the heart muscle or coronary-artery disease.

■ **Cost:** Office, $50; wearable, $200 to $300; stress test, $200 to $300.

■ **Pros:** An EKG recording can be made quickly while resting in a doctor's office. Wearable monitors can detect problems that occur over a day or more.

■ **Cons:** Resting EKG's can miss evidence of heart disease, since abnormal patterns often don't appear until the heart muscle is stressed. When symptoms are present, doctors may order a treadmill stress test, in which the EKG is recorded during and after exercise. This test, though, fails to detect disease half the time and mistakenly announces it 30 percent of the time.

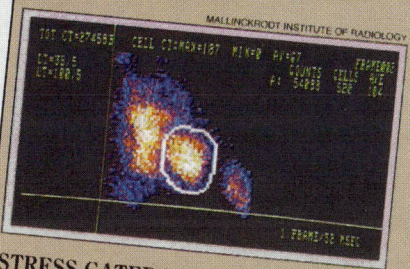

MALLINCKRODT INSTITUTE OF RADIOLOGY

STRESS-GATED BLOOD-POOL SCAN

This test reveals how much blood the heart's left chamber (circled above) holds and pumps. Done during and after exercise, it provides computer-enhanced pictures of the heart muscle in motion.

■ **Cost:** $800 to $1,000.

■ **Pros:** Little discomfort, except that blood is drawn intravenously and reinjected after being tagged with a radioactive tracer.

■ **Cons:** The test typically takes 90 minutes. Much of the time, patients must sit motionless while a gamma camera snaps 32 pictures a second. (Areas with the most blood, above, appear white and yellow.) Some experts consider these scans less accurate than thallium stress tests, right, for detecting coronary-artery disease.

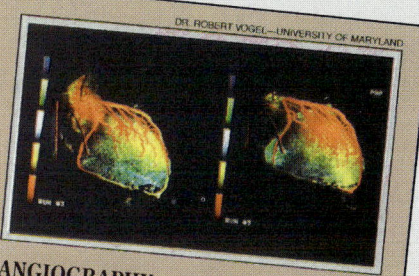

DR. ROBERT VOGEL—UNIVERSITY OF MARYLAND

ANGIOGRAPHY

A catheter is threaded through a vein in the groin or arm into the heart. A dye is injected that produces X-ray images of the coronary arteries.

■ **Cost:** $5,000 to $6,000.

■ **Pros:** Angiography shows more detail than any other test. A computer-assisted version called digital angiography allows "quantitative" measurements using less dye and a smaller catheter. (Above left, a normal heart at rest. At right, blood flow improves after the heart is stressed.)

■ **Cons:** Because catheterization may disturb the heart rhythm, it carries a small risk of death, especially among weaker patients. And interpretations of conventional angiograms must be done visually, producing results that vary from doctor to doctor. A new study shows that only digital angiography accurately determines an artery's narrowings.

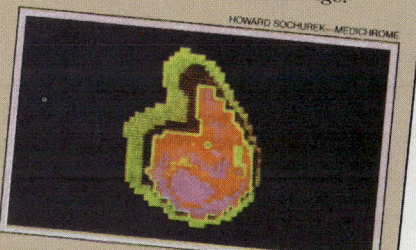

HOWARD SOCHUREK—MEDICHROME

THALLIUM STRESS TEST

This imaging technique identifies impaired blood flow to the heart muscle.

■ **Cost:** $1,000 to $1,200.

■ **Pros:** Safe. Helps determine whether bypass or angioplasty is warranted. The current test requires one injection of radioactively tagged thallium during exercise and another at rest. If coronary arteries are clogged, less thallium gets through and a gamma camera detects less radiation than in surrounding muscle. (In the color-enhanced scan of a healthy man, above, pink and red areas show the most blood flow.)

■ **Cons:** The test incorrectly identifies nearly half the regions with decreased blood supply as irreversibly damaged. New test methods may dramatically improve the accuracy.

5 10 15 20 25 30 35 40 45 50 55 60 65 70 75 80

TEXT BASED EXERCISES

VOCABULARY

Study the meaning of the following words and expressions as used in the text.

1 rough
   - approximate
1 to screen
   - to examine in order to identify changes
2 to trace
   - to track
6 wearable
   - able to be worn
8/12 the pros and cons
   - the arguments for and against
10 to detect
   - to discover; to notice
12 to miss
   - to fail to notice or find
20 mistakenly
   - wrongly
29 to draw (drawn- p.p.)
   - to extract
30 to tag
   - to fix a tag
35 to snap
   - to take a photograph
42 a dye
   - a substance used for colouring
58 to vary
   - to be different
66 to warrant
   - to justify
67 current
   - present
70 to clog
   - to block
78 to damage
   - to injure

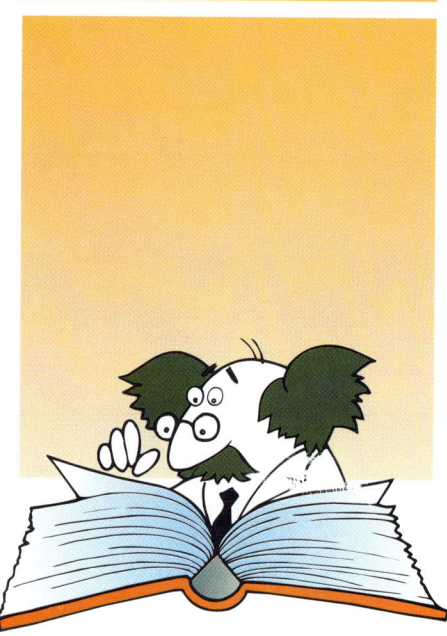

1 WORD CHECK

Give other words or expressions to explain the meaning of the words below.

22 reveals
24 done
26 in motion
28 discomfort
29 intravenously
34 motionless
35 snaps
65 safe
65 whether
70 clogged

2 COMPREHENSION

Read the following sentences. Say whether they are *TRUE* or *FALSE*. Correct the false statements.

1 An EKG can be carried out with a wearable monitor.
2 Resting EKG's always show up heart disease.
3 An EKG recorded during a treadmill stress test is very accurate.
4 A stress-gated blood-pool scan reveals how much blood the heart's left chamber holds and pumps.
5 The angiography is the cheapest of the four tests.
6 Every doctor gives the same interpretation of a conventional angiogram.
7 All versions of angiography accurately determine an artery's narrowings.
8 The thallium stress test identifies impaired blood flow to the heart muscle.
9 The thallium stress test is safe.
10 The current thallium stress test requires several injections of radioactively tagged thallium during exercise and at rest.

3 NOUNS FROM VERBS

Give *nouns* from the following verbs as used in the text.

Verb	Noun
to screen	
to trace	
to record	
to monitor	
to measure	
to dye	
to bypass	
to interpret	
to inject	
to radiate	
to flow	
to scan	

4 NOUNS

Fill in the blanks with the *nouns* below as used in the text.

✔ disease
✔ test
✔ tracer
✔ version
✔ rhythm
✔ pictures
✔ activity
✔ patterns
✔ monitors
✔ scan

a abnormal ....
b the heart ....
c electrical ....
d coronary-artery ....
e a radioactive ....
f the color-enhanced. ....
g a treadmill stress ....

h computer-enhanced ....
i a computer-assisted ....
j wearable ....

5 ADVERBS

Fill in the blanks with the following *adverbs* as used in the text.

✔ mistakenly
✔ intravenously
✔ especially
✔ visually
✔ nearly
✔ quickly
✔ accurately
✔ radioactively
✔ incorrectly
✔ irreversibly
✔ typically
✔ dramatically

1 The test .... takes 90 minutes.
2 A new study shows that only digital angiography .... determines an artery's narrowings.
3 Because catheterization may disturb the heart rhythm, it carries a small risk of death, ... among weaker patients.
4 New test methods may .... improve the accuracy.
5 Little discomfort, except that blood is drawn .... and reinjected after being tagged with a radioactive tracer.
6 The test .... identifies .... half the regions with decreased blood supply as .... damaged.
7 An EKG recording can be made .... while resting in a doctor's office.
8 Interpretations of conventional angiograms must be done .... , producing results that vary from doctor to doctor.
9 This test fails to detect disease half the time and .... announces it 30 percent of the time.
10 The current test requires one injection of .... tagged thallium during exercise.

Notes

6

Fill in the blanks with the words below as used in the text.

✓ interpretations
✓ scans
✓ narrowings
✓ technique
✓ tracings
✓ flow
✓ recording
✓ screening

1 Some experts consider these .... less accurate than thallium stress tests for detecting coronary-artery disease.
2 A new study shows that only digital angiography accurately determines an artery's ....
3 Designed as a rough ...., the EKG provides .... of the heart's electrical activity.
4 This imaging .... identifies impaired blood .... to the heart muscle.
5 An EKG .... can be made quickly while resting in a doctor's office.
6 .... of conventional angiograms must be done visually, producing results that vary from doctor to doctor.

7 VERBS

Fill in the blanks with the *verbs* below in the form used in the text.

✓ thread   ✓ draw
✓ decrease   ✓ clog
✓ stress   ✓ tag
✓ warrant   ✓ impair
✓ damage   ✓ inject
✓ reinject   ✓ record

1 A catheter is .... through a vein in the groin or arm into the heart.
2 A dye is .... that produces x-ray images of the coronary arteries.
3 Little discomfort, except that blood is .... intravenously and .... after being .... with a radioactive tracer.
4 If coronary arteries are .... , less thallium gets through and a gamma camera detects less radiation than in surrounding muscle.
5 The thallium stress test helps determine whether bypass or angioplasty is ....
6 This imaging technique identifies .... blood flow to the heart muscle.
7 The test incorrectly identifies nearly half the regions with .... blood supply as irreversibly ....
8 When symptoms are present, doctors may order a treadmill stress test, in which the EKG is .... during and after exercise.
9 Resting EKG's can miss evidence of heart disease, since abnormal patterns often don't appear until the heart muscle is ....

Notes

EXTENSION EXERCISES

8 REVISION OF IDIOMS

Fill in the missing words in the following idiomatic expressions.

1 He wasn't a .... bit of use.
2 I was ill for a few days and I was .... my food.
3 We didn't know if the patient would pull through. For several days it was .... and go.
4 Eric is very kind. He is always willing to .... someone a favour.
5 Eric's brother is useless. In fact, he does more .... than good.
6 You have to be .... to be kind.
7 When I was a young doctor, I used to get some jobs I didn't like. I felt I was always doing the .... work.
8 Doctor Brent starts work in his surgery at eleven o'clock. First, he visits his patients who are at home. He tries to finish his .... by ten thirty.
9 Susan is a good nurse. She does her .... to help the patients.
10 Every time there is a football match on television, shouts and laughter can be heard coming from the men's ward. The doctors say that watching the match always does the patients a .... of good.

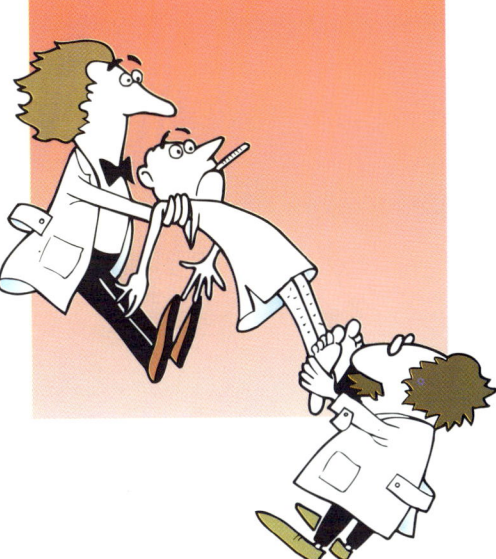

9 PHRASAL VERBS WITH GET

Study the meanings of the verbs below. They are all formed with the verb *TO GET*. Make sentences *in your own words* for each of the verbs. The first one is done for you.

e.g. to get back

I am very busy today. I can only spare a few minutes as I must get back to my surgery by three o'clock.

Phrasal verb	Meaning
to get back	to return to the place one has left e.g. home, office etc.
to get on	to make progress
to get on with	to have a good relationship with someone
to get on someone's nerves	to annoy or irritate someone
to get out of hand	to become uncontrollable
to get over	to recover from an illness or disappointment
to get to	to arrive; to reach
to get to work on	to start working
to get through (1)	to finish a piece of work
to get through (2)	to get into telephone communication

PAST PERFECT CONTINUOUS TENSE

a This tense is formed with the Past Perfect of the verb to be + the present participle.

affirmative John had been working all day.

negative John hadn't been working all day.

interrogative Had John been working all day?

b The Past Perfect Continuous (i.e. *I had* been studying) is the past of the Present Perfect Continuous (i.e. *I have* been studying).

GRAMMAR POINT

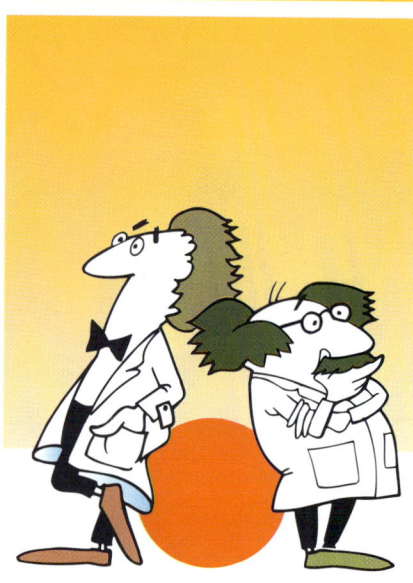

Scintiangiocardiography

c The Past Perfect Continuous can be used to say how long something had been happening before something else happened.

e.g. *He had been waiting* for the bus for half an hour before realizing there was a strike.

10 GRAMMAR CHECK

Read the sentences below. Write sentences of explanation in your own words using the *Past Perfect Continuous*.

e.g. Jack came home dog tired. *He had been working hard all day.*

1 Jane fell asleep at work.
2 Doctor Bell arrived late.
3 Everyone was happy with the news.
4 Peter had a pain in his stomach.
5 The policeman stopped the driver and fined him for speeding.
6 Nobody had seen Mary.
7 Mr. Douglas went to see his doctor.
8 David broke his leg.
9 The patients were bored waiting for their turn.
10 Doctor Bridges decided to have a short holiday.

Read the following passage.

VOCABULARY

Coming Soon: Safer Blood

A new test can detect an elusive and dangerous hepatitis virus

Many people who get blood transfusions these days are understandably nervous. Transfusions have saved countless lives, but they have sometimes transmitted serious blood-borne diseases, including AIDS. While public health officials point out that careful testing has all but eradicated the AIDS virus from the blood supply, they have not been able to claim that transfusions are perfectly safe. Reason: about 5% of patients who receive transfusions are exposed to a virus that can cause a potentially deadly liver infection called non-A, non-B hepatitis.

The mysterious malady is so named because it is not caused by the widely recognized A and B strains of hepatitis viruses. Symptoms include fever, nausea and fatigue and, in chronic cases, cirrhosis of the liver. About 5% of the U.S. population harbors non-A, non-B viruses. The majority of those who are exposed show no symptoms, but of the patients who come down with chronic liver disease, an estimated 10% die within five years. About 150,000 new infections occur each year because of blood transfusions.

This last major threat in the U.S. blood supply may soon be greatly reduced. After six years of research, scientists at Chiron, a genetic-engineering firm in Emeryville, Calif., have developed a test for the presence of a non-A, non-B hepatitis virus in blood samples. According to papers published last week in the journal *Science,* trials have shown that Chiron's test is highly reliable. It can now help eliminate the virus from the blood supply. The inexpensive test (about $2 per blood sample) is expected to be approved by the Food and Drug Administration this year and marketed early in 1990 by Chiron and Ortho Diagnostics Systems, a subsidiary of Johnson & Johnson. Said Dr. S. Gerald Sandler, medical director for blood services of the American Red Cross: "This is a very significant scientific achievement that virtually closes the chapter on post-transfusion hepatitis."

Chiron's initial breakthrough was to isolate a viral protein from blood samples taken from patients with non-A, non-B hepatitis. By cloning large quantities of the protein, the company was able to develop a test to detect its presence in blood. Chiron called the pathogen the "hepatitis-C virus." In clinical studies done at the National Institutes of Health, the Centers for Disease Control and laboratories in Italy and Japan, blood samples from patients thought to have non-A, non-B hepatitis were screened using Chiron's test. At least 80% of the samples tested positive for the hepatitis-C virus.

The fact that the test did not detect non-A, non-B hepatitis 100% of the time suggests that there may be still more viruses at large that can cause hepatitis. But the A, B and C viruses seem to cause the

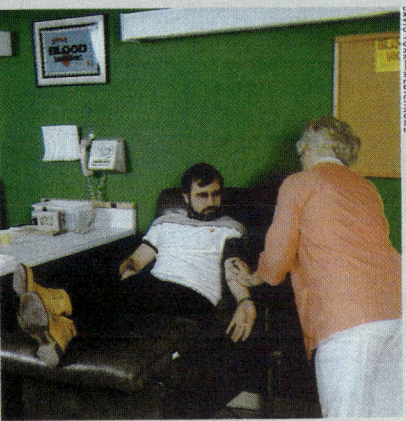

Giving a pint: the donation will be carefully screened

The next step for the researchers is to find a vaccine.

large majority of cases, and so researchers are confident that they can now almost eliminate the risk of contracting hepatitis from a blood transfusion.

Eradicating the disease is another matter. Like the AIDS and hepatitis-B viruses, hepatitis C is spread by sexual contact and, among drug addicts, through contaminated needles. But Chiron's work offers hope that the disease can be controlled. Isolating a protein from the hepatitis-C virus has made it possible to develop a vaccine to ward off the infection. Chiron biochemist Michael Houghton cautions that hepatitis C could be "one of those awkward viruses like herpes and AIDS" for which vaccines are elusive. But, he says, the C virus resembles the one that causes German measles, which can be prevented by one of the "best vaccines ever developed."

—By John Langone

title elusive
   - difficult to understand or catch
8 all but
   - almost
15 malady
   - illness
89 to ward off
   - to avert; to prevent from happening

Notes

WRITING

11 WRITING NOTES

Complete the following table.
Write notes on the pros and cons
of the following tests.

ELECTROCARDIOGRAM

Pros:

Cons:

ANGIOGRAPHY

Pros:

Cons:

STRESS-GATED BLOOD-POOL
SCAN

Pros:

Cons:

THALLIUM STRESS TEST

Pros:

Cons:

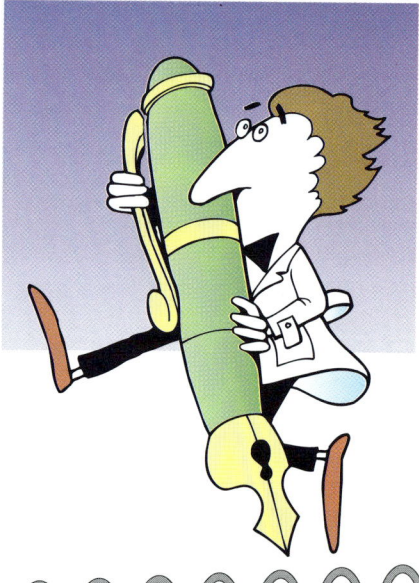

12 NON-A, NON-B HEPATITIS

Write a short paragraph about
non-A, non-B hepatitis. The words
below will help you.

- not caused by A and B strains
- fever, nausea, fatigue
- cirrhosis of the liver
- about 5% of the U.S. population
- the majority - no symptoms
- chronic liver disease - 10% die
within five years
- 15,000 new infections - blood
transfusions

Notes

SPEAKING

13 TEST FOR NON-A, NON-B HEPATITIS VIRUS

Explain the following in your own words:

- the importance of the test that has been developed for the presence of a non-A, non-B hepatitis virus in blood samples
- the initial breakthrough and how the genetic-engineering firm was able to develop the test
- the clinical studies conducted at the National Institutes of Health, the Centers for Disease Control and laboratories in Italy and Japan
- the conclusion the researchers

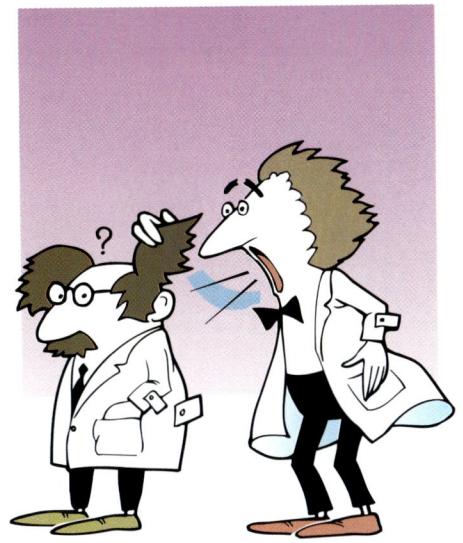

came to when the test did not detect non-A, non-B, hepatitis 100% of the time.

14 DOCTOR/PATIENT DIALOGUE

Work in pairs.
Conduct the following doctor/patient dialogue.

A patient goes to his doctor to ask for advice. He is shortly due to undergo a major operation. He is concerned that he may need a blood transfusion and is worried about the risk of contracting the AIDS or hepatitis viruses.

UNDERSTANDING IDIOMATIC ENGLISH

Explain the idiom.

She has a heart of gold

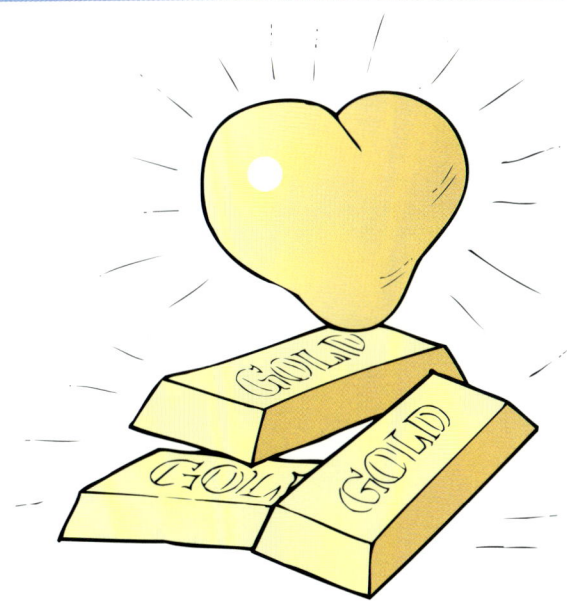

UNIT 15

The physical effects of stress on healthy hearts

The pressure-cooker factor

The stresses of daily life can harm even healthy hearts

Too much to do, too little time. Work deadlines, traffic jams, financial pressure, family tiffs. You probably sense that all this stress is not good for your health, and researchers back you up. "The evidence is stronger than ever," says Dr. Kenneth Pelletier, a stress expert at the University of California at San Francisco, that life's aggravations, large and small, contribute in very real ways to heart disease.

Recent studies have shown that mental stress raises blood pressure, squeezes the heart's coronary arteries and makes them go into spasms and increases levels of chemicals in the blood that cause clots. Over time, these effects can weaken the coronary arteries and the heart muscle. In people who already have some clogging in their arteries or who have had a heart attack, stress can kill. Numerous studies show that heart-attack victims who continue to lead stressful lives have two to three times the incidence of repeat heart attacks of survivors who learn to control their stress.

But even people with clean arteries may suffer damaging physical effects because of stress. And they may not appreciate their danger, since the initial stages of heart disease don't reveal themselves with pain or other symptoms. Doctors now believe, in fact, that stress may trigger undetected, or "silent," mini-heart attacks when spasms in the coronary arteries reduce the oxygen reaching the heart muscle and weaken it. In people with or without clogged arteries, these mini attacks set the stage for life-threatening heart attacks later on.

The new Type A. Stress has been fingered for decades as a suspect in the progression of heart disease, as anyone labeled a "Type A" personality no doubt knows. In the 1960s and 1970s, several major studies and an onslaught of books popularized the notion that Type A's, especially white-collar Type A men— aggressive, competitive, impatient and easily angered—were twice as likely to

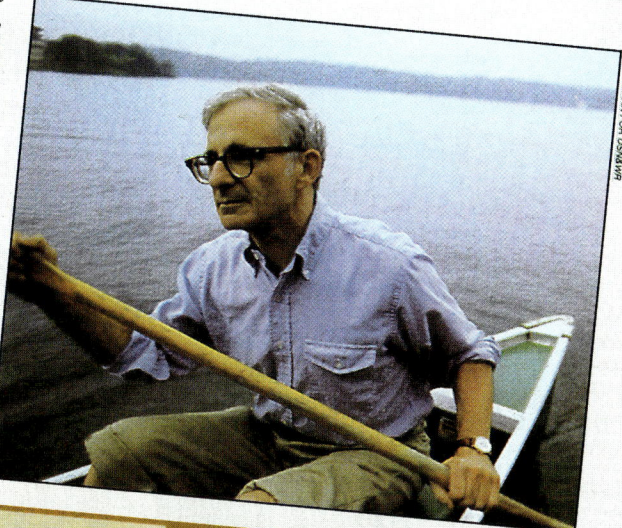

JOE ROSEN, 60

History: Heart attack in February, high blood pressure, stressful job

Strategy: Reduce stress, cut intake of fats and cholesterol, exercise faithfully

To date: Blood pressure, cholesterol and stress all lower. Takes regular walks

Rosen's main challenge is to control the pressures of his consulting job. He now meditates and takes on only work he can handle. Keep it up, say his doctors, and he has an excellent chance of avoiding another attack.

have heart attacks as their laid-back Type B colleagues. But later studies have refined that concept. Dr. Redford Williams, for example, a behavioral-medicine specialist at Duke University, has found that most components of Type A behavior do not predispose people to heart disease. The hard-driving, competitive businessman who thrives on constant activity and feels in control of his destiny, Williams found, is at no greater risk of heart disease unless he smokes or has other risk factors, such as a family history of heart disease. By contrast, salesmen who must meet weekly quotas, or clerical and blue-collar workers laboring under the twin burdens of constant pressure and lack of control over their work and workloads, *are* two to four times likelier than the average person to develop heart disease.

Aggressiveness and competitiveness, it seems, don't necessarily cause stress.

The bad guys, rather, are chronic hostility, anger and powerlessness. Furthermore, says Pelletier, "What is stressful for one person may be easily handled by another. It's all in how someone copes."

One experience stressful to virtually everyone, apparently, is loneliness. A large body of evidence now shows that people who feel alone in the world, uninvolved with other people and their community, run a higher risk of illness, including heart disease. Heart-attack survivors are at especially high risk. In one study, people who were found through questionnaires and interviews to be socially isolated and to have a high degree of psychosocial stress— unhappiness with job or marriage, for example—were four times more likely to die from a second heart attack than those with the lowest levels of stress and isolation.

Almost all recovery programs for heart patients now include stress-reduction techniques such as daily meditation, yoga or relaxation exercises. Patients also are taught how to overcome hostility and anxiety about time pressure, and the importance of group and community activities. One popular technique to reduce hostility, for example, is to have patients keep a log of what makes them angry; realizing how trivial many of their gripes are can help them control their anger. The sense of being imprisoned by the clock eases as people learn to schedule their lives more carefully and to lower expectations about how much they "should" get done in a day or a week.

No one knows whether stress reduction might be enough, at least for some people, to prevent or reverse heart disease, even without a healthy diet and exercise program. The evidence strongly suggests that easing the pressure or learning to cope with it certainly can't hurt. And whatever the benefit to your heart, life should be sunnier. ∎

by Steven Findlay

VOCABULARY

Study the meaning of the following words and expressions as used in the text.

title   **a pressure cooker**
- a cooking utensil in which food is cooked under steam pressure

title   **to harm**
- to injure; to damage

2   **a deadline**
- the time by which some task has to be completed

4   **a tiff**
- a little quarrel or disagreement

7   **to back up**
- to support; to provide arguments in favour of

13   **an aggravation**
- something irritating or annoying

34   **a survivor**
- one who remains alive after experiencing some danger

48   **to set the stage**
- to prepare the way

51   **to finger**
- to indicate; to point to

55   **an onslaught**
- a vigorous attack

60   **laid-back**
- relaxed

74   **a quota**
- a limited quantity of goods to be sold in a stated period

76   **a burden** (fig.)
- something heavy to carry or endure

TEXT BASED EXERCISES

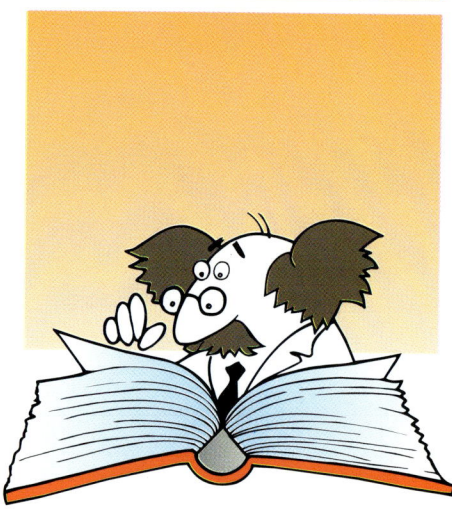

88   **to handle**
- to control

89   **to cope**
- to deal successfully with a difficulty

123   **a log**
- a daily record

124   **a gripe** (sl.)
- a cause of discontent

126   **to imprison**
- to put in prison; to restrict

127   **to ease**
- to relieve; to loosen

1   COMPREHENSION

Answer the following questions.

1   Why is "The pressure-cooker factor" a good title for the text?

2   What have recent studies shown are the physical results of mental stress?

3   What effects can these physical results have over the years?

4   Why do people with clean arteries not realize that they may suffer damaging physical effects because of stress?

5   What does the writer mean by a "silent" mini-heart attack?

6   Do all Type A personality businessmen run a greater risk of having a heart attack?

7   What are the twin burdens that some occupation groups work under that makes them two to four times likelier than the average person to develop heart disease?

8   What do heart patients learn on a recovery programme?

9   In what way does keeping a log of what makes them angry help the patients?

10   What effect does learning to schedule their lives have on these patients?

2   WORD CHECK

Explain the following expressions in your own words.

13   life's aggravations
20   spasms
22   a clot
37   damaging physical effects
44   mini-heart attacks

47 clogged arteries
53 Type A personality
61 Type B colleagues
63 a behavioral-medicine
     specialist
114 stress-reduction techniques

3 NOUNS FROM VERBS

Give a *noun* formed from the following verbs.

Verb	Noun
to aggravate	
to relax	
to meditate	
to survive	
to compete	
to isolate	
to expect	
to question	
to experience	
to reduce	

4 NOUNS

Fill in the blanks with the following *nouns* as used in the text.

✔ factors
✔ specialist
✔ colleagues
✔ studies
✔ disease
✔ personality
✔ progression
✔ risk
✔ notion
✔ concept
✔ activity
✔ lack
✔ destiny
✔ history
✔ person

The new Type A. Stress has been fingered for decades as a suspect in the .... of heart .... as anyone labled a "Type A" .... no doubt knows. In the 1960's and 1970's, several major .... and an onslaught of books popularized the .... that Type A's, especially white-collar Type A men – aggressive, competitive, impatient and easily angered – were twice as likely to have heart attacks as their laid-back Type B .... But later studies have refined that .... Dr. Redford Williams, for example, a behavioral-medicine .... at Duke University, has found that most components of Type A behavior do not predispose people to heart disease. The hard-driving, competitive businessman who thrives on constant .... and feels in control of his ...., Williams found, is at no greater .... of heart disease unless he smokes or has other risk ...., such as a family .... of heart disease. By contrast, salesmen who must meet weekly quotas, or clerical and blue-collar workers laboring under the twin burdens of constant pressure and .... of control over their work and workloads, are two to four times likelier than the average .... to develop heart disease.

5 VERBS

Fill in the blanks with the *verbs* below in the form used in the text.

✔ set   ✔ increase
✔ learn   ✔ reveal
✔ raise   ✔ show
✔ lead   ✔ appreciate
✔ weaken   ✔ believe
✔ trigger   ✔ cause
✔ reduce   ✔ squeeze
✔ suffer

Recent studies have (1) .... that mental stress (2) .... blood pressure, (3) .... the heart's coronary arteries and makes them go into spasms and (4) .... levels of chemicals in the blood that (5) .... clots. Over time, these effects can (6) .... the coronary arteries and the heart muscle. Numerous studies show that heart-attack victims who continue to (7) .... stressful lives have two to three times the incidence of repeat heart attacks of survivors who (8) .... to control their stress.

But even people with clean arteries may (9) .... damaging physical effects because of stress. They may not (10) .... their danger, since the initial stages of heart disease don't (11) .... themselves with pain or other symptoms. Doctors now (12) .... , in fact, that stress may (13) .... undetected or "silent" mini-heart attacks when spasms in the coronary arteries (14) .... the oxygen reaching the heart muscle and weaken it. In people with or without clogged arteries, these mini attacks (15) .... the stage for life-threatening heart attacks later on.

6 PREPOSITIONS

Fill in the blanks with a *preposition* as used in the text.

1 You probably sense that all this stress is not good for your health, and researchers back you ....
2 Life's aggravations, large and small, contribute .... very real ways .... heart disease.

3 .... people who already have some clogging .... their arteries or who have had a heart attack, stress can kill.
4 What is stressful .... one person may be easily handled .... another.
5 A large body .... evidence now shows that people who feel alone .... the world, uninvolved .... other people and their community, run a higher risk .... illness, including heart disease.
6 Heart-attack survivors are .... especially high risk.
7 The sense .... being imprisoned .... the clock eases as people learn to schedule their lives more carefully and to lower

expectations .... how much they "should" get done .... a day or week.
8 Rosen's main challenge is to control the pressure .... his consulting job.
9 He now meditates and takes .... only work he can handle.
10 Keep it ...., say his doctors, and he has an excellent chance .... avoiding another attack.

7

Find the expressions in column B *that best describe* those in column A.

A	B
Dr. Kenneth Pelletier	hard driving
recovery programmes for heart patients	unhappiness with job or marriage
Type A personality	a stress expert
Dr. Redford Williams	white-collar; blue-collar
a competitive businessman	laid-back
workers	a behavioral-medicine specialist
Type B personality	aggressive, competitive, impatient and easily angered
psychosocial stress	stress-reduction techniques such as daily meditation, yoga or relaxation exercises

EXTENSION EXERCISES

8

Make sentences *in your own words*. Use each of the words given below.

a Aggressiveness.
b Competitiveness.
c Powerlessness.
d Loneliness.
e Dizziness.
f Unhappiness.
g Stiffness.
h Willingness.

9 PAST PERFECT WITH JUST AND WHEN

Join the following sentences together to form one complete sentence.
Use the Past Perfect. Add the words *just* and *when* as in the example.

e.g. He went out. John called.
He had *just* gone out *when* John called.

1 He finished eating. He started to feel sick.
2 They washed the car. The rain started.
3 Steve began his daily meditation. The door bell rang.
4 Dr. Peterson told his colleague that he would stand in for him.

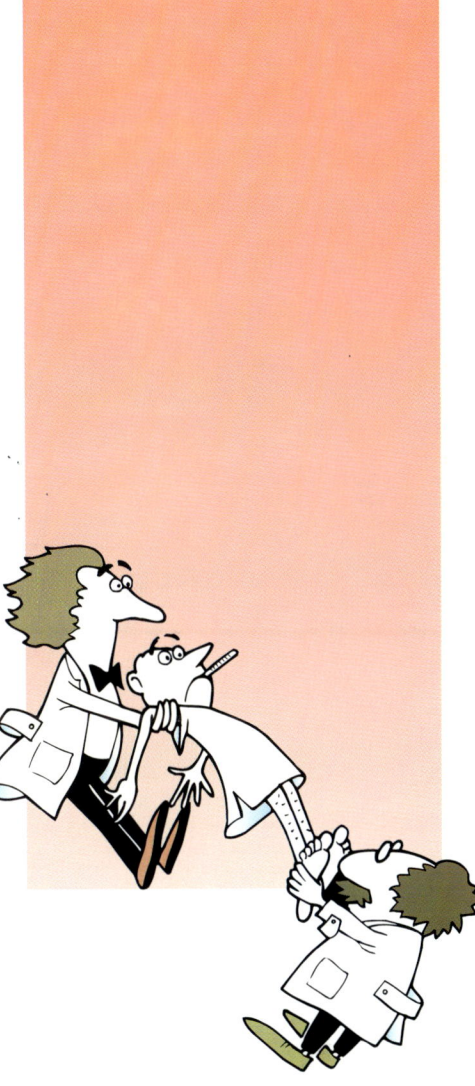

He received an emergency call and he had to go out.
5 I started to work. I was interrupted.
6 They arrived at the airport.

They heard their flight being called.
7 We got to the bus stop. We saw the bus leaving.
8 Mike started a course on coping with anger and hostility. His wife came home and told him she had crashed their new car.

10 REVISION PHRASAL VERBS

Fill in the missing part of the phrasal verb in the sentences below.

1 Bill is coming back next week. He is .... for a fortnight.
2 He can't go to the cinema this week. He has to stay at home as he is doing .... his appartment.
3 I'm bored. I don't know what to do .... myself.
4 Some patients have strange reactions when they come .... after a general anaesthetic.
5 She'll look for a new job at the end of the year when her contract is ....
6 They are out at the moment but I'll tell them about it when they get ....
7 We are out .... coffee so we will have to drink tea.
8 I'll speak to my wife about it. The decision is really .... to her.

GRAMMAR POINT

QUESTION TAGS

a This is a common form of asking questions in English. A tag is added to the end of a statement. The subject of the tag is always a pronoun.

e.g. The doctor's coming, *isn't he*? (*question tag*)

b Following the rule of *only one negative per sentence*, these sentences are constructed as shown below.

affirmative sentence
– negative tag
Mary will be late, *won't she*?

negative sentence
– positive tag
They didn't go, *did they*?

c Every *tag* corresponds to the tense of the first part of the sentence using the respective auxiliary.

e.g. *Present – Present*
He wants to see them, *doesn't he*?

Future – Future
They won't try to operate, *will they*?

Past – Past
She has been to London, *hasn't she*?
She didn't telephone, *did she*?

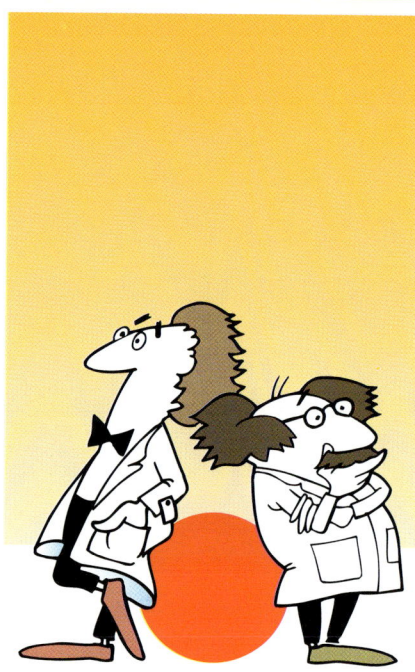

Conditional – Conditional
They would like to be specialists, *wouldn't they*?

d *How you say the sentence is important to the meaning.*
If the voice goes *down on the tag question,* then you are really only asking the listener to agree with you.

e.g. He is a good doctor, isn't he?

If the voice goes *up* then you are asking for information.

e.g. He is a good doctor, isn't he?

GRAMMAR CHECK

Finish these sentences with the appropriate question tag.

1 She is going to pass her exam, ... ?
2 You were at school with him, ... ?
3 Tim hasn't a dog, ... ?
4 You haven't seen him yet, ... ?
5 I can come when I like, ... ?
6 It won't break when I use it, ... ?
7 There are many treatments available, ... ?
8 You don't like it, ... ?
9 He should start to do some exercise, ... ?
10 Everyone could do it if they tried, ... ?
11 Paul would like to go too, ... ?
12 There weren't many applicants for the job, ... ?
13 Patients keep a log of what makes them angry, ... ?
14 Aggressiveness and competitiveness don't necessarily cause stress, ... ?
15 Joe Rosen has to cut his intake of fats, ... ?
16 It isn't going to rain, ... ?
17 You've posted it already, ... ?
18 They'll send it tomorrow, ... ?

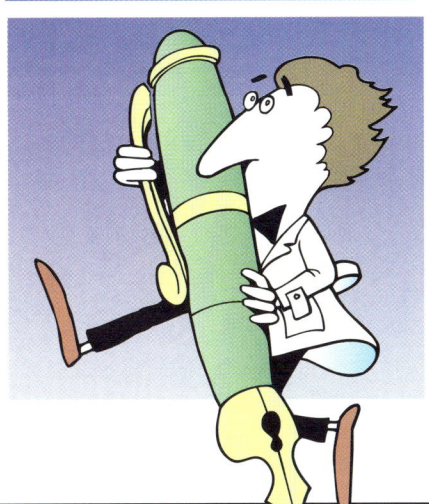

WRITING

Notes

12 STRESS TEST

Try the following Stress Test.
Answer YES or NO to each of the questions.
Check your score at the end of the test.

YOUR PSYCHOLOGICAL RESILIENCE: do you have an 'at risk' personality type?

Some personality traits have been shown to be more likely to lead to stress-related ill health than others. Of two 'at risk' personality types, the first predisposes to excessive stress by inviting it, and the second by allowing it to become too important. Do you recognize yourself in either profile?

1. Are achievement and personal success extremely important to you?

2. Do you thrive on competitions, sports and games where you are pitting your wits or your physical strength against others?

3. Do you find other people's failings (inefficiency, incompetence, unpunctuality) infuriating?

4. Are you time conscious and do you expect others to be so too?

5. Do you tend to do everything in a rush, including walking, talking and eating?

6. Are you easily bored?

7. If your life is relatively quiet, do you tend to crave excitement?

8. Do you feel most stimulated when under pressure, such as trying for a deadline, starting a new job or undertaking something that you feel may be beyond your capabilities?

9. Do you consider sleep a waste of time?

10. Do you always wake to an alarm and/or do you feel guilty if you 'oversleep'?

11. Do you find it difficult to relax and 'switch off'?

12. When you have finished an important task or project, do you plunge into the next without savouring a sense of achievement?

13. If you have a problem at work or at home, do you tend to rehearse the scene endlessly in your head?

14. If 'yes' to the above, do you find yourself unable to act it out without becoming angry, tearful or self-effacing?

15. Do you find it difficult to express your feelings for others?

16. Would you find it difficult to ask for a raise in salary at work?

17. If something you do is criticized, do you accept the criticism, even if you feel it was unjustified?

18. Do you find it difficult to turn down invitations that you are being pressed to accept when there is something that is more urgent or that you would prefer to do?

19. Do you find it difficult to express an opinion with which others might not agree and/or to speak up when someone else is expressing an opinion with which you strongly disagree?

20. Do you find it difficult to ask for money that is owed you?

21. Would you find it difficult to take a new and faulty item back to the shop and to ask for a repair or your money back?

22. Do you feel that you have achieved nothing in life and have very little to be proud of?

Questions 1 to 12. Six or more 'yes' answers indicate very definite type 'A' personality traits. While type A tend to be 'achievers', they also tend to be more prone to the negative effects of stress than the more easy-going type 'B'. So, learn how to relax and find creative rather than competitive activities outside your immediate sphere of work. You will then be extending your potential and substantially reducing your chances of succumbing to stress-related ill health.

Questions 13-22. Four or more 'yes' answers indicate that your self-confidence is low and that you find it difficult to assert yourself. In addition, the difficulty you find in expressing what you feel may result in prolonged psychological stresses. Try to assert yourself, to build up more self-esteem, by finding things in yourself and in what you do that you like and feel are worthwhile. You may well find that your relationships — at home, at work and socially — improve as a result.

Read the following information about a heart attack survivor who has had bypass surgery.

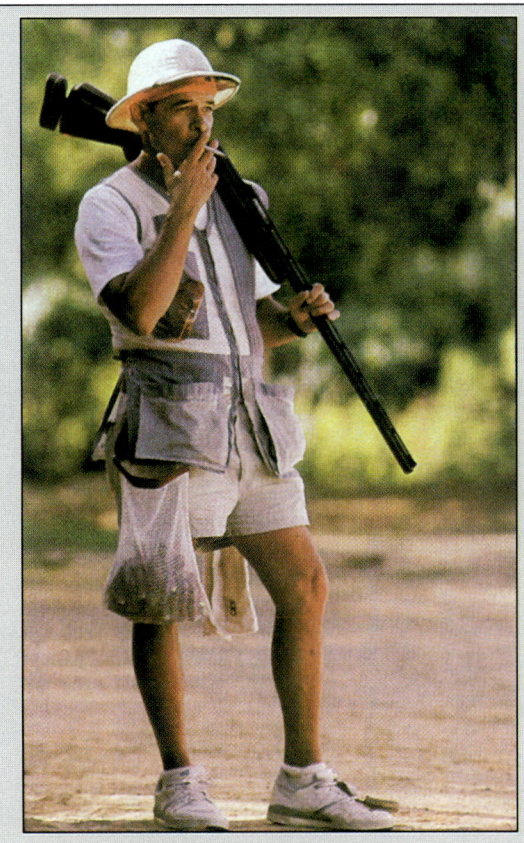

DERAL HART, 52

History: Heart attack in 1976, bypass surgery in 1977, second attack in 1987. Was overweight, with cholesterol level of 270

Strategy: To lose weight and lower cholesterol level by revamping his diet

To date: Lost 65 pounds; cholesterol at 165

5

Ordered to diet, exercise and stop smoking, Hart now weighs 150 and watches every molecule of fat. But he doesn't exercise and still smokes. Given 10 his history, his risk of another heart attack is high unless he quits. "I have no excuses," he says.

VOCABULARY

5 to revamp (sl.)
- to make better or more efficient
12 to quit (coll.)
- to stop; to give up

a pound = 454 grams

Notes

SPEAKING

13 DOCTOR PATIENT DIALOGUE

Work in pairs.
Conduct the following doctor/patient dialogue.

You are Deral Hart's doctor. He comes to you for his regular check-up. Ask him some questions about his diet and his habits e.g. smoking and exercise. Explain the risks he is running unless he follows your advice closely.

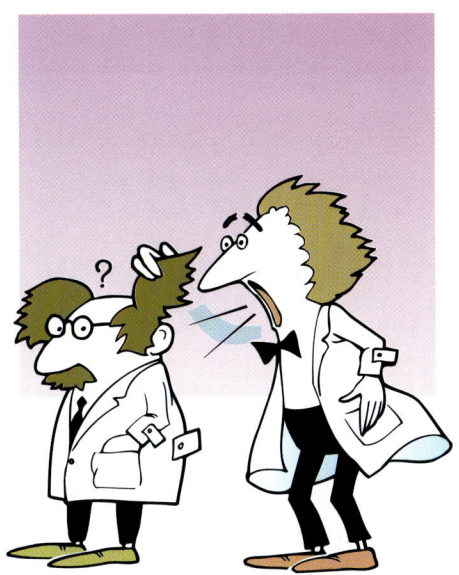

14

Group work.
Make a list of situations in life which you consider to be very stressful. Begin with the following:

Death of husband or wife
Divorce
Separation
Being sent to prison
Death of a family member
Illness or accident

Add to the list. Compare your list with those of other groups.

UNDERSTANDING IDIOMATIC ENGLISH

Explain the idiom.

You've got a nerve!

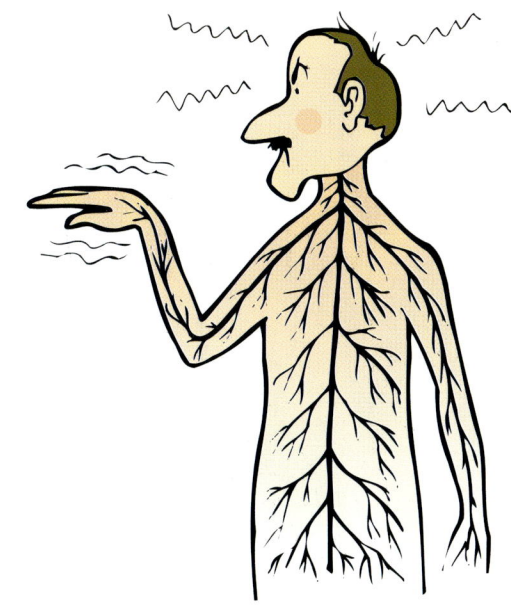

UNIT 16

A book that helps plan
exercise programmes
for patients with
special needs

VOCABULARY

Study the meaning of the following words and expressions as used in the text.

1 to prescribe
  - to order (especially medical treatment)
3 a wealth
  - an abundance
8 pregnant
  - expecting a baby
8 elderly
  - approaching old age
8 wheelchair
  - invalid's chair on wheels
8 to confine
  - to restrict; to limit
9 to pose
  - to put forward
12 to benefit
  - to do good to
18 to train
  - to educate or instruct by systematic practice
22 to outline
  - to summarize
24 compliance
  - disposition to do as you are asked
26 a table
  - a set of facts or figures arranged in lines or columns
28 a glance
  - a quick look
30 superb
  - excellent
32 renowned
  - famous
39 to employ
  - to make use of

40 a practice
  - the professional activity of a doctor or lawyer etc.
43 to keep fit
  - to stay in good condition by exercising
44 a dividend
  - a profit

TEXT BASED EXERCISES

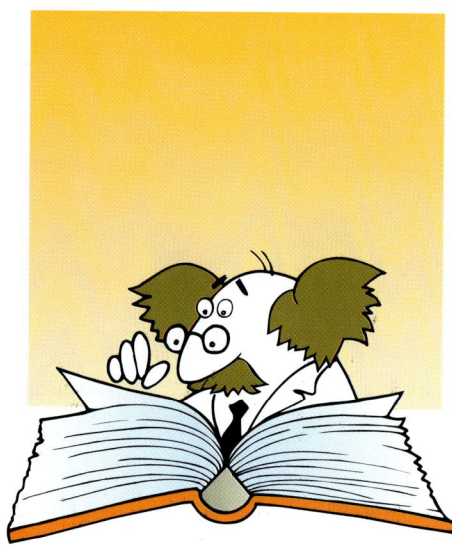

1

Say what the following expressions *refer to* in the text.

e.g. Not a simple task.
Prescribing an exercise program for your healthy patients.

a 8 wheelchair-confined
b 10 an interesting challenge
c 15 fast and easy
d 22 practical and effective
e 30 superb
f 38 safe and effective
g 38 one-of-a-kind
h 42 sick and well
i 42 a growing series
j 44 health and longevity

2 WORD CHECK

Explain these expressions in your own words.

e.g. An authority
  An authority is an expert in a specific field.

a 7 obesity
b 13 an option
c 18 a precaution
d 18 limitations
e 18 dialysis
f 23 strategies
g 34 contributors
h 38 a reference

3 VERBS FROM NOUNS

Give the *verbs* from which the following nouns are formed.

e.g. Contributor → to contribute

Noun	Verb
training	
illustration	
adaptions	
compliance	
a quotation	
prescription	
a summary	
options	
reference	
limitations	
a dividend	
requirements	
consultation	
practice	

4 ADJECTIVES

Fill in the blanks with the *adjectives* below as used in the text.

- ✔ special
- ✔ growing
- ✔ valuable
- ✔ scientific
- ✔ respective
- ✔ simple
- ✔ renowned
- ✔ interesting
- ✔ healthy
- ✔ important
- ✔ appropriate
- ✔ sick
- ✔ superb
- ✔ well
- ✔ distinguished

1 Their limitations and .... requirements pose

an .... challenge.

2 You'll find .... chapters by .... contributors.

3 Prescribing an exercise program for your .... patients may not be a .... task, yet there is a wealth of information available to provide the guidelines you need to design an .... plan.

4 Each chapter of this .... text is written by a .... authority in their .... fields.

5 Order today and get the facts you need to employ these .... principles in your practice.

6 We doctors can now state from our experience with people, both .... and .... , and from a .... series of .... researches that "keeping fit" does pay richly in dividends of health and longevity.

5 PREPOSITIONS

Fill in the blanks with *prepositions* as used in the text.

1 Prescribing an exercise program .... your healthy patients may not be a simple task, yet there is a wealth .... information available to provide the guidelines you need to design an appropriate plan.

2 But what .... your patients .... special needs?

3 The text includes unique chapters .... non-ischemic heart disease, chronic dialysis and exercise physiology.

4 The final chapter outlines practical and effective strategies .... enhancing patient compliance .... the exercise program you've developed .... them.

5 Figures, tables and illustrations summarize principles .... a glance.

6 Each chapter .... this superb text is written .... a renowned authority .... their respective fields.

7 Guide your patients .... an exercise plan that is safe and effective .... this one- .... -a-kind reference.

8 Order today and get the facts you need to employ these valuable principles .... your practice.

9 We doctors can now state .... our experience .... people, both sick and well, and .... a growing series .... scientific researches that "keeping fit" does pay richly .... dividends .... health and longevity.

10 Ordering is as easy as picking .... your phone.

EXTENSION EXERCISES

6 OPPOSITES

Give the *opposite* of the following words by adding the prefix *UN or IN*.

- ✔ healthy
- ✔ structured
- ✔ appropriate
- ✔ effective
- ✔ frequent
- ✔ soluble
- ✔ interesting
- ✔ distinguished
- ✔ expensive
- ✔ direct
- ✔ suited
- ✔ scientific
- ✔ accurate
- ✔ active

7 ADJECTIVES

Give *adjectives* related to the nouns below.

e.g.　　　health → healthy

- ✔ wealth
- ✔ response
- ✔ protection
- ✔ provocation
- ✔ obesity
- ✔ effect
- ✔ danger
- ✔ selection
- ✔ tragedy
- ✔ defect

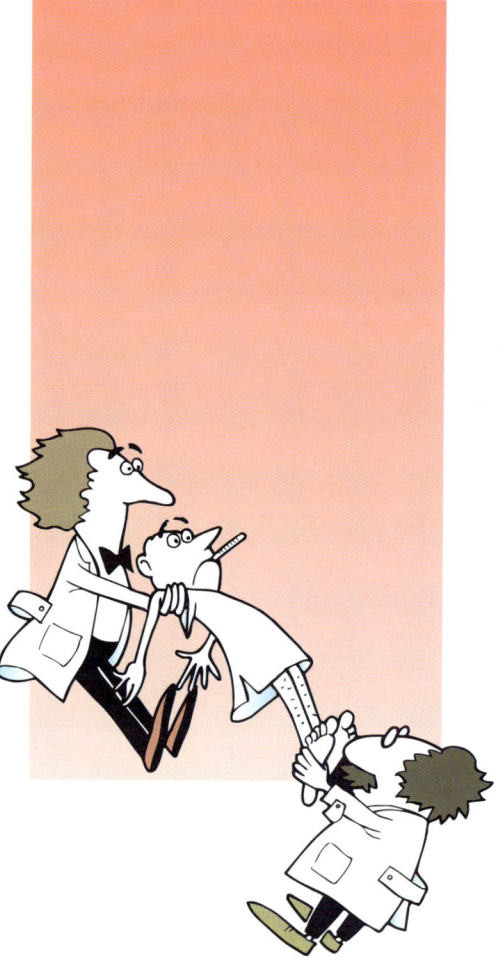

8 DO/DOES/DID IN AFFIRMATIVE SENTENCES

Study the following sentence.

43 Keeping fit *does pay* richly in dividends of health and longevity.

The auxiliaries DO, DOES, DID can be used in affirmative sentences for emphasis. They are usually used when another speaker has already expressed *doubt* about the situation being discussed.

Reply to the following sentences. Use DO, DOES, DID in the answer in affirmative sentences. DO, DOES, DID should be *emphasized* when speaking.

e.g. You didn't go.
　　　I *did* go.

1　It doesn't tell you how to choose a programme to benefit these patients.
2　The text doesn't include a chapter on non-ischemic heart disease.
3　The final chapter didn't outline practical and effective strategies for enhancing patient compliance.
4　The figures, tables and illustrations don't summarize principles at a glance.
5　A wheelchair-confined patient doesn't need an exercise programme.
6　You don't need to design an appropriate plan.
7　Their special limitations didn't pose an interesting challenge.
8　Don't order today.

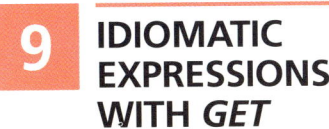

IDIOMATIC EXPRESSIONS WITH *GET*

Study the idiomatic expressions with the verb *TO GET* in column 1. Try to join them to their corresponding meaning in column 2.

Column 1	Column 2
1 to get going	a to achieve little
2 to get the idea	b to become tense
3 to get uptight	c to become too self-important
4 to get the sack	d to start to move
5 to get nowhere	e to achieve one's aim
6 to get there	f to understand what someone has explained
7 to get too big for one's boots	g to get revenge for something done to one's disadvantage
8 to get even	h to be dismissed from one's job

Notes

CONDITIONALS – TYPE 1

There are three main types of conditional sentences in English.

TYPE 1 - The meaning is future. The result *PROBABLE*.

a *Basic construction.*
IF + PRESENT TENSE + FUTURE

N.B. The verb in the IF clause is in the Present Tense

e.g. *If it rains*, you'll get wet.

b The above sentence can also be expressed as follows.
FUTURE + IF + PRESENT TENSE
You'll get wet if it rains.

GRAMMAR POINT

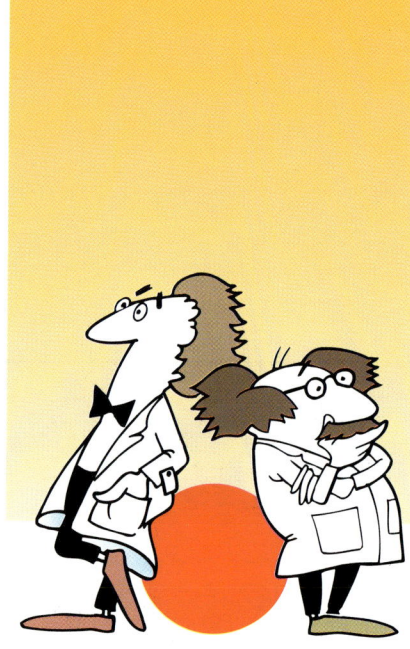

c *LEARN BY HEART*

ONLY ONE FUTURE PER SENTENCE.

(WRONG: You'll get wet if it'll rain).

10 GRAMMAR CHECK

Complete the following sentences.

1 If he goes to hospital...
2 He'll be ill if...
3 If you're late for work...
4 She won't undergo an operation if...
5 The doctor will see him if...
6 What will happen if...?
7 If they need help...
8 If you don't mind waiting...
9 You'll feel much better if...
10 If he doesn't come soon …

Notes

WRITING

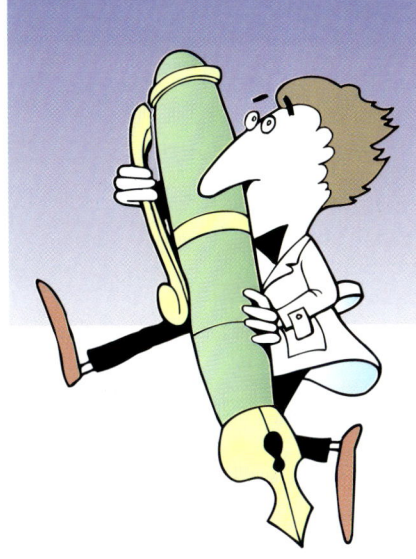

11 WHAT SPECIFIC PATIENTS CAN AND *CAN'T* DO

Say what the following groups of patients *can* and *cannot* do in an exercise programme.

CARDIAC PATIENTS

can

can't

EXTREMELY OBESE PATIENTS

can

can'

WHEELCHAIR - DEPENDENT INDIVIDUALS

can

can't

PREGNANT PATIENTS

can

can't

THE ELDERLY

can

can't

12 WRITING AN APPLICATION

You have just read the advertisement for a team physician for the California State University. Write a short letter of application.

TEAM PHYSICIAN

Part-time. Provides primary diagnosis and treatment for CSUN athletes and to all students in sports medicine. Valid California license; current board certification or eligibility in family practice and completion of Sports Medicine fellowship preferred. Completion of residency program. Salary: $3176.50-3844.50/mo. Position open until filled.

Submit letter of application and resume to the:

Personnel Department
California State University, Northridge
18111 Nordhoff Street
Admin 515-4
Northridge, CA 91330

Notes

Read the following passage.

GUIDELINES FOR EXERCISE TRAINING AFTER CARDIAC TRANSPLANTATION

Cardiac transplantation began at the Mayo Clinic in 1981, and at present an active program continues with transplant surgeon Dr. Christopher G. A. McGregor and a team of cardiologists, anesthesiologists, infectious disease specialists, nephrologists, nurse clinicians, physical medicine specialists, and social workers. The exercise portion of rehabilitation includes the services of physical and occupational therapists, cardiac rehabilitation nurses, exercise physiologists, and exercise specialists.

Our current clinical practice includes graded exercise testing with full electrocardiographic, expired air, and blood pressure monitoring as part of the pre-transplant evaluation for patients who are able to exercise. Based upon the test results, a medically supervised low-level exercise training program of treadmill walking and cycle ergometry is initiated for the purposes of preparing the patient for the post-transplant exercise regimen and maintenance of fitness prior to surgery. Patients may exercise in a supervised cardiac rehabilitation setting or at home, depending upon their clinical status.

After surgery, mobilization from bed and initiation of low-level range of motion exercises begin once the patient is extubated. Inpatient physical rehabilitation after cardiac transplantation has been detailed previously (35a). The occurrence of an episode of moderate to severe acute rejections results in a reduction or elimination of physical activity (other than passive range of motion) until the rejection has resolved. Cycle ergometry in the patient's room is performed while the patient remains in reverse isolation to reduce the risk of infection. When out of isolation, the exercise program continues with walking, cycling, and mild muscle strengthening activities. As outpatients, transplant recipients continue exercise at the cardiac rehabilitation facility at the medical center. Full graded exercise with expired air analysis testing is performed 1-2 months after surgery.

35a. SQUIRES R. W. Cardiac rehabilitation issues for heart transplantation patients. J. Cardiopulmonary Rehabil. 10:159-168, 1990.

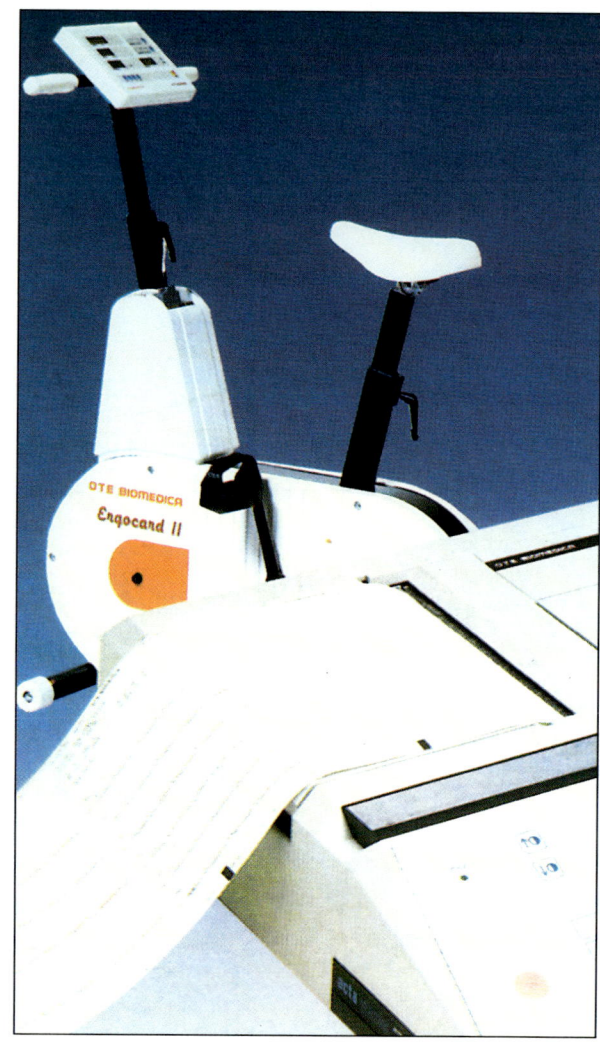

VOCABULARY

10 to grade
- to arrange according to difficulty

18 prior
- before

23 to extubate
- to remove tubes

13 EXERCISE AFTER CARDIAC TRANS-PLANTATION

Explain, in your own words, some of the guidelines for exercise training after cardiac transplantation that you have just read. The words below will help you.

- cardiac transplantation - Mayo Clinic 1981
- active program - transplant surgeon - Dr. McGregor
- cardiologists, anesthesiologists, infectious disease specialists, nephrologists, nurse clinicians, physical medicine specialists and social workers
- exercise portion - physical and occupational therapists, cardiac

SPEAKING

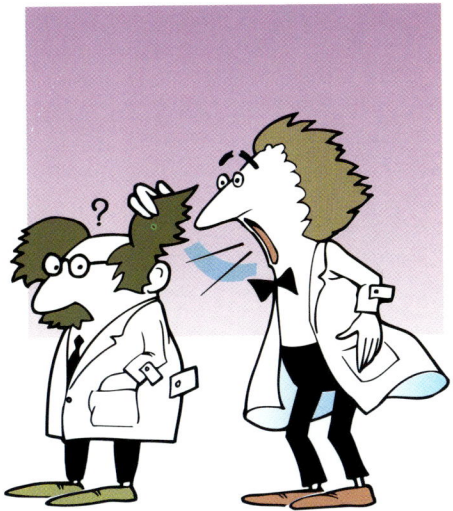

rehabilitation nurses, exercise physiologists and exercise specialists
- graded exercise testing - electrocardiographic, expired air and blood pressure

monitoring - pre-transplant evaluation
- low-level exercise program - treadmill - walking - cycle ergometry - preparing the patient for the post-transplant exercise regimen
- after surgery - low-level range of motion exercises - extubated
- moderate to severe acute rejections - reduction or elimination of physical activity
- cycle ergometry - patient's room - reverse isolation - reduce the risk of infection
- out of isolation - walking, cycling and mild muscle strengthening activities
- outpatients - transplant recipients - exercise - cardiac rehabilitation facility
- full graded exercise - expired air analysis - 1-2 months after surgery

UNDERSTANDING IDIOMATIC ENGLISH

Explain the idiom.

On the morning of the examination he got cold feet

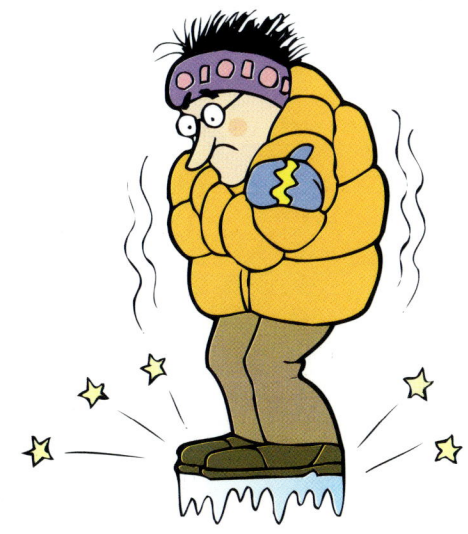

UNIT 17

The factors causing diabetes

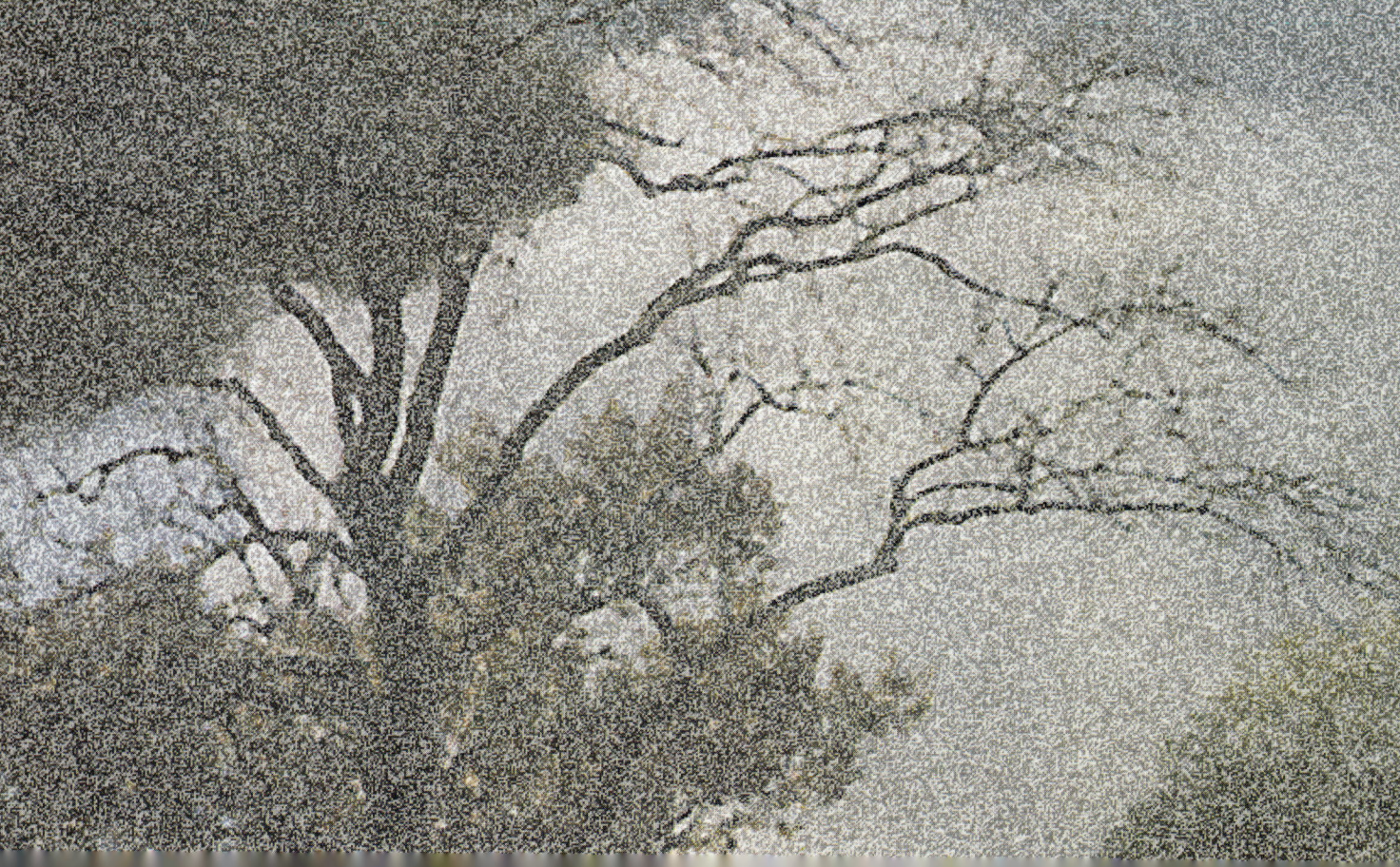

What Causes Diabetes?

For insulin-dependent diabetes, the answer is an autoimmune ambush of the body's insulin-producing cells. Why the attack begins and persists is now becoming clear

by Mark A. Atkinson and Noel K. Maclaren

People stricken with what is today called insulin-dependent, or type I, diabetes once faced certain death within about a year of diagnosis. They died because the pancreas lost its ability to make insulin, which is required for normal metabolism. Isolation of the hormone from animals in 1921 made treatment possible and has since meant survival for millions of diabetics.

Yet neither animal insulin nor the more modern, human, form offers a cure. Injections must be taken once or more a day for life. Moreover, many diabetics eventually suffer from devastating complications. As the disease persists, blood vessels can be damaged, leading to heart disease, stroke, blindness or kidney failure. Nerve damage is also common.

Improved techniques for delivering insulin might slow the development of complications, but the ideal solution is to prevent diabetes itself. To do that, however, investigators must uncover the root causes. Recently, research into that problem has advanced with remarkable speed. It is now clear that insulin-dependent diabetes stems from an autoimmune, or self-directed, attack on the pancreas. Dozens of laboratories in the U.S. and abroad—including our own at the University of Florida—are currently attempting to clarify the details of that process. We are trying to determine which components of the immune system are the major agents of attack, what triggers the autoimmune reaction and what allows it to persist.

On the basis of such work, physicians should soon be able to identify the one person in 300 who will acquire insulin-dependent diabetes, so that treatment can be initiated at the very first sign of disease. By the turn of the next century, it should also be possible to offer such individuals safe preventive therapy.

The autoimmune process that causes insulin-dependent diabetes is highly selective and frequently begins before adulthood (which is why the disease was formerly called juvenile-onset diabetes). The attack does not affect the majority of pancreatic cells, which secrete digestive enzymes. Instead it restricts itself to the hormone-producing cells. These are clustered in spherical groupings—the islets of Langerhans—scattered throughout the pancreas. Even in the islets, three out of the four cell types are spared; only the insulin-producing beta cells, which make up the large core of an islet, are targeted.

Insulin helps most cells of the body take up biological fuels, including the sugar glucose. As the beta cells are killed and the pancreas stops producing this crucial hormone, glucose accumulates in the blood, giving rise to the abnormally high glucose levels that are a hallmark of diabetes. Then the body becomes dehydrated as the kidneys overwork to filter the excess glucose into the urine. Meanwhile body cells starve in a sea of plenty, and so they uncontrollably break down their stores of fat and protein to provide more fuel.

If the breakdown of fat continues unchecked, acidic by-products called ketones build up. These, combined with dehydration, can induce coma and, finally, death.

Insulin injections can halt this lethal sequence and prevent it from recurring, but they cannot mimic the normal pattern of insulin release by the pancreas. Nor can they normalize metabolic functioning well enough to prevent the long-term complications of diabetes. These are generally believed to be caused or exacerbated by chronically elevated blood glucose levels.

MARK A. ATKINSON and NOEL K. MACLAREN are, respectively, assistant professor and professor in the department of pathology and laboratory medicine at the University of Florida College of Medicine in Gainesville. Atkinson received a B.S. from the University of Michigan and a Ph.D. in pathology from the University of Florida. He is currently focusing his attention on the pancreatic proteins involved in the development of insulin-dependent diabetes. Maclaren, who chairs his department, received much of his training in New Zealand, earning an M.D. at the University of Otago Medical School in 1963 and then specializing in internal medicine at Wellington Hospital. He also received training in pediatric endocrinology at Johns Hopkins University before moving to Florida in 1978 to pursue research into the genetics and pathogenesis of autoimmune endocrine diseases.

ISLETS OF LANGERHANS house the hormone-producing cells of the pancreas and include the beta cells, which make insulin. This islet was made visible in a slice of a normal pancreas by fluorescently labeled antibodies that bind to a component of the islet-cell cytoplasm. The antibodies came from the blood of an insulin-dependent diabetic, and their recognition of a healthy islet indicates that an autoimmune attack of normal tissue contributes to diabetes. The disease emerges after most of the pancreatic beta cells are destroyed.

TEXT BASED EXERCISES

VOCABULARY

Study the meaning of the following words and expressions as used in the text.

1 stricken
- afflicted
10 survival
- act of surviving; being alive after and in spite of a danger
16 devastating
- that destroys or damages greatly
27 root
- basic
29 speed
- rapidity
30 to stem from
- to originate from
36 to clarify
- to make clear; to make more easily understandable
46 to initiate
- to begin
47 a sign
- an indication
47 by the turn of
- at the beginning
54 adulthood
- adult life
55 onset
- beginning
60 to cluster
- a number of things grouped together or growing together
60 spherical
- shaped like a sphere
61 an islet
- a small island
62 to scatter
- to disperse

64 to spare
- not to kill
65 to make up
- to form
66 a core
- central part
66 to target
- to direct a weapon or blow towards an object to be hit
68 a fuel
- any substance used to produce heat by burning it

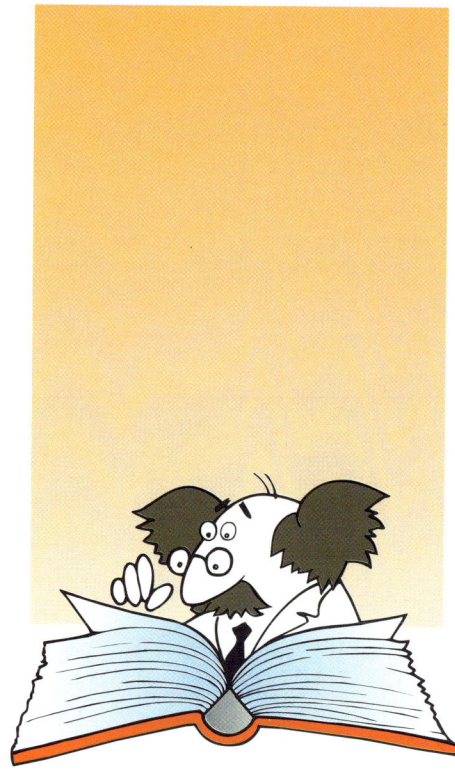

72 to give rise to
- to cause
74 a hallmark (fig.)
- a mark of genuineness
78 to starve
- to die of hunger
78 plenty
- abundance
79 a store
- provisions kept for future need
86 to halt
- to stop
94 to exacerbate
- to make worse
96 to house
- to provide a house or shelter for
100 a slice
- a thin, broad piece
101 to bind
- to fix

1 COMPREHENSION

Answer the following questions.

1 What was once the destiny of sufferers of type I diabetes?
2 What effect has the improved techniques for delivering insulin had on these patients?
3 What must investigators first find in order to be able to prevent diabetes?
4 What does insulin-dependent diabetes stem from?
5 In what way is the University of Florida attempting to clarify

the details of what causes diabetes?

6 What will be the benefit of being able to identify those who will acquire insulin-dependent diabetes?

7 When do the researchers estimate that preventive therapy will be available?

8 What type of cells are attacked in cases of insulin-dependent diabetes?

9 Are all types of cells in the islets of Langerhans attacked?

10 What causes the high glucose levels in the blood that indicate the presence of diabetes?

11 What are insulin injections not able to do?

a the insulin-producing ....
b a self-directed ....
c the hormone-producing ....
d insulin-dependent ....
e acidic ....
f the long-term ....
g preventive ....
h biological ....
i this crucial ....
j this lethal ....

2 NOUNS

Fill in the blanks with *the nouns* below as used in the text.

✔ diabetes
✔ complications
✔ fuels
✔ therapy
✔ sequence
✔ cells
✔ beta cells
✔ by-products
✔ attack
✔ hormone

3 ADJECTIVES

Fill in the blanks with *the adjectives* below as used in the text.

✔ remarkable
✔ digestive
✔ normal
✔ spherical
✔ devastating
✔ metabolic
✔ ideal
✔ major

a .... complications
b the .... solution
c with .... speed
d .... functioning
e .... enzymes
f the .... pattern
g in .... groupings
h the .... agents

4 ADVERBS

Fill in the blanks with *the adverbs* below as used in the text.

✔ chronically
✔ generally
✔ abnormally
✔ recently
✔ highly
✔ currently
✔ uncontrollably
✔ frequently

a The autoimmune process that causes insulin-dependent diabetes is .... selective and .... begins before adulthood.

b .... , research into that problem has advanced with remarkable speed.

c Dozens of laboratories in the U.S. and abroad are .... attempting to clarify the details of that process.

d The long-term complications of diabetes are .... believed to be caused or exacerbated by .... elevated blood glucose levels.

e As the beta cells are killed and the pancreas stops producing this crucial hormone, glucose accumulates in the blood, giving rise to the ....

high glucose levels that are a hallmark of diabetes.

f Meanwhile body cells starve in a sea of plenty, and so they .... break down their stores of fat and protein to provide more fuel.

5

Fill in the blanks with the words below as used in the text.

- ✓ diagnosis
- ✓ insulin
- ✓ heart
- ✓ causes
- ✓ type 1
- ✓ dehydration
- ✓ breakdown
- ✓ disease
- ✓ metabolism
- ✓ pancreas
- ✓ stroke
- ✓ ability
- ✓ attack
- ✓ death
- ✓ glucose
- ✓ failure
- ✓ ketones
- ✓ fat
- ✓ coma
- ✓ vessels

a People stricken with what is today called insulin-dependent or (1) .... diabetes, once faced certain (2) .... within about a year of (3) .... They died because the (4) .... lost its (5) .... to make (6) .... , which is required for normal (7) ....

b Investigators must uncover the root (8) ....

c If the (9) .... of (10) .... continues unchecked, acidic by-products called (11) .... build up. These combined with (12) .... can induce (13) .... and, finally, death.

d As the (14) .... persists, blood (15) .... can be damaged, leading to (16) .... disease (17) .... , blindness or kidney (18) ....

e Insulin helps most cells of the body take up biological fuels, including the sugar (19) ....

f The (20) .... does not affect the majority of pancreatic cells, which secrete digestive enzymes.

6 PREPOSITIONS

Fill in the blanks with *prepositions* as used in the text.

1 If the breakdown .... fat continues unchecked, acidic by-products called ketones build ....

2 The hormone-producing cells are clustered .... spherical groupings, the islets .... Langerhans, scattered .... the pancreas.

3 Only the insulin producing beta cells, which make .... the large core .... an islet are targeted.

4 It is now clear that insulin-dependent diabetes stems .... an autoimmune or self-directed attack .... the pancreas.

5 Dozens .... laboratories .... the U.S. and abroad, including our own .... the University .... Florida, are currently attempting to clarify the details .... that process.

6 .... the turn .... the next century, it should be possible to offer such individuals safe preventive therapy.

7 Meanwhile body cells starve .... a sea .... plenty, and so they uncontrollably break .... their stores .... fat and protein to provide more fuel.

8 Improved techniques .... delivering insulin might slow the development .... complications, but the ideal solution is to prevent diabetes itself.

EXTENSION EXERCISES

7

Add *should* to the following sentences and give the opposite of the words *in italics*. Make any other necessary changes in the sentence. As in the use of DO, DOES, DID in the affirmative (see Unit 16), should is *emphasized* when spoken.

e.g. It is *impossible* to offer such individuals safe preventive therapy.
It *should be possible* to offer such individuals safe preventive therapy.

a The new operation was *unsuccessful*.
b Discomfort is *common*.
c Investigators are working on *few* projects.
d It is a *time-consuming task*.
e The technique is very *complicated*.
f Severe flexion contracture of the hips was corrected by *partial* hip replacement.
g Establishing guidelines is *tricky*.
h The treatment is very *expensive*.

8

Read the following imperative sentences. Make sentences beginning with the words *my*

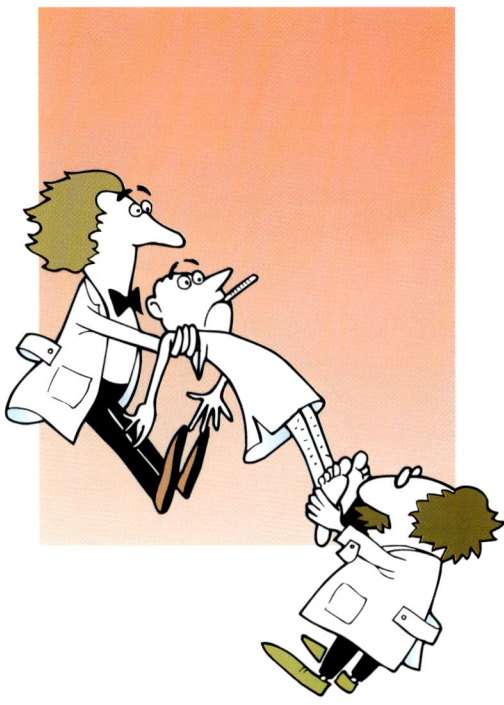

doctor as in the example. Use the verbs *recommended*, *suggested* or *insisted* and *should*.

e.g. Stop smoking.

My doctor *recommended* that I *should* stop smoking.

1 Change your diet.
2 Work less.
3 Take a holiday.
4 Walk more.
5 Drink less coffee.
6 Relax more.
7 Take up a sport.
8 Worry less.
9 Go to bed earlier.
10 Come for a check-up more often.

9 REFLEXIVE PRONOUNS

Fill in the blanks with a suitable *reflexive pronoun*.

e.g. The ideal solution is to prevent diabetes ....
The ideal solution is to prevent diabetes *itself*.

a As Watson .... concedes, establishing guidelines for sequencing data may be trickier.
b Dr. Blackburn has identified a key enzyme that is necessary for chromosomes to make copies of .... before cell division.
c During cell division, the DNA arranges .... into 23 pairs of complementary chromosomes.
d I try to keep .... fit by walking for an hour each day.
e Jane was tired of waiting for her husband to put up a shelf, so she decided to do it ....
f Thank you for a lovely evening. We really enjoyed ....
g You'll hurt .... if you aren't careful.
h Let's all sit down to eat. Would you like to help .... ?

10 PHRASAL VERBS WITH LOOK

Study the phrasal verbs with *TO LOOK* in column 1. Try to join them to their corresponding meaning in column 2.

Column 1	Column 2
a to look after	1 to admire; to regard with respect
b to look back (1)	2 to search; to try to find
c to look back (2)	3 to find in a book (e.g. a word, a telephone number)
d to look for	4 to consider the future
e to look forward to	5 to investigate
f to look in	6 to take care of
g to look up	7 to consider the past
h to look up to	8 to expect with pleasure
i to look ahead	9 to pay a short visit
j to look into	10 to look behind

Notes

CONDITIONALS - TYPE 2

TYPE 2

a The meaning is present or future.
The result is *possible but improbable*.

> e.g. If I had time, I'd go out this evening.

b *Construction*
IF + SIMPLE PAST + SIMPLE CONDITIONAL

> e.g. *If you studied* hard, *you'd pass* your Biology exam.

c N.B. *You'd* is the contracted form of *you would*.
Note the final letter 'd. Do not confuse this with the contracted future auxiliary will.

d *IF* is followed by a verb in the Simple Past.

> e.g. If *I went* to London, I'd visit my English friends.
>
> I'd buy a new car if *I had* enough money.

11 GRAMMAR CHECK

Complete the following sentences *in your own words*.

1   If I had more time
....

GRAMMAR POINT

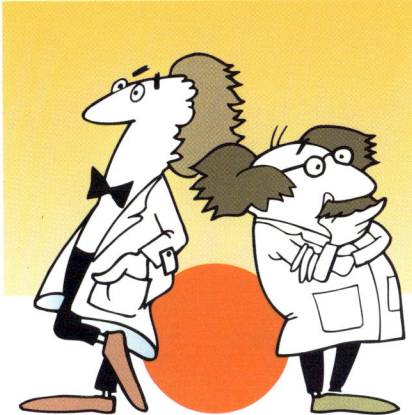

2 What would you do if
.... ?
3 If we had fewer patients in the ward ....
4 If he went to see his doctor
....
5 They'd be happy to help us if
.... ?
6 Would you attend the conference if .... ?
7 Mr. Blake would sleep better if
....
8 We'd all live longer if
....
9 He wouldn't come even if
....
10 If you took the medicine
....

12 GRAMMAR CHECK

Give advice. Reply to the following sentences using the construction "*If I were*" as in the example.

A I'm not going to the meeting.
B *If I were you, I'd go.*

1 I've been offered the job but I'm not going to accept it.
2 He isn't going to tell them what happened.
3 Jack doesn't want to take his injections.
4 They aren't going to improve the technique.
5 I'm not going to try the test.
6 She won't clarify the details.
7 They don't want to ask for help.
8 She isn't going to read the report.
9 He doesn't want to start the treatment.
10 They aren't going to reveal their findings.

Notes

WRITING

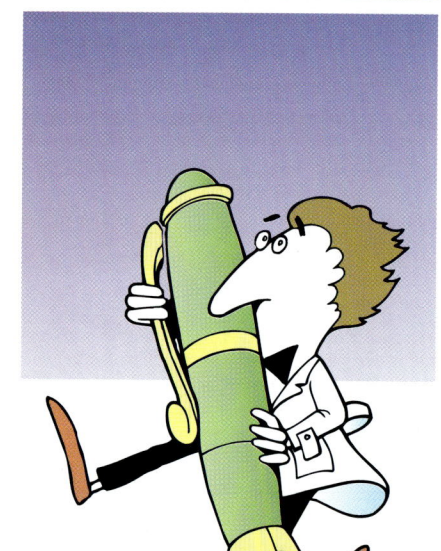

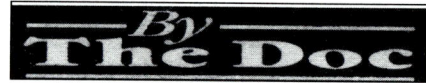

13 "THE DOCTOR ANSWERS"

Your local newspaper has invited you to write for their weekly column "The Doctor Answers". Write short replies to the following questions sent in by some of the readers.

1 What are the symptoms of Diabetes?
2 Is it true there is no known cure for type I diabetes?

3 I am a 55 year old male. I run three times a week for an hour each time and I take part in half marathons two or three times a year. I have just been told that I have insulin-dependent diabetes. Should I modify my life-style?

Notes

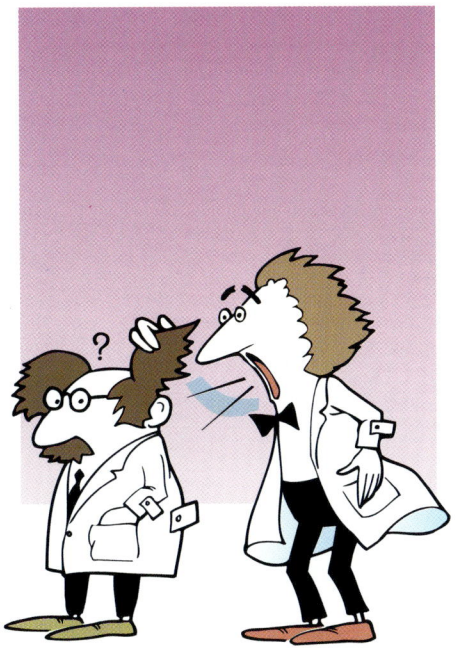

SPEAKING

14 PREVENTIVE THERAPY

Describe, in your own words, the possibility of offering preventive therapy for insulin-dependent diabetes. The words below will help you.

- improved techniques - slow development of complications
- ideal solution - prevent diabetes itself
- investigators must uncover the root causes
- research - advanced - remarkable speed
- insulin-dependent diabetes -

autoimmune attack - pancreas
- dozens of laboratories - currently attempting - details of that process
- determine - components of the immune system - major agents of attack - triggers the autoimmune reaction - what allows it to persist
- basis of such work - soon able to identify - one person in 300 - acquire insulin-dependent diabetes
- treatment - initiated - first sign of the disease
- by the turn of the next century - should be possible - such individuals - safe preventive therapy

UNDERSTANDING IDIOMATIC ENGLISH

Explain the idiom.

He has a sweet tooth

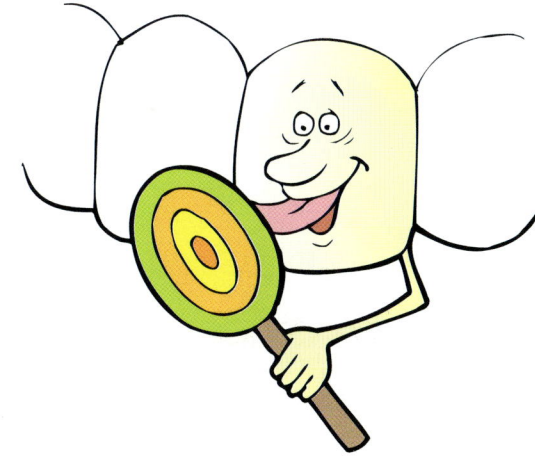

UNIT 18

Immunology: a rapidly progressing field

Stop That Germ!

Rapid-fire discoveries are revealing how the body's immune system endlessly fights off disease—and occasionally goes awry

It's a jungle out there, teeming with hordes of unseen enemies. Bacteria, viruses, fungi and parasites fill the air. They cluster on every surface, from the restaurant table to the living-room sofa. They abound in lakes and in pools, flourish in the soil and disport themselves among the flora and fauna. This menagerie of microscopic organisms, most of them potentially harmful or even lethal, has a favorite target: the human body. In fact, the tantalizing human prey is a walking repository of just the kind of stuff the tiny predators need to survive, thrive and reproduce.

Humans are under constant siege by these voracious adversaries. Germs of every description strive tirelessly to invade the comfortably warm and bountiful body, entering through the skin or by way of the eyes, nose, ears and mouth. Fortunately for man's survival, most of them fail in their assault. They are repelled by the tough barrier of the skin, overcome by the natural pesticides in sweat, saliva and tears, dissolved by stomach acids or trapped in the sticky mucus of the nose or throat before being expelled by a sneeze or a cough. But the organisms are extraordinarily persistent, and some occasionally breach the outer defenses. After entering the bloodstream and tissues, they multiply at an alarming rate and begin destroying vital body cells.

The invaders soon receive a rude shock, for they encounter one of nature's most incredible and complex creations: the human immune system. Inside the body, a trillion highly specialized cells, regulated by dozens of remarkable proteins and honed by hundreds of millions of years of evolution, launch an unending battle against the alien organisms. It is high-pitched biological warfare, orchestrated with such skill and precision that illness in the average human being is relatively rare.

Early-warning cells constantly monitor the bloodstream and tissues for signs of the enemy. With the gusto of Pac-Man, they gobble up anything that is foreign to

the body. They envelop dust particles, pollutants, microorganisms and even the debris of battle: remnants of invaders and infected or damaged body cells. Other early warners direct the production of unique killer cells, each designed to attack and destroy a particular type of intruder. Some of the killers, alerted to body cells

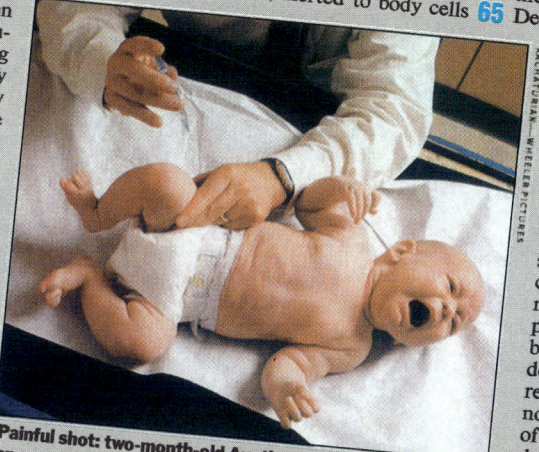

Painful shot: two-month-old Austin Reed is inoculated with an experimental vaccine against meningitis.

that have become cancerous, may annihilate these too.

Endowed with such specialized weapons, the properly functioning immune system is a formidable barrier to disease. Even when an infection is severe enough to overcome the system's initial response and cause illness, the immune cells are usually able to regroup, call up reinforcements and eventually rout the invaders. But when the system is weakened by previous illness or advancing age, for example, the body becomes more vulnerable to cancers and a host of infectious diseases. And should the system overreact or go awry, it can cause troublesome allergies and serious disorders called autoimmune diseases.

As they probe the intricate workings of the immune system, scientists are awestruck. "It is an enormous edifice, like a cathedral," says Nobel Laureate Baruj Benacerraf, president of Boston's Dana-Farber Cancer Institute. The immune system is compared favorably with the

most complex organ of them all, the brain. "The immune system has a phenomenal ability for dealing with information, for learning and memory, for creating and storing and using information," explains Immunologist William Paul of the National Institutes of Health (NIH). Declares Dr. Stephen Sherwin, director of clinical research at Genentech: "It's an incredible system. It recognizes molecules that have never been in the body before. It can differentiate between what belongs there and what doesn't."

Knowledge about the inner workings of the immune system has undergone an astonishing explosion in the past five years. Although researchers began to pry loose its secrets in the late 19th century, it was not until after World War II that the pace of discovery began to quicken, boosted by such achievements as the deciphering of the genetic code and recombinant DNA technology. But no early advances can match those of recent years, which have enabled doctors to devise ingenious new treatments for a host of disorders. Says Immunologist John Kappler, of the National Jewish Center for Immunology and Respiratory Medicine in Denver: "The field is progressing so rapidly that the journals are out of date by the time they are published."

Kappler is not exaggerating. In the past few months alone, dozens of new immune discoveries and promising therapies have been reported. Researchers announced in March that by activating certain immune cells, they had increased by 20% the five-year survival rate of patients in the early stages of lung cancer. In the same month, European scientists reported eliminating the need for insulin shots in some diabetic children by administering a drug that suppresses the immune system. Researchers in Colombia have tested a malaria vaccine that, unlike previous efforts, seems to provide protection against the disease. Advances have come so fast, says Dana-Farber's Benacerraf, that "we're now on the threshold of being able to activate the different components of the immune system at will to provide

KACHATURIAN—WHEELER PICTURES

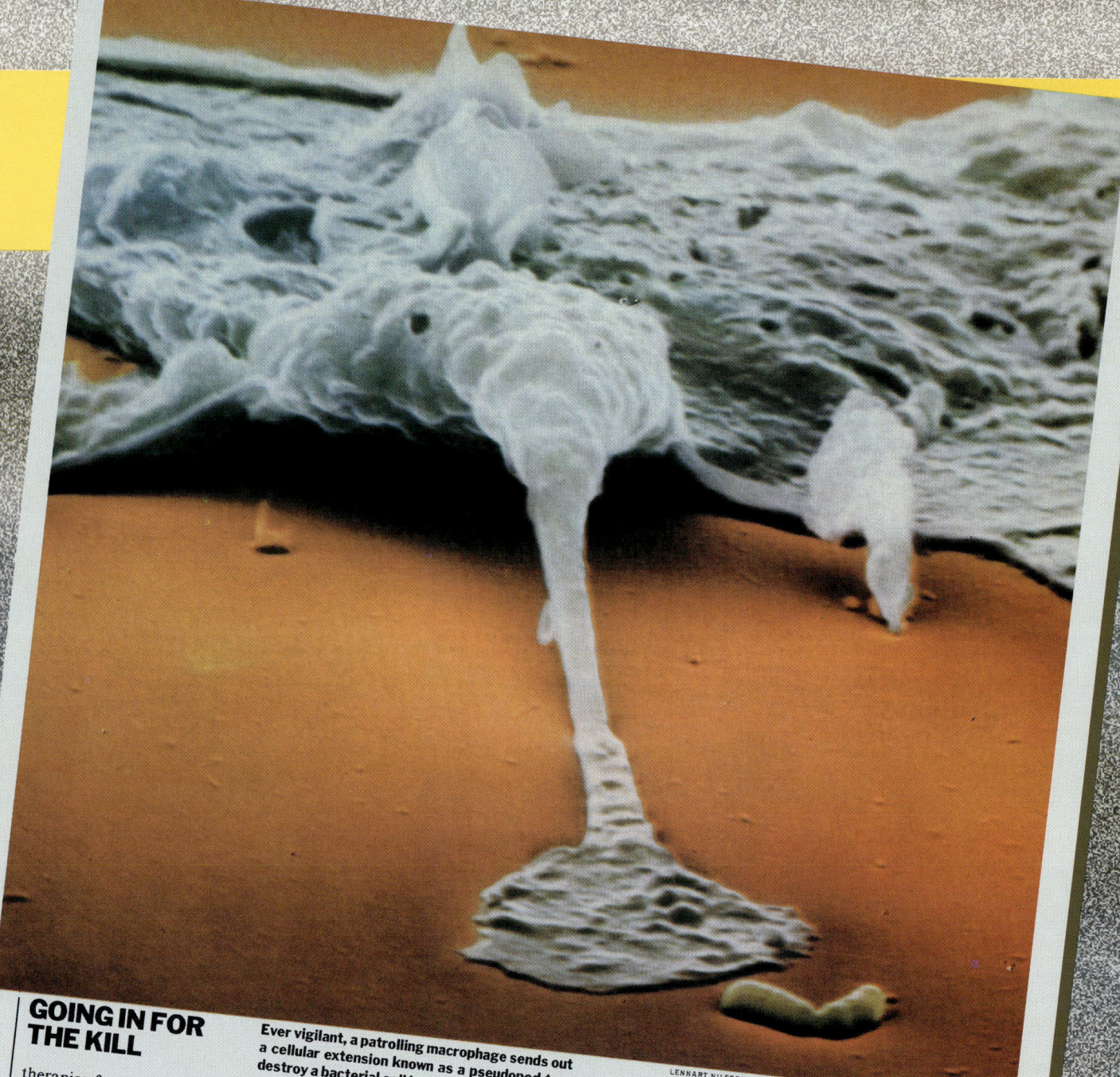

GOING IN FOR
THE KILL

Ever vigilant, a patrolling macrophage sends out a cellular extension known as a pseudopod to engulf and destroy a bacterial cell before alerting more defenders.

LENNART NILSSON—©BOEHRINGER INGELHEIM INTERNATIONAL GMBH

therapies for cancer and even for AIDS."

In fact, it is the AIDS epidemic that has spurred much of the recent interest in immunology. The AIDS virus strikes a key component of the immune system, destroys it, and in so doing virtually knocks out the entire system. Nothing illustrates the importance of a healthy immune system more dramatically than the disastrous consequences of its loss. AIDS sufferers become vulnerable to many kinds of invading organisms. Fungal growths corrode the skin and lungs. Normally dormant parasites in the lungs become active, causing *Pneumocystis carinii* pneumonia. As viruses and bacteria multiply out of control, competing for body cells and destroying them far faster than they can be replaced, victims can be stricken with severe cases of herpes and tuberculosis. What is more, they lose their resistance to some types of cancer, particularly Kaposi's sarcoma.

Tragic as it is, says Dr. Anthony Fauci, the AIDS research coordinator for the National Institutes of Health, the AIDS epidemic has provided important new insights into the immune system.

"AIDS is the perfect disease for studying the immune system," he explains. "The virus destroys one of the major cells of the system. So now nature is doing the experiment. It has just pulled out a major chip, and we're watching everything else go haywire." On the other hand, AIDS Expert Robert Gallo of the National Cancer Institute believes that much of the progress in AIDS research would have been impossible without discoveries about the immune system made shortly before the epidemic bloomed. "If AIDS had come along in the 1970s," he says, "we'd still be looking under rocks for the cause."

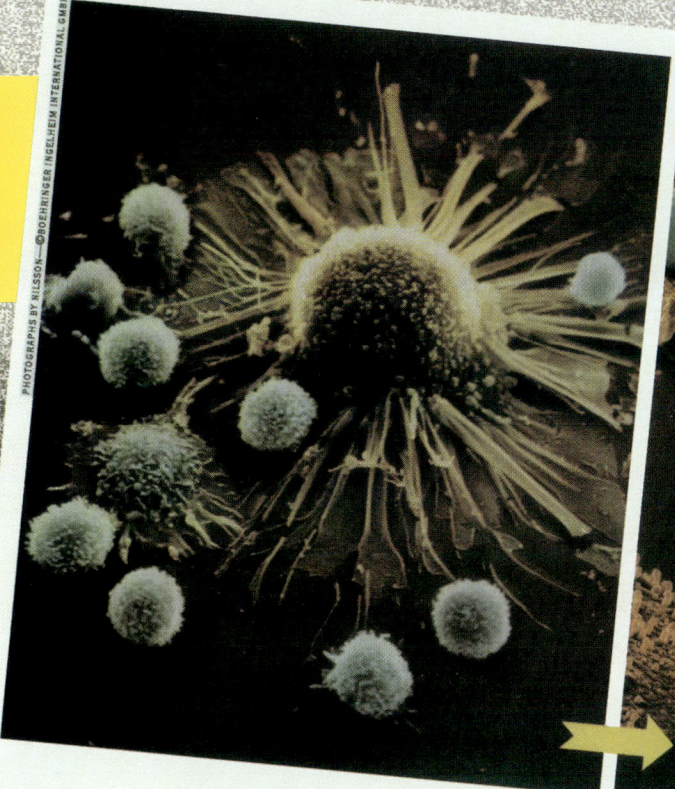

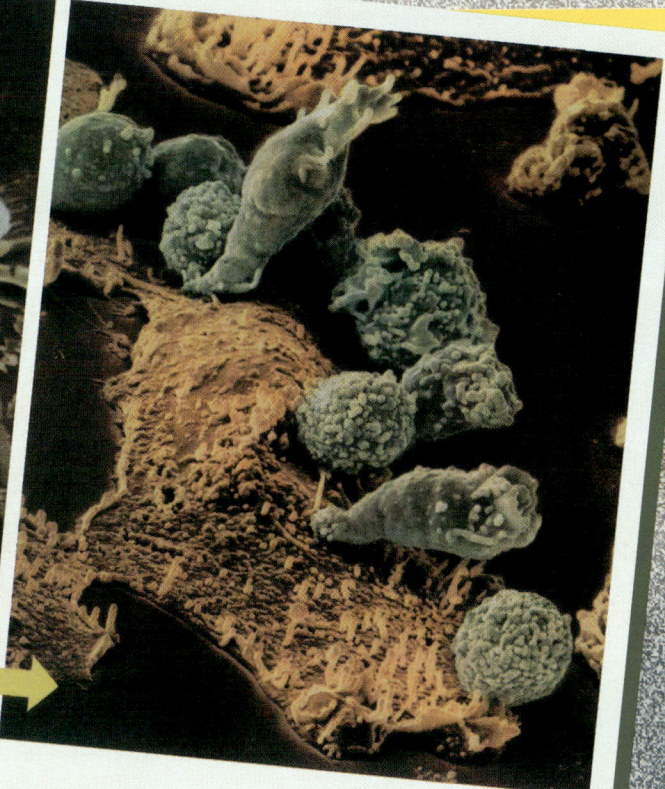

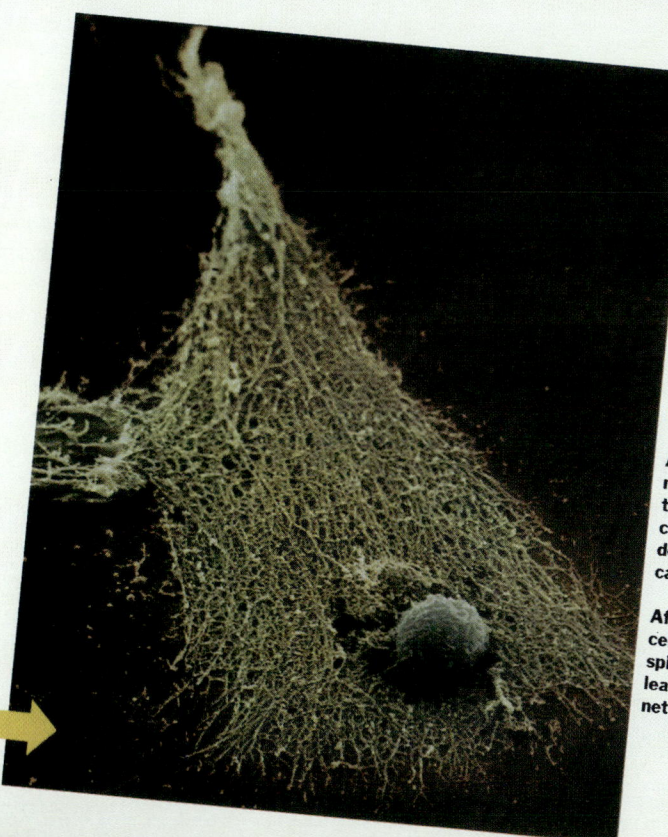

DEATH OF A CANCER CELL

A squad of killer T cells surround a cancerous cell, move in for the kill, and leave behind nothing but its cellular skeleton.

Recognition: the aroused élite troops, attracted to the abnormal cell by its telltale surface antigens, begin to take lethal action.

Attack: the killer cells, normally round, change their shape as they wage chemical warfare to break down the membrane of the cancer cell.

Aftermath: the cancer cell, once it has ruptured, spills its innards and dies, leaving only a collapsed network of fibers behind.

TEXT BASED EXERCISES

VOCABULARY

Study the meaning of the following words and expressions as used in the text.

2 to fight off
- not allow to approach
2 awry
- distorted
3 to teem
- to be full of
4 hordes
- great numbers
8 to abound
- to be existing in great quantities; abundant
9 to flourish
- to thrive; to be active
9 soil
- earth
12 harmful
- causing damage
14 to tantalize
- to torment by presenting some desirable but unattainable object
15 a prey
- an animal hunted for food by another
20 a siege
- a persistent attack
21 to strive
- to try hard
28 tough
- strong; not easily damaged
30 sweat
- perspiration
32 to trap
- to catch in a trap
32 sticky
- adhesive; glutinous

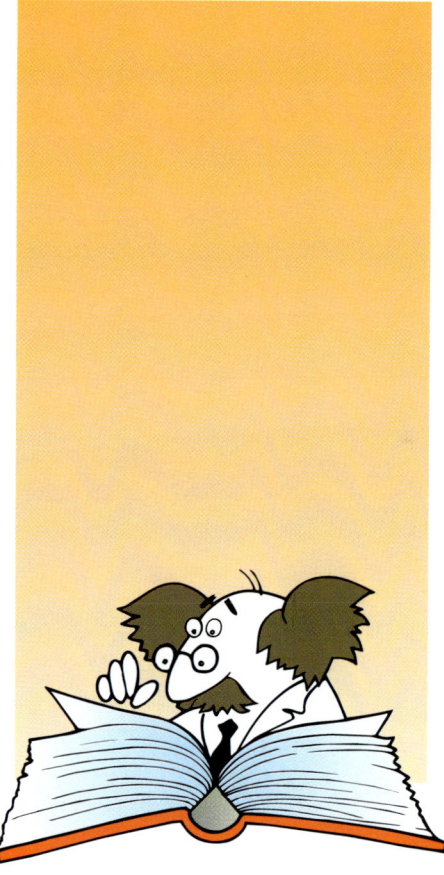

36 to breach
- to break through
41 rude
- violent
42 to encounter
- to be confronted by; to meet
47 to hone
- to intensify
48 to launch
- to initiate

48 unending
- ceaseless; without coming to an end
49 alien
- foreign
51 skill
- practical ability
57 to gobble up
- to eat quickly
68 endowed
- given talents or natural qualities
75 to rout
- to completely defeat
79 a host
- a large number; an army
83 to probe
- to investigate
84 awestruck
- astonished (awe-reverential fear)
108 to pry loose
- to investigate and release
112 to boost
- to help forward (coll.)
115 to match
- to be equal to
117 to devise
- to invent
134 a shot
- (coll.) an injection
142 threshold
- beginning (fig.)
144 at will
- as and when desired
147 to spur
- to incite; to stimulate
157 to corrode
- to gradually destroy
179 haywire (coll.)
- disorganized; crazy
185 to bloom
- to flourish

1 WORD CHECK

Explain the following expressions *in your own words*.

- 3 teeming with hordes of unseen enemies
- 48 launch an unending battle
- 50 high pitched biological warfare
- 62 early warners
- 68 such specialized weapons
- 70 a formidable barrier
- 117 ingenious new treatments for a host of disorders
- 127 promising therapies
- 132 early stages
- 148 a key component

2

Say what the following refer to *in the text*.

- 12 them
- 27 them
- 58 they
- 83 they
- 85 it
- 115 those
- 130 they
- 150 it
- 162 them
- 165 they
- 174 he
- 177 it
- 186 we

3 SYNONYMS

Find *synonyms* from the text for these words and expressions.

- 4 enemies
- 37 the outer defenses
- 54 early-warning cells
- 60 the debris of battle
- 63 killer cells
- 66 to annihilate
- 83 intricate
- 154 AIDS sufferers

4 ADVERBS

Fill in the blanks with the following *adverbs* as used in the text.

- ✓ usually
- ✓ tirelessly
- ✓ occasionally
- ✓ relatively
- ✓ comfortably
- ✓ extraordinarily
- ✓ fortunately
- ✓ eventually
- ✓ potentially

1 This menagerie of microscopic organisms, most of them .... harmful or even lethal, has a favorite target: the human body.

2 .... for man's survival, most of them fail in their assault.

3 But the organisms are .... persistent and some .... breach the outer defenses.

4 It is high-pitched biological warfare, orchestrated with such skill and precision that illness in the average human being is .... rare.

5 Germs of every description strive .... to invade the .... warm and bountiful body, entering through the skin or by way of the eyes, nose, ears and mouth.

6 Even when an infection is severe enough to overcome the system's initial response and cause illness, the immune cells are .... able to regroup, call up reinforcements and .... rout the invaders.

5 MIXED VERBAL FORMS

Put the verbs in brackets into the verbal form used in the text. Look back at the text only to check your answers.

a Knowledge about the inner workings of the immune system (undergo) an astonishing explosion in the past five years.

b No early advances can (match) those of recent years, which have (enable) doctors (devise) ingenious new treatments for a host of disorders.

c Kappler (not exaggerate). In the past few months alone, dozens of new immune discoveries and promising therapies (report). Researchers (announce) in March that by (activate) certain immune cells, they (increase) by 20% the five-year survival rate of patients in the early stages of lung cancer.

d The field (progress) so rapidly that the journals (be) out of date by the time they (publish).

e Robert Gallo of the National Cancer Institute (believe) that much of the progress in the AIDS research (be) impossible without discoveries about the immune system (make) shortly before the epidemic bloomed. "If AIDS (come) along in the 1970's," he says, "we'd still (look) under rocks for the causes."

6 ADJECTIVES

Fill in the blanks with the following *adjectives* as used in the text.

✔ new	✔ alarming
✔ sticky	✔ dormant
✔ tough	✔ troublesome
✔ vital	✔ vulnerable
✔ natural	✔ invading
✔ serious	✔ intricate

1 They are repelled by the .... barrier of the skin, overcome by the .... pesticides in sweat, saliva and tears, dissolved by stomach acids or trapped in the .... mucus of the nose or throat before being expelled by a sneeze or cough.

2 After entering the bloodstream and tissues, they multiply at an .... rate and begin destroying .... body cells.

3 AIDS sufferers become .... to many kinds of .... organisms.

4 Should the system overreact or go awry, it can cause .... allergies and .... disorders called autoimmune diseases.

5 As they probe the .... workings of the immune system, scientists are awestruck.

6 Normally .... parasites in the lungs become active, causing Pneumocystis Carinii Pneumonia.

7 The AIDS epidemic has provided important .... insights into the immune system.

7 NOUNS

Fill in the blanks with the following *nouns* as used in the text.

✔ system	✔ brain
✔ epidemic	✔ cancers
✔ illness	✔ allergies
✔ bloodstream	✔ tissues
✔ disorders	✔ organ
✔ lungs	✔ cells
✔ protection	✔ vaccine
✔ diseases	

a When the system is weakened by previous (1) .... or advancing age, for example, the body becomes more vulnerable to (2) .... and a host of infectious diseases. Should the (3) .... overreact or go awry, it can cause troublesome (4) .... and serious (5) .... called autoimmune (6) ....

b Researchers in Colombia have tested a malaria (7) .... that, unlike previous efforts, seems to provide (8) .... against the disease.

c The AIDS (9) .... has provided important, new insights into the immune system.

d After entering the (10) .... and (11) ...., they multiply at an alarming rate and begin destroying vital body (12) ....

e The immune system is compared favourably with the most complex (13) .... of them all, the (14) ....

f Fungal growths corrode the skin and (15) ....

8 DESCRIBING BODY SYSTEMS

Study this sentence.

91 *"The immune system has a phenomenal ability for* dealing with information, for learning and memory, for creating and storing and using information.

This is immunologist William Paul's description of *the immune system.*

Give a sentence *in your own words* to describe each of the following systems. Begin each sentence as above.

e.g. *The respiratory system* has a phenomenal ability for ....

a The respiratory system
b The circulatory system
c The digestive system
d The excretory system
e The nervous system
f The muscular system
g The skeletal system
h The sensory system

9

Study this sentence.

107 Although researchers began to pry loose its secrets in the late

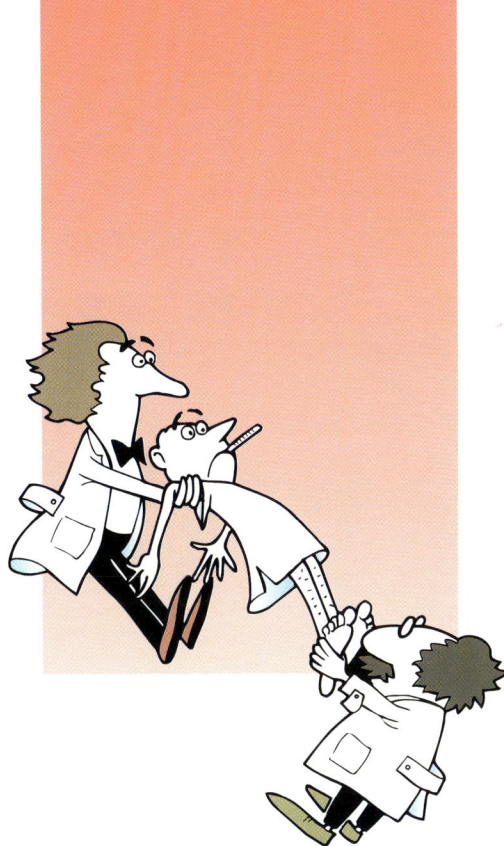

EXTENSION EXERCISES

19th century, *it was not until* after World War II *that* the pace of discovery began to quicken.

Complete the following sentences in your own words. Use the expression *it was not until* followed by the word *that* in order to explain the consequence as in the above sentence.

1 Although he smoked too much ....
2 Although she liked her job ....
3 Although we had studied English ....
4 Although she had thought about becoming a blood donor ....
5 Although Mike skied very well ....
6 Although he had suffered from the complaint for many years ....

Notes

CONDITIONALS - TYPE 3

a *Study this sentence.*

181 Much of the progress in AIDS research *would have been* impossible without discoveries about the immune system made shortly before the epidemic bloomed.

WOULD HAVE BEEN is an example of the PERFECT CONDITIONAL.

This conditional is formed by using:

the subject + the conditional auxiliary would + have + the past participle

Affirmative   It would have been

Negative   It wouldn't have been

Interrogative Would it have been?

b *Type 3 conditional* is formed by using:

IF + the PAST PERFECT + the PERFECT CONDITIONAL

c *In type 3 conditionals*, it is *impossible* to carry out the condition as the time is passed and the action in the IF clause didn't happen.

   e.g. If I had taken the medicine, I'd have felt better.

d The IF is followed by a verb in

GRAMMAR POINT

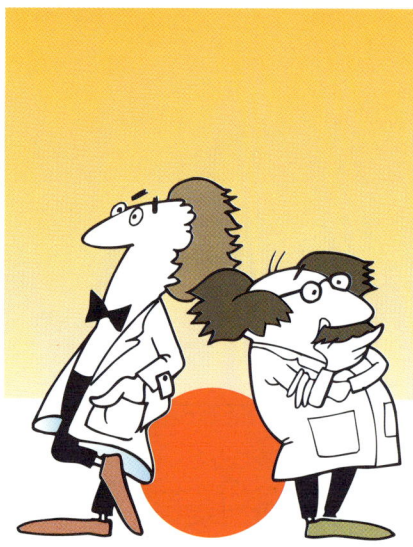

the PAST PERFECT not the conditional.
IF + the PAST PERFECT

e *HAD* can be placed first and the if omitted.

   e.g. If you had arrived on time, you'd have seen him.
   Had you arrived on time you'd have seen him.

10 GRAMMAR CHECK

Put the verbs in brackets into the *Past Perfect* or the *Perfect Conditional*.

1 If Jack (apply) for the job, he (get) it.
2 You (ask) me for advice I (give) you it.
3 I (not lend) him my car if I (know) he was such a bad driver.
4 If you (tell) me that she was in hospital, I (visit) her.
5 Tom (not break) his leg if he (fall) down the stairs.
6 She (attend) all the lectures she (have) no difficulty in passing the exam.
7 If the patient (take) the tablets, his condition (not deteriorate).
8 If I (not lift) that heavy box, I (not hurt) my back.

11 GRAMMAR CHECK

Translate the following sentences into your native language.

1 If I had known he was arriving, I would have met him at the airport.
2 If it had rained yesterday, she wouldn't have gone.
3 The hospital would have phoned me if there had been an emergency.
4 If he hadn't caught a cold, he wouldn't have had to miss the football match.
5 Had I known he was in hospital I would have visited him.

WRITING

12 SENTENCE COMPLETION

The workings of the immune system are described by the writer as a battle.
Form complete sentences from the words below to describe this internal battle. Try to use some of the verbs, adjectives and adverbs you have studied in this unit.

HUMANS: constant seige - adversaries.

GERMS: strive tirelessly - invade - body - skin - eyes - nose - ears - mouth.
Repelled - barrier - skin - natural pesticides - sweat - saliva - tears - stomach acids - sticky mucus - nose - throat - expelled - sneeze - cough.

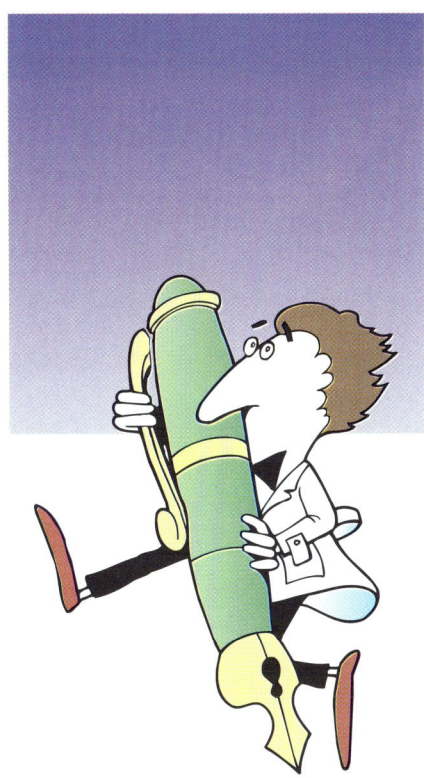

INVADERS: rude shock - encounter - human immune system.

HIGHLY SPECIALIZED CELLS: regulated - proteins - unending battle - alien organisms.

EARLY WARNING CELLS: monitor - bloodstream - tissues - signs - enemy.
Dust particles - microorganisms - debris - battle.

OTHER EARLY WARNERS: production - killer cells - designed - a particular type.

THE PROPERLY FUNCTIONING IMMUNE SYSTEM: formidable barrier - disease.
Even when - infection - severe - overcome - initial response - illness - the immune cells - usually - regroup - reinforcements - rout - invaders.

Notes

179

Study the following article.

Death-Defying Drug Therapy

Colon cancer held at bay

For decades the only true weapon against colon cancer has been surgery. If the scalpel could take out the entire tumor, the patient was cured; if not, the cancer recurred. But now, for the first time, researchers have developed a drug therapy that may reduce the high death rate from this form of cancer, which kills 53,500 Americans each year and is the third most common type of malignancy in the U.S.

In a series of studies coordinated by Dr. Charles Moertel of the Mayo Clinic in Rochester, Minn., researchers tested a combination of two drugs: 5-fluorouracil, a proven anticancer agent, and levamisole, a medication commonly used by veterinarians to clear worms from the intestines of animals. Included in the studies were some 1,700 cancer patients, most of whom had been operated on for Dukes' C colon cancer. In this stage of the cancer, the tumor has penetrated the bowel wall but has not spread to the rest of the body. The results of the first study, which appeared in this month's *Journal of Clinical Oncology,* showed that 49% of patients receiving the treatment were still alive after five years, in contrast to 37% of another group that did not receive the drugs. In a second and much larger study, which has yet to be published, the benefit from the drug therapy "at least matched" the results achieved in the first experiment, said Dr. Moertel.

The researchers caution, however, that the drugs are not effective for patients with more severe colon cancer, in which the malignancy has already spread throughout the body. Nor have studies shown a benefit for those patients whose cancers were detected at an early stage.

Still, Dr. Michael Friedman of the National Cancer Institute called this first success for drug therapy against colon cancer a "terrific intellectual breakthrough." The institute has alerted 35,000 cancer doctors across the country. And some experts are hopeful that the findings will lead to similar therapies for other cancers. ■

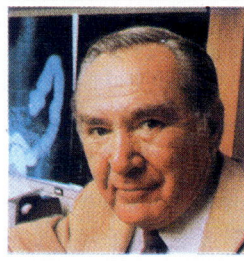

Charles Moertel

PER BREUEHAGEN

VOCABULARY

title	to defy
	- to challenge; to resist strongly
title	to hold at bay
	- to ward off
3	a scalpel
	- a small surgical knife
4	to cure
	- to heal
5	to recur
	- to happen again
10	malignancy
	- quality of being malignant (malignant-likely to be fatal)
16	proven
	- proved
17	a veterinarian
	- a veterinary surgeon
23	bowel
	- colon
24	to spread
	- to extend

Notes

SPEAKING

13 INTERVIEW

Group work.
One student should take the part of Dr. Charles Moertel of the Mayo Clinic in Rochester. Describe the drug therapy used against colon cancer. Begin with the words, "For decades the only true weapon against colon cancer has been surgery".

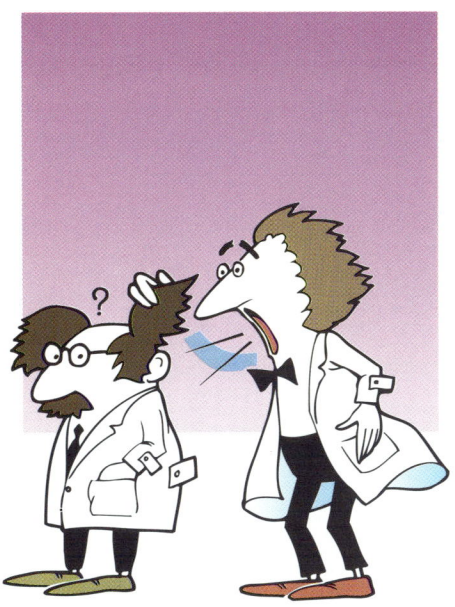

The other students should take the part of journalists from the *Journal of Clinical Oncology*. They should ask questions about the drug therapy and its future possibilities.

e.g. Are the drugs effective for patients with severe colon cancer?

Will your findings lead to similar therapies for other cancers?

UNDERSTANDING IDIOMATIC ENGLISH

Explain the idiom.

He's got nothing between his ears

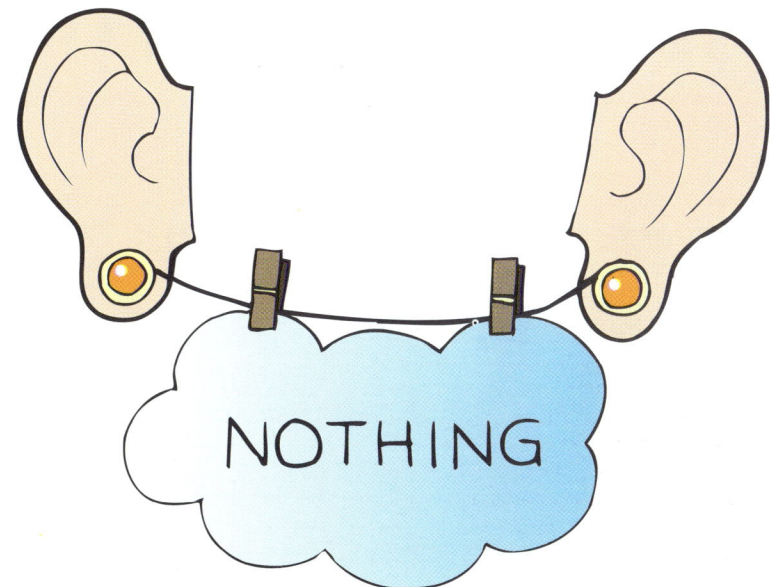

NOTHING

UNIT 19

The immune system's response to infection

BIOLOGICAL WARFARE

Now, however, scientists have a good grasp not only of the broad workings of the immune system but of many of the nitty-gritty details as well. In a typical infection, for example, a flu virus burrows into a cell in the lining of an air passage, takes over the machinery of the cell, and orders it to produce more flu viruses. Quickly engorged, the invaded cell bursts, releasing new viruses to infiltrate other cells and replicate further. Left unchecked, the onslaught would eventually kill enough cells to cause death. But the intruders soon encounter roving scavenger cells called phagocytes, which simply engulf and digest them. These defenders—monocytes, neutrophils and macrophages—secrete substances that dilate nearby blood vessels and make them more permeable, enabling even more defenders to get from the bloodstream to the infection site. Other proteins, those belonging to the complement system, aid in this process.

Upon meeting a virus, the macrophage, which moves about, amoeba-like, on long cellular extensions known as pseudopods (false feet), does more than just ingest the intruder. It has another, even more important function. On its surface, like virtually all body cells, the macrophage carries MHC (for major histocompatibility complex) molecules, protein badges that enable other immune cells to recognize the macrophage as friend, or self, and not attack it. After digesting the virus, the macrophage proudly displays strips of protein from the virus in the grooves of some of its MHC molecules. Once a bit of protein—which is part of the virus's own identity molecule, or antigen—is nestled in the groove of the macrophage's MHC molecule, it acts as a red flag for the immune system, warning it that a particular type of virus is loose in the body.

"At this point, it's still a race between the immune system and the virus," says Dr. Carl Nathan of Cornell University Medical College. "The virus is trying to replicate before the immune system has a chance to gear up." In order to mobilize the system, the macrophage must find—or literally bump into—a helper T cell, the battle manager of the immune system. The catch is that only a tiny fraction of the billions of T cells in the body are capable of attaching to the antigen of this particular flu virus and taking action. To increase its odds of meeting up with an appropriate T cell, the macrophage probably moves from the body tissue into the nearest lymph node, through which helper T cells of all kinds continually pass. Robert Coffman, a scientist at Palo Alto's DNAX Research Institute, likens the site to a busy Manhattan sidewalk. "If you walk the street enough," he says, "pretty soon you'll run into almost everyone who lives in New York City."

When the macrophage finally runs into a compatible helper T cell, it inserts its antigen-bearing MHC molecule into a T-cell receptor shaped to receive it, much as a key would fit into a lock. The macrophage then secretes a protein called interleukin-1, a chemical signal that causes the T cell to begin replicating. Simultaneously, interleukin-1 acts on the body's central thermostat, causing a fever, which may depress viral activity and enhance the immune response.

The rapidly multiplying helper T cells now begin releasing a flood of their own chemical signals, the so-called lympho-

BIOLOGICAL WARFARE

From deliberate exposure to an unguarded sneeze, the threat may come from anywhere. But the body commands a wide assortment of defenders to eliminate the danger and guard against repeat invasions.

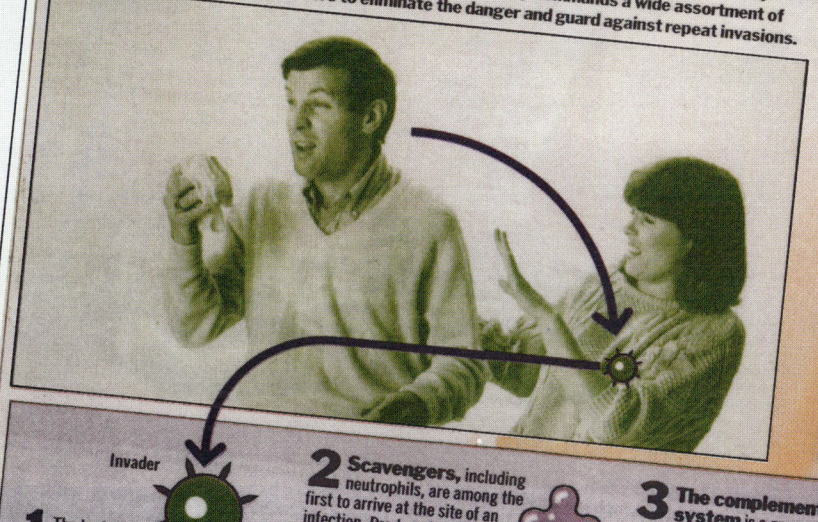

6 **T cells** carry their own array of receptors that can recognize specific invaders' antigens. When recognition occurs, the T cell grows and divides. Three main populations of T cells are known.

Receptor — Antigen

5 Having ingested an invader, the macrophage displays specific markers from the invader on its surface. These markers, or antigens, signal other immune-system cells, called helper T cells.

Invader

1 The body is constantly being bombarded by viruses, bacteria and other microbes. When the body is invaded, the microbe begins its attack by multiplying. Within minutes, the immune system, sensing the invader's presence, sends out its forces.

2 **Scavengers,** including neutrophils, are among the first to arrive at the site of an infection. Produced in the bone marrow, they survive for only a few days.

3 **The complement system** is a group of at least 20 proteins circulating in the blood. The proteins can stick to an invader, setting off a chain reaction that eventually kills it.

4 **Macrophages** are long-lived scavengers that migrate through the body and engulf foreign matter as well as cellular debris. They signal other cells in the immune system to join the fight.

kines, which include gamma interferon and other types of interleukin. These stimulate the defense system even more, spurring the proliferation of phagocytes, including macrophages, and other immune fighters—something like a draft call in wartime. The result is the familiar swelling and inflammation of an infection.

At the same time, other helper T cells in the lymph nodes move to couple with yet another kind of immune fighter, the B cells. Releasing still more chemicals, the helper T cells stimulate the B cells to reproduce. These proliferating B cells then mature into plasma cells, which DNAX's Coffman calls "dedicated antibody factories," that begin to mass-produce antibodies. Antibodies are proteins capable of recognizing and binding specifically to the flu virus that triggered the alarm. Circulating in the blood to seek out their quarry, they begin attaching themselves to the viruses, signaling the macrophages and other immune scavengers to move in for the kill.

Meanwhile, gamma interferon released by the T cells has not only slowed viral replication but also whipped the macrophages into a feeding fury. Their cell membranes become ruffled, their feet more numerous and their appetites ferocious. "They don't necessarily eat faster," notes Dr. Richard Johnston Jr. of the University of Pennsylvania School of Medicine, "but they kill better."

The flu viruses, however, are not finished yet. Those still multiplying inside the body's cells are momentarily safe from scavengers and antibodies, but the free lunch is over quickly. While the B cells are being activated, other helper T cells have been creating an army of killer T cells. These killers recognize the flu-ridden cells because, like macrophages, infected cells display a bit of viral antigen on their outer membranes. Says Coffman: "For many viral infections, the most important response is the killer T cell. Viruses live inside cells, so it's essential to kill not only the viruses themselves but those cells that are infected with the virus."

The killer T cells are relentless. Docking with infected cells, they shoot lethal proteins at the cell membrane. Holes form where the protein molecules hit, and the cell, dying, leaks out its insides. To ensure that the cell and its viral occupants are destroyed, the killer T cells then deliver the coup de grace by transmitting a signal that causes the cell to chew up DNA from both itself and the virus. Explains Dr. Irving Weissman of Stanford: "This is an overlapping, dual system of killing that ensures that the seed of viral production will be eliminated from the body."

When victory over the virus is achieved, the wildly accelerating responses of the immune system slow, then shut down. Scientists believe that still other immune specialists, known as suppressor T cells, call off the battle. As the

130
135
140
145
150
155
160
165

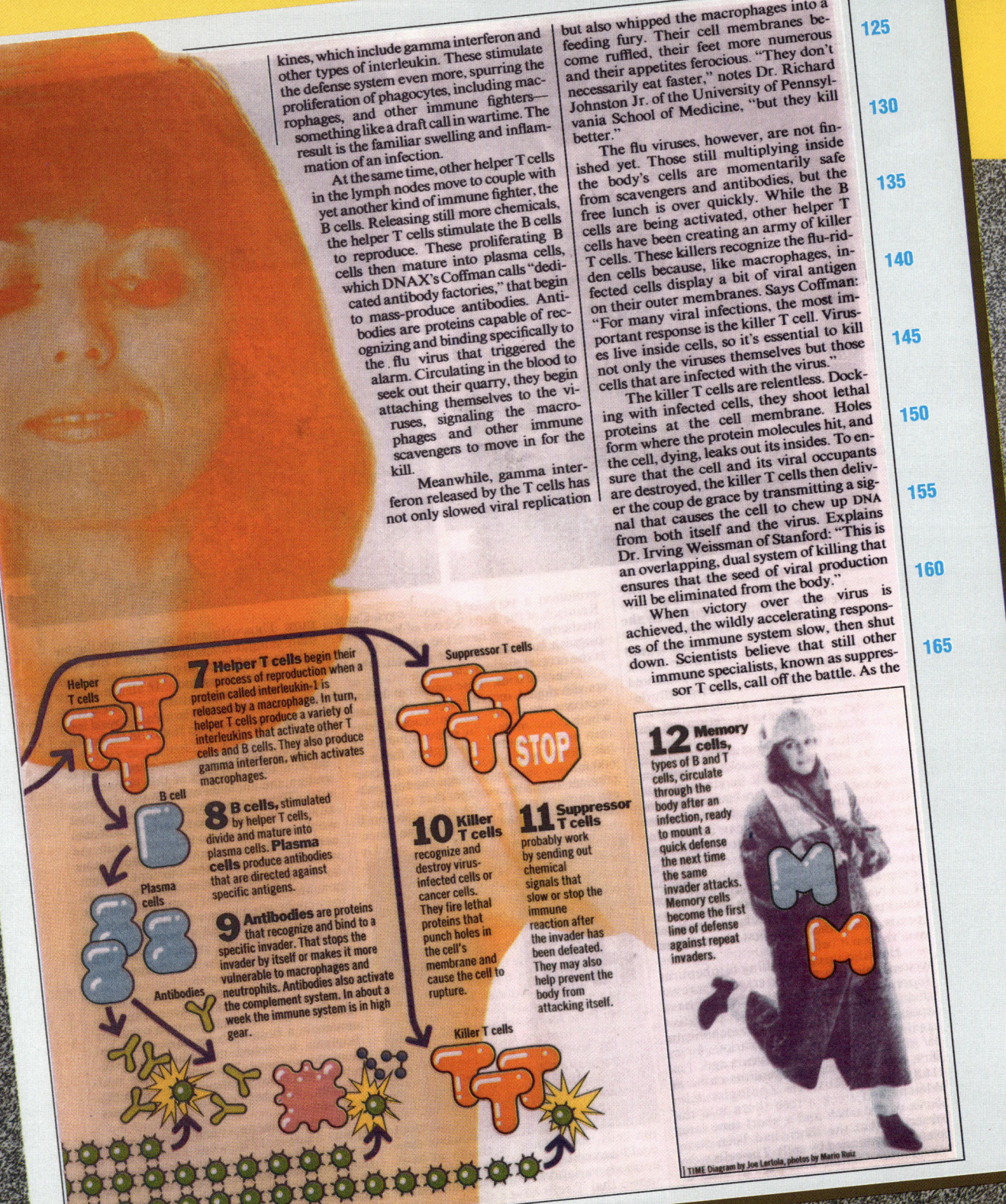

7 **Helper T cells** begin their process of reproduction when a protein called interleukin-1 is released by a macrophage. In turn, helper T cells produce a variety of interleukins that activate other T cells and B cells. They also produce gamma interferon, which activates macrophages.

8 **B cells,** stimulated by helper T cells, divide and mature into plasma cells. **Plasma cells** produce antibodies that are directed against specific antigens.

9 **Antibodies** are proteins that recognize and bind to a specific invader. That stops the invader by itself or makes it more vulnerable to macrophages and neutrophils. Antibodies also activate the complement system. In about a week the immune system is in high gear.

10 **Killer T cells** recognize and destroy virus-infected cells or cancer cells. They fire lethal proteins that punch holes in the cell's membrane and cause the cell to rupture.

11 **Suppressor T cells** probably work by sending out chemical signals that slow or stop the immune reaction after the invader has been defeated. They may also help prevent the body from attacking itself.

12 **Memory cells,** types of B and T cells, circulate through the body after an infection, ready to mount a quick defense the next time the same invader attacks. Memory cells become the first line of defense against repeat invaders.

Helper T cells

B cell

Plasma cells

Antibodies

Suppressor T cells

STOP

Killer T cells

| TIME Diagram by Joe Lertola; photos by Mario Ruiz

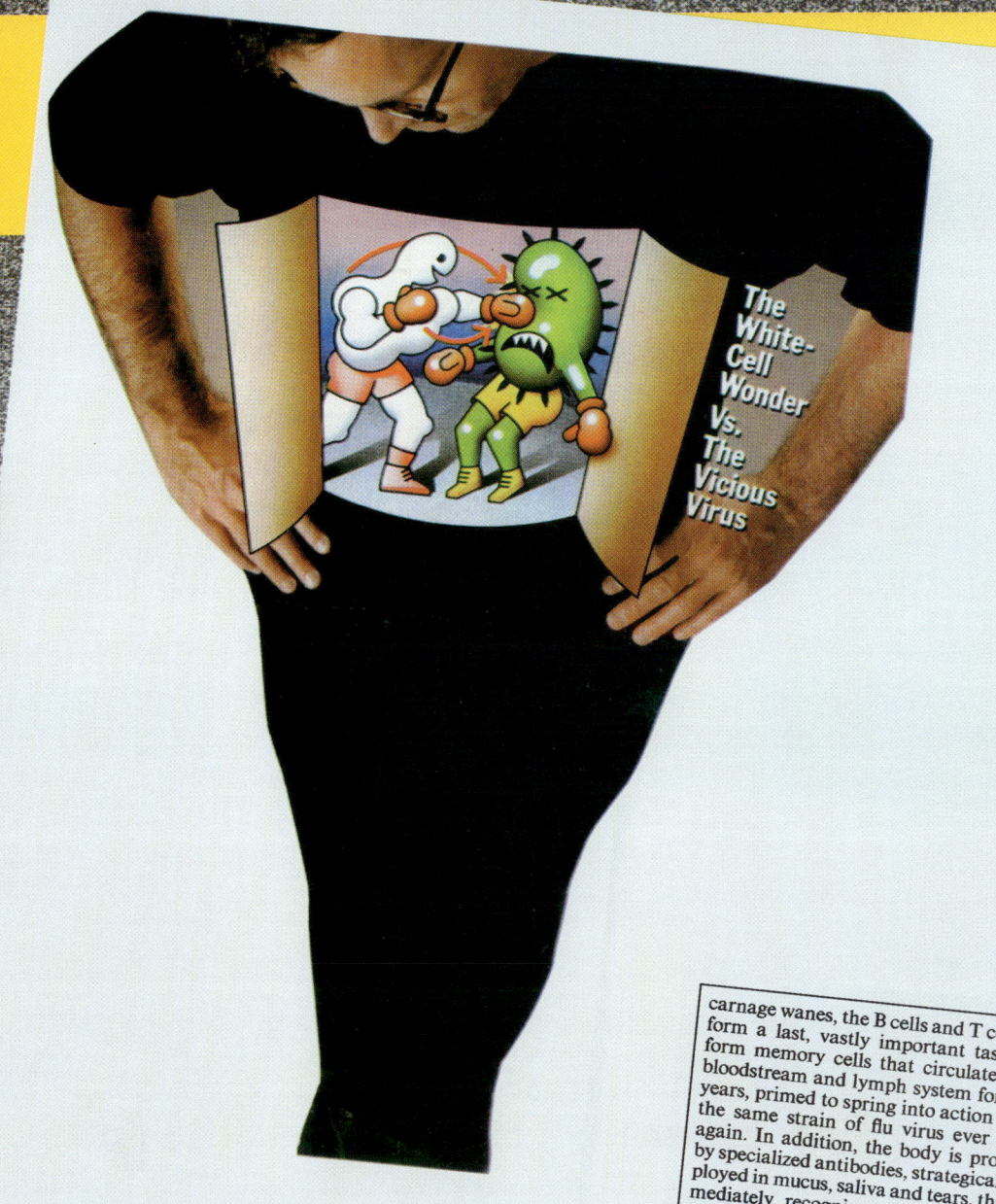

The White-Cell Wonder Vs. The Vicious Virus

carnage wanes, the B cells and T cells perform a last, vastly important task: they form memory cells that circulate in the bloodstream and lymph system for many years, primed to spring into action should the same strain of flu virus ever attack again. In addition, the body is protected by specialized antibodies, strategically deployed in mucus, saliva and tears, that immediately recognize any return of this particular virus.

While a healthy immune system may take as long as three weeks to complete the job against a specific flu virus, its next response to the same viral strain reaches full force immediately, and the invaders are overcome before they can do any significant damage. In other words, the body has become immune—but only to that specific virus. "You probably wouldn't even know you'd been reinfected," says Carl Nathan. "The immune system has a short track and a long track, and it all depends on whether it's a first encounter or you've seen it before."

VOCABULARY

Study the meaning of the following words and expressions as used in the text.

2   a grasp
    - an understanding
3   nitty-gritty (inf.)
    - basic, fundamental
5   to burrow
    - to penetrate
14 to rove
    - to move without purpose or planned route
14 a scavenger
    - one who collects refuse
15 to engulf
    - to swallow up; to make disappear as if taking in food
23 to aid
    - to help; to assist
24 upon
    - on
32 a badge
    - a distinguishing mark or sign
36 to display
    - to exhibit
36 a strip
    - a long, narrow piece
37 a groove
    - a long, narrow hole or channel
40 to nestle
    - to place in a comfortable position
43 to warn
    - to give information of approaching danger
51 to gear up
    - to increase in operational efficiency

TEXT BASED EXERCISES

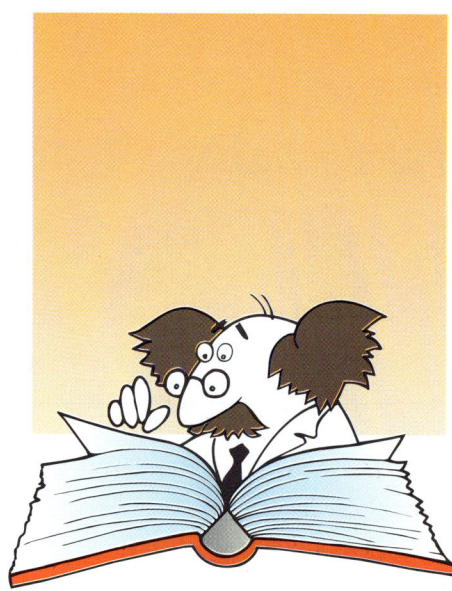

53 to bump into
    - to meet by chance
55 a catch
    - a surprise or trick in an apparently advantageous situation
57 to attach
    - to join, to stick
59 odds
    - probability; chance
59 to meet up with
    - to make contact with
66 to liken
    - to compare
69 to run into
    - to meet
76 to fit
    - to be the correct size and shape for

89 a flood
    - (fig.) a profuse flow
97 a draft call
    - a call to go to war
98 a swelling
    - an unnatural enlargement of a part of the body
101 to couple
    - to connect; to link
114 to seek out
    - to search for; to look for
114 a quarry
    - one being hunted or persued
123 to whip
    - to beat with a whip
125 to ruffle
    - to disturb, discompose
138 ridden
    - attacked and full of
147 relentless
    - without pity
151 to leak out
    - to exude slowly
151 insides
    - inner parts
158 dual
    - double
166 to call off
    - to give the order to stop
167 carnage
    - massacre
167 to wane
    - to decrease
171 to prime
    - to prepare esp. an explosive charge
172 a strain
    - a type
174 to deploy
    - to put into a specific position

1 WORD CHECK

Explain the meaning of the following expressions in your own words.

11   left unchecked
34   friend or self
42   a red flag
54   the battle manager
91   so-called
107 dedicated antibody factories
109 mass-produce
118 to move in for the kill

2 WORD CHECK

Explain the meaning of the words *in italics* as used in the text.

2   the *broad* workings
11   replicate *further*
12   *eventually* kill
15   *simply* engulf and digest
20   *even more* defenders
27   does more than *just* ingest
     the intruder
71   *finally* runs into
77   *then*
80   *simultaneously*
84   which *may* depress
168 *vastly* important task
174 *strategically* deployed

3 COMPREHENSION

Read the following sentences and choose *the most appropriate answer* as applied to the text.

1 *Scientists*
   a Have a good understanding of how the particular components of the immune system function.
   b Understand only the general workings and not the details.
   c Don't yet have a good understanding of the workings of the immune system.

2 *When a flu virus enters a cell in the lining of an air passage it*
   a Stops the machinery of the cell.
   b Helps the machinery of the cell.
   c Controls the machinery of the cell.

3 *The macrophage*
   a Ingests the intruder.
   b Is an amoeba.
   c Does not ingest the intruder.

4 *The helper T cells*
   a Release only a few lymphokines.
   b Release a great number of lymphokines.
   c Release three types of lymphokines.

5 *The killer T cells*
   a Try to penetrate the cell membranes.
   b Try to repair the holes in the cell membranes.
   c Shoot proteins that infect the cell membranes.

4 ASKING QUESTIONS

Write questions to which the following are the answers.

1   It takes over the machinery of the cell and orders it to produce more flu viruses.
2   It would eventually kill enough cells to cause death.
3   In order to try to improve the chances of meeting an appropriate T cell.
4   It inserts its antigen-bearing MHC molecule into a T-cell receptor.
5   It may depress viral activity and enhance the immune response.
6   The result is the familiar swelling and inflammation of an infection.
7   They mature into plasma cells.
8   They display a bit of viral antigen on their outer membranes.
9   In order to ensure that the cell and its viral occupants are destroyed.
10 No, only to that specific virus.

5

Fill in the blanks with the words below.

> ✔ flu virus   ✔ strain
>
> ✔ antibodies   ✔ blood vessels
>
> ✔ memory cells   ✔ fever
>
> ✔ viral activity   ✔ infection
>
> ✔ bloodstream   ✔ substances
>
> ✔ immune response   ✔ process

a These defenders – monocytes, neutrophils and macrophages – secrete (1) .... that dilate nearby (2) .... and make them more permeable, enabling even more defenders to get from the (3) .... to the (4) .... site. Other proteins, those belonging to the complement system aid in this (5) ....

b Simultaneously, interleukin-I acts on the body's central thermostat, causing a (6) .... , which may depress (7) .... and enhance the (8) ....

c As the carnage wanes, the B cells and T cells perform a last, vastly important task:

they form (9) .... that circulate in the bloodstream for many years, primed to spring into action should the same (10) .... of (11) .... ever attack again. In addition, the body is protected by specialized (12) .... , strategically deployed in mucus, saliva and tears, that immediately recognize any return of this particular virus.

6   VERBS

Fill in the blanks with the *verbs* below in the form used in the text.

> ✔ begin
>
> ✔ carry
>
> ✔ activate
>
> ✔ kill
>
> ✔ digest
>
> ✔ secrete
>
> ✔ call
>
> ✔ enable
>
> ✔ aid
>
> ✔ cause
>
> ✔ produce
>
> ✔ stick
>
> ✔ engulf
>
> ✔ survive
>
> ✔ mature

a On its surface, like virtually all body cells, the macrophage (1) .... MHC molecules, protein badges that (2) .... other immune cells to recognize the macrophage as friend, or self, and not attack it.

b Produced in the bone marrow, scavengers (3) .... for only a few days.

c The macrophage then (4) .... a protein called interleukin-I, a chemical signal that (5) .... the T cell to begin replicating.

d The intruders soon encounter roving scavenger cells called phagocytes, which simply (6) .... and (7) .... them.

e These proliferating B cells then (8) .... into plasma cells, which DNAX'S Coffman (9) .... "dedicated antibody factories" that (10) .... to mass-produce antibodies.

f Plasma cells (11) .... antibodies that are directed against specific antigens.

g Antibodies also (12) .... the complement system.

h Other proteins, those belonging to the complement system, (13) .... in this process.

i The proteins can (14) .... to an invader, setting off a chain reaction that eventually (15) .... it.

7

Before completing this exercise, study the detailed diagram describing *the biological warfare*. Join the names in column 1 with an appropriate description in column 2.

Column 1	Column 2
a Plasma cells	1 They divide and mature into plasma cells
b A helper T cell	2 Scavengers that engulf foreign matter and signal other cells to join the fight
c Phagocytes	3 Proteins that recognize and bind to a specific invader; they activate the complement system
d B cells	4 Antibody factories
e The complement system	5 They send out chemical signals that slow or stop the immune reaction after the invader has been defeated
f Macrophages	6 A group of at least 20 proteins circulating in the blood
g Antibodies	7 The battle manager
h Killer T cells	8 They circulate through the body after an infection, ready to mount a quick defense the next time the same invader attacks
i Suppressor T cells	9 They recognize and destroy virus infected or cancer cells
j Memory cells	10 Roving scavenger cells

8 PHRASAL VERBS

Several phrasal verbs have been used in the text. Fill in the missing part of the phrasal verbs in the following sentences.

1 In a typical infection, for example, a flu virus burrows into a cell in the lining of an air passage, takes .... the machinery of the cell and orders it to produce more flu viruses.

2 The virus is trying to replicate before the immune system has a chance to gear ....

3 When the macrophage finally runs .... a compatible helper T cell, it inserts its antigen-bearing MHC molecule into a T cell receptor shaped to receive it.

4 Simultaneously, interleukin-I acts .... the body's central thermostat causing a fever.

5 Circulating in the blood to seek .... their quarry, antibodies begin attaching themselves to the viruses, signaling the macrophages and other immune scavengers to move .... for the kill.

6 To ensure that the cell and its viral occupants are destroyed, the killer T cells transmit a signal that causes the cell to chew .... DNA from both itself and the virus.

7 When victory over the virus is achieved, the wildly accelerating responses of the immune system slow, then shut ....

8 Scientists believe that still other immune specialists, known as suppressor cells, call .... the battle.

EXTENSION EXERCISES

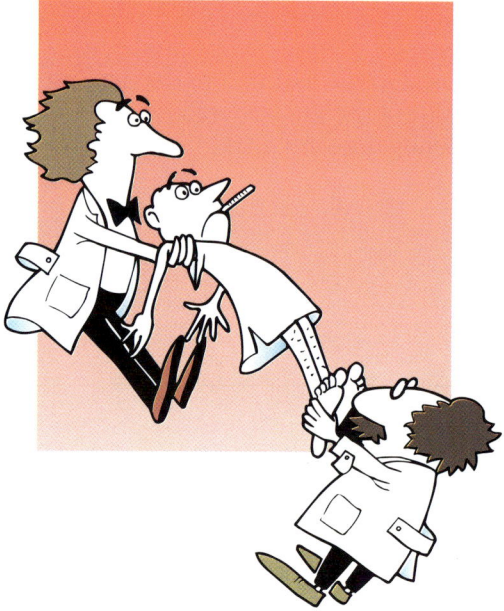

9 DEFINING

Study the following sentence.

109 *Antibodies* are proteins capable of recognizing and binding specifically to the flu virus that triggered the alarm.

Following the above example, *define the terms below* in your own words.

a Capillaries.
b A stethoscope.
c The oesophagus.
d The kidneys.
e A protein.
f An electrocardiogram.
g Insulin.
h Enzymes.
i Fibrinogen.
j A virus.

10 HAVING + PAST PARTICIPLE

Study this sentence.

"*Having ingested* an invader, the macrophage displays specific markers from the invader on its surface."

In this sentence, we find more than one action and more than one clause.
When one action happens before another, it is possible to use *having + the past participle* for the first action.

e.g. He finished studying. He went home.
Having finished studying, he went home.

Join the following sentences as in the above example. Begin each sentence with *having*.

1 He broke his leg. He decided to give up skiing.
2 She had a hard day at work. She went home to relax.
3 Mike woke up late. He missed the bus.
4 Mr. Foster felt ill. He went to see his doctor.
5 She wrote the letter. She went out to post it.
6 They checked that the train strike had been called off. They went to the station.
7 We drove all day. We were very tired when we arrived.
8 He was told that he had been promoted. He phoned his wife to tell her the news.
9 They saw the accident. They telephoned for an ambulance.
10 Carol read the book. She lent it to her friend.

Notes

VARIATIONS OF CONDITIONALS

a *IF + 2 PRESENT TENSES*

  e.g. If you freeze water,
       it turns to ice.

FOR HABITUAL OR
AUTOMATIC RESULTS

b IF + PRESENT +

+ MAY
  MIGHT   possibility

+ CAN   permission

+ MUST   request
  SHOULD   advice
               command

e.g. If the results of your tests are
    good, you *may*
    be able to go home.
                    POSSIBILITY

   If the results of your tests
   aren't good, you *might* be
   admitted to hospital.
                    POSSIBILITY

   If the doctor agrees, you *can*
   go home.
                    PERMISSION

   You *must* stop smoking, if you
   want to get better.
                    COMMAND

   If you want to live longer, you
   should try to keep yourself fit.
                    ADVICE

c *COULD* or *MIGHT* may be
   used instead of would.

GRAMMAR POINT

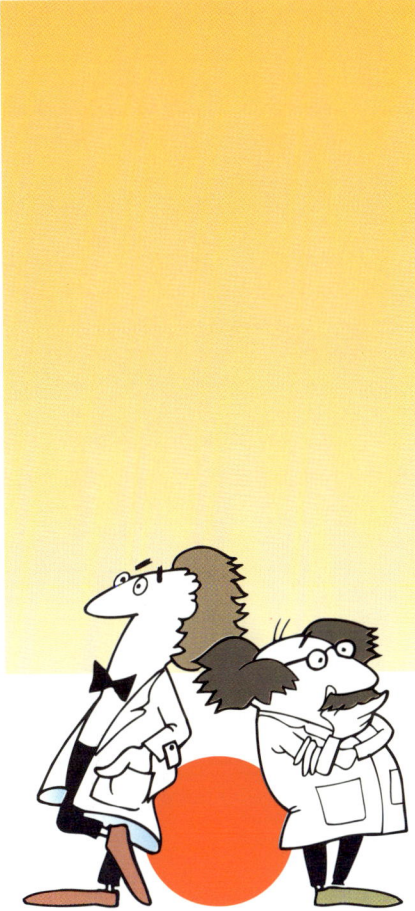

e.g. If he had come sooner, we
    could have helped him.
                    ABILITY

   If he had come sooner, we
   might have been able to help
   him.
                    POSSIBILITY

11 GRAMMAR CHECK

Complete the following sentences
in your own words.

1 If the heart stops beating
   ....
2 We could have arrived earlier
   if ....
3 You lose weight if ....
4 She must have the operation if
   ....
5 The patient might have been
   able to go home sooner if
   ....
6 They may be able to go away
   next weekend if ....
7 I should really study harder if
   ....
8 He might have passed the
   examination if ....

12 GRAMMAR CHECK

Translate the following sentences
into your native language.

1 She may come today if you
   ask her.
2 You must study if you want to
   pass the exam.
3 If he had told me the truth, I
   might have been able to do
   something.
4 I could come tomorrow
   afternoon if that suits you.
5 If you want to be more health
   conscious, you should eat less
   fatty foods.

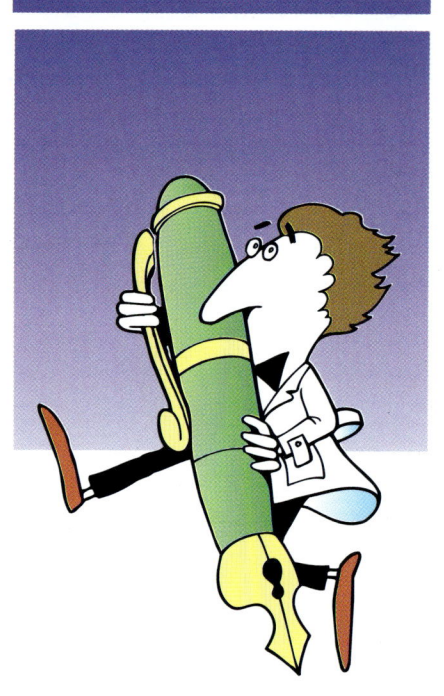

WRITING

13 DESCRIPTION FROM DIAGRAM

Follow the diagram below. Explain, *in your own words*, the nature and function of the various components of the immune system.

Notes

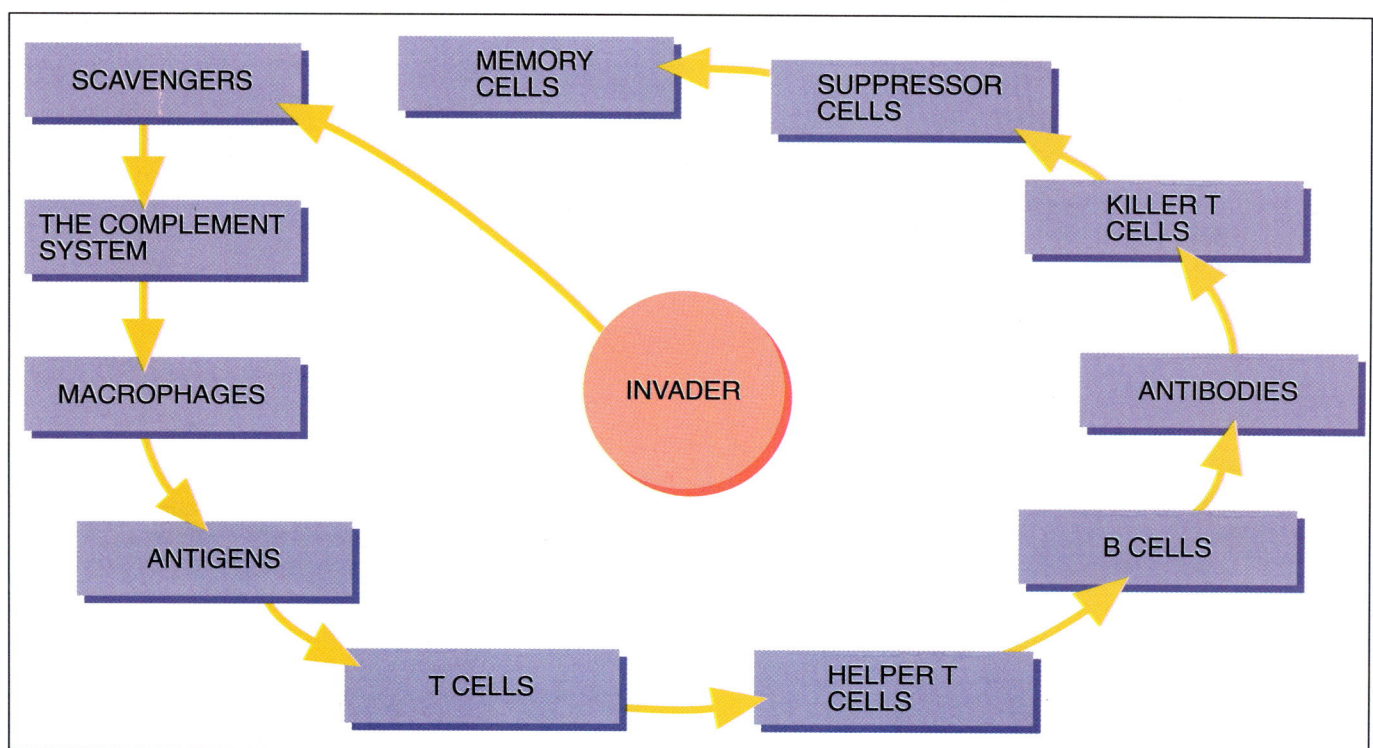

SPEAKING

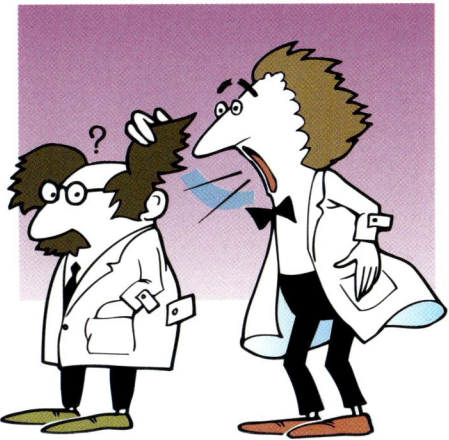

14 AIDS RISK

Read the following passage.

Medical experts currently maintain that the risk of getting AIDS from a doctor or dentist is extremely low. Catching it requires expo- [5] sure to an infected person's bodily fluids. As a precaution, all health-care workers today are encouraged to wear gloves and masks in [10] any situation where infection might occur. CDC statistics indicate that AIDS afflicts at least 144 dentists and hygienists and 668 physicians, including 40 surgeons. Some AIDS victims [15] have been fired from hospitals, some have been sued by patients and others have continued to practice. Last week, the *Journal of the American Medical Association* offered some reassurance in a report [20] about a surgeon with AIDS. Researchers tested 616 of his patients and found that only one was infected with the virus and that the infection had occurred before his surgery. Still, a 1988 poll indicated that [25] 56 percent of Americans would switch doctors if theirs had AIDS, and one fourth said they would switch if their doctors treated AIDS patients.

AIDS virus

14 VOCABULARY

12 CDC
    centers for disease control
16 to fire
    - (coll.) to dismiss from a post
17 to sue
    - to take legal proceedings against
25 a poll
    - an unofficial estimate of public opinion on specific points by questioning a random selection of persons
26 to switch
    - to change

Comment on the passage you have just read.

UNDERSTANDING IDIOMATIC ENGLISH

Explain the idiom.

As he was feeling very generous, he offered to foot the bill

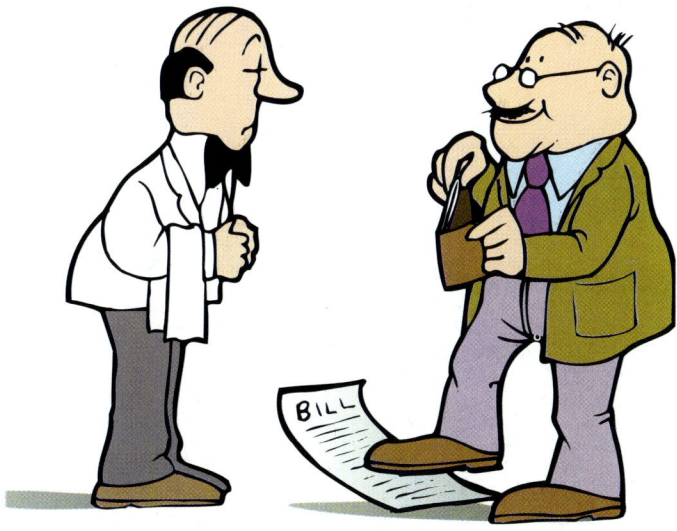

UNIT 20

Difficulties in creating
new vaccines

These days the explosive growth of both molecular biology and immunology has enabled vaccine makers to take a safer and more effective approach to their work. Instead of using dead or attenuated bacteria or viruses, they remove from the bug's surface the marker protein, or antigen, that provokes the immune response. Employing gene-splicing techniques, they mass-produce the antigen, or a portion of it, and use it as the prime ingredient of the vaccine.

Researchers are also creating vaccines that consist largely of antigens synthesized from chemicals on the laboratory shelf. When these vaccines prove ineffective, scientists can now usually determine why. Says M.I.T. Molecular Biologist Malcolm Gefter: "Today, when a vaccine doesn't elicit a protective response, it is possible to detect what is or is not working—the B cells, the T cells, the lymphokines, whatever." Scientists can then "fix" the vaccine. For example, the 1985 vaccine against *Hemophilus influenzae* Type B, which causes bacterial meningitis, was only partially effective; although it protected older children, it did not work for babies under two years, who are most at risk. The antigen used to make the original vaccine has been re-engineered to make it more potent, and the new vaccine is being tested in infants.

Despite such advanced techniques, it seems tougher than ever to create new vaccines. Some viruses, bacteria and parasites are so complex and well evolved in their defenses against an immune reaction that no vaccine strategy has yet been entirely effective. Flu viruses, for example, mutate rapidly, continually changing their antigens in the process. As a result, an immune system strengthened by a flu shot against last year's predominant strain of flu will probably not be helped by it this year. The common cold virus is also troublesome, because it comes in at least 100 identifiable varieties. The parasite that causes malaria poses still other problems: it penetrates cells so quickly that it is hidden from antibodies. To complicate matters, it goes through three stages of life, displaying different antigens in each stage. Because none of the malaria vaccines yet developed can cope with these diverse strategies, the affliction is still rampant in the tropics.

Such challenges to the vaccine makers, however, pale in comparison with that presented by the AIDS virus. Says M.I.T.'s Gefter: "We're looking at a strong, well-evolved, well-designed organism that is doing whatever it can to protect itself." The AIDS virus mutates twice as fast as the flu bug. It can lie dormant in body cells, where antibodies cannot attack it, without revealing its telltale antigen (a dead giveaway to killer cells). New findings indicate that the virus also uses immunological decoys that provoke impotent immune responses. Worst of all, the AIDS virus is unique in that it can mount a speedy and lethal attack on helper T cells, which cripples the immune system before it can counterattack. This means that to prevent an AIDS infection from taking hold, a vaccine must stimulate the immune system to incapacitate the AIDS virus immediately after exposure, before it can penetrate the helper T cells.

Scientists are scrutinizing the AIDS virus for any sections of its outer coat that remain unchanged during its rapid mutations. With antigens from these sections, they hope to produce a vaccine that will remain effective despite many mutations. A group led by Dr. Daniel Zagury at the Pierre and Marie Curie University in Par-

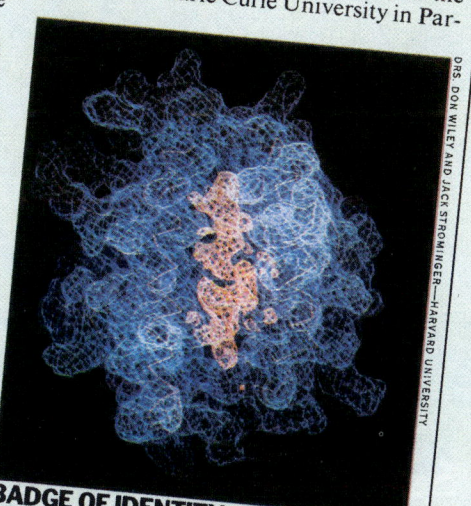

DRS. DON WILEY AND JACK STROMINGER—HARVARD UNIVERSITY

BADGE OF IDENTITY

X-ray image of a major histocompatibility complex (MHC) protein, the key to the body's ability to distinguish its own cells from others.

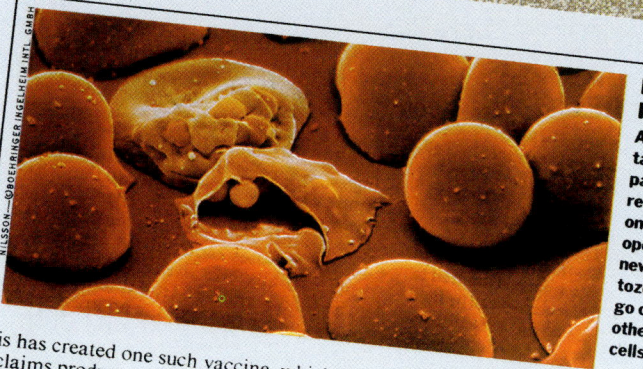

DEADLY INVADERS
After being attacked by malaria parasites, stricken red blood cells, one of them burst open, teem with newly formed protozoans that will go on to infect other healthy cells.

is has created one such vaccine. which he claims produces a weak immune reaction. Zagury and several volunteers went so far as to inoculate themselves with the vaccine last year. Even so. many researchers. Merck's Hilleman among them. believe the prospects for an AIDS vaccine are dismal. Others disagree. "We've known about the tricks of this virus for only a year or so." says Gefter. "With a better understanding of its strategems and with the genetic-engineering tools we have, we can design sophisticated vaccines tailor-made to the life cycle of the AIDS virus."

Even without provocation by the AIDS virus or other infectious organisms. the immune system can sometimes go awry. Often. entirely on its own. it can over-respond. fail to respond or turn against the body it is designed to protect with the same lethal fury it directs against invaders and cancerous cells. Some 80 immune-system deficiencies have been identified so far. About one in 400 people has at least one immune-system component missing or malfunctioning, usually for genetic reasons. In one in 10,000 people, the deficiency leads to serious disorders. Perhaps the most tragic example is severe combined immunodeficiency disease. a rare condition in which both B cells and T cells are lacking. The most famous SCID victim. a Texas boy named David. lived for twelve years in a germ-free bubble while doctors searched in vain for a cure for his disease. He died in 1984. four months after receiving a bone-marrow transplant that doctors hoped would supply his missing immune cells.

As hay fever and other allergy sufferers will testify. the immune system can sometimes react to pollen. animal dander.

molds and drugs that are normally harmless. In allergy victims. however. the immune system goes into high gear at the appearance of these substances. or allergens. It begins producing antibodies called immunoglobulin E. which attach themselves to mast cells located in the tissues of the skin. in the linings of the respiratory and intestinal tracts. and around the blood vessels. The mast cells promptly begin to release a number of chemical signals. including histamine. a substance that dilates blood vessels and makes it easier for cells to pass through the capillary walls. These changes. meant to expedite the arrival of immune cells. cause the inflammation and swelling associated with allergic reactions.

Allergy sufferers are now treated with antihistamines. which temporarily block the immune response, as well as steroid nasal sprays and inhalers. which reduce inflammation. But more effective help may be on the way. Scientists have synthesized bits of protein molecules that prevent immunoglobulin E antibod-

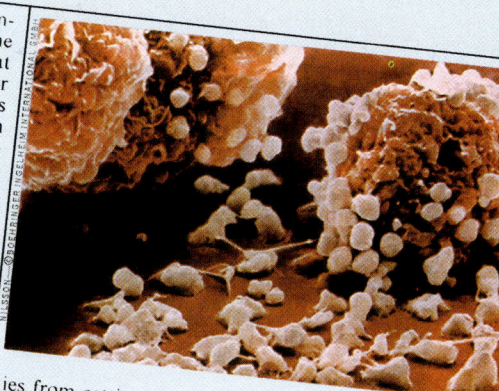

SNEEZE COMING ON?
Exploding mast cell releases granules full of histamines that cause sneezing and watery eyes; allergy sufferers overproduce antibodies that assault mast cells when allergens like pollen enter the body.

ies from setting off an allergic reaction.

One of the more devastating errors of the immune system involves its failure to distinguish between self and nonself. resulting in so-called autoimmune diseases. which can be crippling and sometimes fatal. Dozens of disorders that once mystified doctors are now thought to be autoimmune. Among them: Type 1 diabetes. myasthenia gravis. multiple sclerosis. rheumatoid arthritis and systemic lupus erythematosus. In these and other autoimmune diseases. the immune system mounts a selective and ferocious assault against parts of the body. destroying cells or cell components that it mistakenly identifies as alien.

Type 1 diabetes. for example. which afflicts 1.5 million Americans and is brought on by an insufficient supply of insulin. was for years believed to be caused by a virus. Researchers have now shown that it probably results from a defective immune system. For reasons that are not yet clear, immune cells invade the pancreas and destroy the beta cells, which produce insulin. When this happens, the body cannot convert sugar into the energy that cells need to function. The cells starve. and the unconverted sugar builds up in the bloodstream. damaging the fragile lining of blood vessels. Complications associated with Type 1 diabetes include heart and kidney disease. poor circulation, eye problems and stroke.

VOCABULARY

Study the meaning of the following words and expressions as used in the text.

5   to attenuate
    - to make thin; to diminish the force
6   a bug
    - (coll.) a virus
9   to splice
    - to join
16 to prove
    - to turn out to be; to result
20 to elicit
    - to evoke
28 to work
    - to function
57 rampant
    - found in many places; widespread
59 pale
    - less important
67 dead
    - complete; sure
67 a giveaway
    - a disclosure; a telltale sign
72 speedy
    - quick; rapid
76 to take hold
    - to acquire power over
82 a coat
    - outer layer; membrane
90 to claim
    - to affirm
91 so far as
    - to the extent of
95 dismal
    - gloomy; pessimistic

TEXT BASED EXERCISES

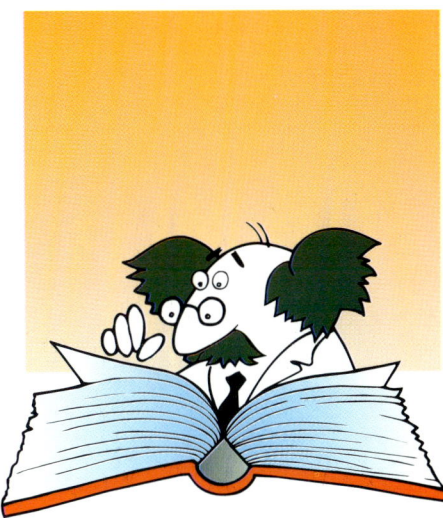

97   a trick
     - a personal and curious habit; a cunning act used to deceive another
100 tools
     - instruments; implements used by workmen
101 tailormade (fig.)
     - precisely adapted to suit a particular need
114 missing
     - not present
122 a bubble
     - a globular film of liquid filled with air or gas; a small pocket of air or gas in a liquid or solid
125 marrow
     - soft, fatty substance in the cavities of bones

128 hay fever
     - an allergic catarrh of nose and throat caused by inhaling pollen, dust or other irritants
130 pollen
     - fine dust composed of the microspores of seed plants
131 a mold
     - a fungus
145 to mean
     - to intend (meant p.t.)
145 to expedite
     - to help on; to accelerate
152 an inhaler
     - an apparatus for inhaling medicated vapour
163 to mystify
     - to puzzle; perplex
176 to bring on (brought p.t.)
     - to cause
189 fragile
     - delicate; easily destroyed
193 poor
     - not good; inadequate

1   WORD CHECK

Explain the meaning of the following words and expressions.

3   a vaccine
29   at risk
43   a flu shot
83   mutations
91   volunteers
114 malfunctioning
118 an immunodeficiency disease
125 a bone-marrow transplant
150 antihistamines
194 a stroke

2 WORD CHECK

Give words or expressions which have the same meaning as the words below.

10   a portion
16   ineffective
43   strengthened
47   troublesome
55   to cope with
81   scrutinizing
90   weak
92   to inoculate
139   tracts
150   temporarily

3 COMPREHENSION

Correct the following statements.

1   Synthesized antigens are not used in creating vaccines.
2   Flu viruses mutate slowly and do not change their antigens in the process.
3   The malaria parasite has hidden antibodies.
4   The AIDS virus mutates as fast as the flu bug.
5   Once the AIDS virus has taken hold, helper T cells assist in the counterattack against the virus.
6   It is only the AIDS virus that causes the immune system to go wrong.
7   Immunoglobulin E antibodies stop an allergic reaction.

8   In the case of autoimmune diseases, the immune system correctly identifies the enemy and mounts an attack against the infected parts of the body.
9   When the beta cells are destroyed, too much insulin is produced.
10   Fortunately, there are no complications associated with type I diabetes.

4 PREFIXES

Join the words in column B to their relative prefixes in column A to form words found in the text.

A	B
anti	immune
anti	agree
auto	sufficient
dis	vocation
dis	respond
in	functioning
in	engineered
in	bodies
mal	changed
over	capacitate
pre	converted
pro	histamines
re	dominant
un	effective
un	orders

5 NOUNS

Fill in the blanks with the nouns below as used in the text.

✓ condition   ✓ approach
✓ response   ✓ ingredient
✓ varieties   ✓ growth
✓ stages   ✓ supply
✓ reaction   ✓ techniques

a   a safe and more effective ....
b   gene-splicing ....
c   the prime .... of the vaccine
d   an insufficient .... of insulin
e   the explosive .... of molecular biology
f   it comes in at least 100 ....
g   a weak immune ....
h   a protective ....
i   three .... of life
j   a rare .... in which both B cells and T cells are lacking.

6 NOUNS FROM VERBS

Find nouns in the text that are formed from the following verbs.

e.g. to grow → growth.

Verb	Noun
✔ to suffer	
✔ to mutate	
✔ to provoke	
✔ to respond	
✔ to afflict	
✔ to inflame	
✔ to mark	
✔ to vaccinate	
✔ to react	
✔ to fail	
✔ to circulate	
✔ to arrive	
✔ to appear	

7

Join the *adjectives* in column 1 with *nouns* in column 2 to form expressions used in the text.

Column 1	Column 2
intestinal	sclerosis
bacterial	organisms
immunological	reactions
multiple	meningitis
nasal	cells
infectious	signals
cancerous	sprays
allergic	tract
chemical	decoys

8

Fill in the blanks with the following words and expressions as used in the text.

✔ for example
✔ seems
✔ as
✔ so
✔ also
✔ still
✔ each
✔ at least
✔ ever
✔ strengthened
✔ yet
✔ despite
✔ against
✔ because
✔ well

(1) .... such advanced techniques, it (2) .... tougher than (3) .... to create new vaccines. Some viruses, bacteria and parasites are so complex and (4) .... evolved in their defences (5) .... an immune reaction that no vaccine strategy has (6) .... been entirely effective. Flu viruses, (7) .... , mutate rapidly, continually changing their antigens in the process. (8) .... a result, an immune system (9) .... by a flu shot against last year's predominant strain of flu will probably not be helped by it this year. The common cold virus is (10) .... troublesome, (11) .... it comes in (12) .... 100 identifiable varieties. The parasite that causes malaria poses (13) .... other problems: it penetrates cells (14) .... quickly that it is hidden from antibodies. To complicate matters, it goes through three stages of life, displaying different antigens in (15) .... stage.

Notes

EXTENSION EXERCISES

9 ACTIVES TO PASSIVES

Turn the following *active* sentences into *passives*. Remember that it is not always necessary to repeat the agent.

e.g. active   They are testing the new vaccine.
   passive   The new vaccine *is being tested*.

1 They remove from the bug's surface the marker protein that provokes the immune response.

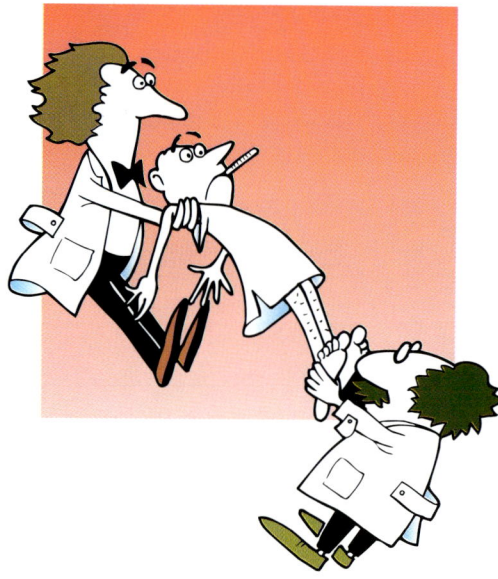

2 They mass-produce the antigen.

3 The parasite that causes malaria poses still other problems.

4 It can mount a speedy and lethal attack on helper T cells.

5 Scientists have synthesised bits of protein molecules.

6 A group in Paris has created one such vaccine.

7 These changes cause the inflammation and swelling.

8 Scientists are scrutinizing the AIDS virus.

10 IDIOMATIC EXPRESSIONS WITH *LOOK*

Study this sentence.

61 We're *looking at* a strong, well-evolved, well-designed organism.

Many idioms are also formed with the verb *TO LOOK*. Read the sentences in column 1. Follow each sentence with the most appropriate sentence from column 2.

Column 1	Column 2
1 You are as white as a sheet.	a Things are *looking* very black.
2 Don't rush into it.	b You *look* as if you've seen a ghost.
3 There is no sign of hope.	c He wanted *to look* the part.
4 The man had seen the fight, but he didn't want to get involved.	d He wanted *to look* his best.
5 He looks like an angel but he is really a terrible child.	e You should *look* before you leap.
6 When he became a doctor, he always wore his stethoscope round his neck.	f He always *looks* as if butter wouldn't melt in his mouth.
7 Jack is never fussy about his appearance.	g He pretended *to look* the other way.
8 As he was getting married the following week, Tom decided to buy himself a new suit.	h He always *looks* as if he has slept in his clothes for a week.

WANT+INDIRECT OBJECT

Study these examples.

a The verb want can be followed by *an object*.
   e.g. I want a job.

b It can be followed by *an infinitive*.
   e.g. I want to go.

c N.B. When the verb *want* is followed by an indirect object *do not* use a construction with that.

(wrong I want that you come.)

The correct construction is:
I want you to come.
AFFIRMATIVE
indirect object + infinitive with to

We didn't want him to go.
NEGATIVE
indirect object + infinitive with to

Did you want them to come?
INTERROGATIVE
indirect object + infinitive with to

 11 GRAMMAR CHECK

Now correct the following sentences. Correct the part *in italics*.

GRAMMAR POINT

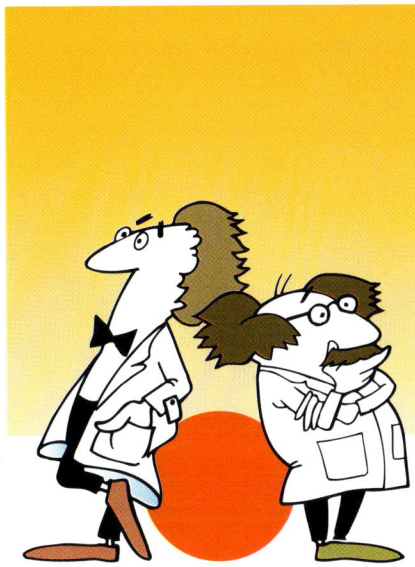

1 I wish it would stop raining. *I want that they go out.*
2 We are going to watch our team play on Saturday. *We want that they win.*
3 *She didn't want that we told you.*
4 John has been offered a good job. *I want that he accepts it.*
5 Barbara's father is a lawyer. *He wants that she becomes a lawyer too.*
6 *I want that you tell me the truth.*
7 *They wanted that she went to the cinema with them.*
8 *Everyone wanted that he told them about his experiences.*
9 *Do you want that I make some coffee?*
10 *We all wanted that it was the best holiday we had ever had.*

12 GRAMMAR CHECK

Translate the following sentences into your native language.

1 I want him to study molecular biology.
2 They want me to telephone them.
3 Does he want her to wait?
4 He wanted me to lend him my car.
5 Did you want us to begin?
6 She wanted him to scrutinize the results.

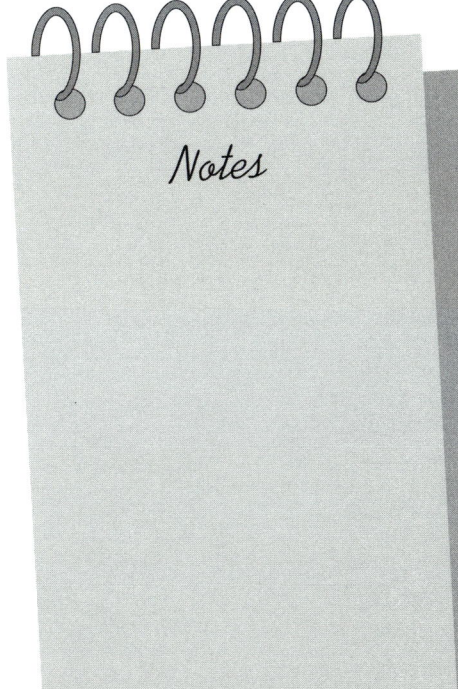

Notes

Study the following passages.

AIDS
WHAT EVERYBODY NEEDS TO KNOW

WHAT CAUSES AIDS?

AIDS is caused by a virus called HIV (previously called HTLV-III).

When you catch a virus, the virus makes its way into your blood. Certain white blood cells then
5 produce *antibodies* which attack and kill the virus. But when the HIV virus gets into the blood, it can actually destroy those white blood cells, leaving the body wide open to attack from other infections.

10 Anyone who has the HIV virus could pass the virus on to someone else. They could pass it on *either* if they have intimate sexual contact with another person, *or* if their infected blood gets into another person's body.

15 Experts think that up to 40,000 people in the UK may already have been infected with HIV.

But just because somebody gets HIV virus, it doesn't automatically follow that he or she will get AIDS. Of the 40,000 people in the UK
20 thought to have been infected with HIV virus, fewer than 600 had developed AIDS by the end of September 1986. Where this has happened, it has taken anything between 6 weeks and 5 years, and sometimes longer.

25 The majority of the 40,000 have remained fit and well. No-one yet knows why the HIV virus affects different people in such different ways.

Notes

VOCABULARY

8 wide
- fully

WHAT ARE THE SYMPTOMS OF AIDS?

When you begin to read this list of symptoms, you might start thinking, "Yes, I've got that ... and that ... and that. Oh, no ..., I must have AIDS ...." But remember:

5 ☐ AIDS is rare.

☐ It's only if you have many of these symptoms together and they last for a long time that AIDS might possibly be the cause.

☐ There can be lots of other reasons for nearly all
10 these symptoms. For example, swollen glands can be a sign of glandular fever. Tiredness, fever and weight loss are much more likely to be signs of worry or going without sleep, or a sign of flu coming on.

15 The symptoms which *may* suggest AIDS are:

Swollen glands, especially in the neck and armpits.

Profound fatigue, which lasts for several weeks, with no obvious cause.

20 **Unexpected weight loss** – more than 10 pounds (4.5 kg) in two months.

Fever and night sweats, lasting for several weeks.

Diarrhoea which lasts for more than a week, with no obvious cause.

25 **Shortness of breath and a dry cough** lasting longer than it would if it were just from a bad cold.

Skin disease – newly formed pink to purple blotches, appearing on the skin, including in the mouth or on the eyelids. They are usually hard,
30 and look a bit like a bruise or a blood blister.

Remember – some of these symptoms are very common, so don't jump to the conclusion that you have AIDS just because you have one of them. Being over-anxious about getting AIDS
35 could even cause some of the symptoms. But, if you *are* worried, talk it over with your own doctor ,

Notes

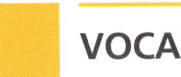

VOCABULARY

10 swollen
   - p.p. of swell
17 armpit
   - hollow under the arm where it joins the body
28 a blotch
   - a spot or discoloured mark on the skin
29 eyelids
   - lids or covers of the eyes
30 a bruise
   - a contusion; a discoloured lump
36 to talk over
   - to discuss

WRITING

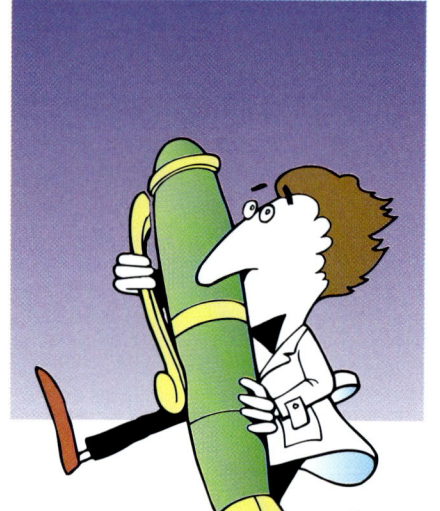

13

Explain the following sentence in your own words, "Just because somebody gets HIV virus, it doesn't automatically follow that he or she will get AIDS".

14

Describe, in your own words, the symptoms which may suggest AIDS.

Notes

SPEAKING

15 DOCTOR/PATIENT DIALOGUE

Work in groups.
Three patients ask their doctor questions. The doctor should try to answer their questions using simple terms.

Patient A asks why he needs a flu injection this year as he had one last year.

Patient B is an allergy sufferer. She wants to know why she has to take an antihistamine.

Patient C has a son who has AIDS. He wants to know why it is so difficult to find a vaccine.

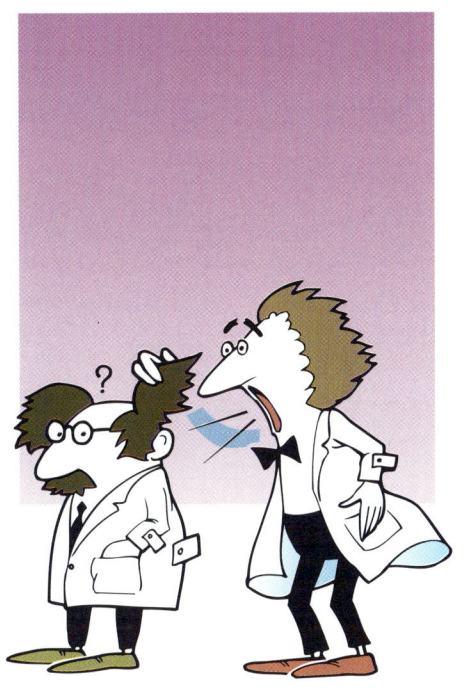

Notes

UNDERSTANDING IDIOMATIC ENGLISH

Explain the idiom.

He's got a skeleton
in the cupboard

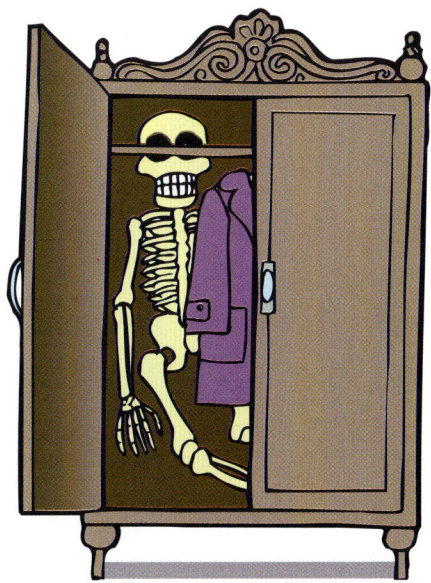

UNIT 21

Reverse genetics

Antisense RNA and DNA

Molecules that bind with specific messenger RNA's can selectively turn off genes. Eventually certain diseases may be treated with them; today antisense molecules are valuable research tools

by Harold M. Weintraub

It takes about 100,000 genes to make a human being. What exactly do they do, and how do they do it? To answer these questions, biologists must tinker with individual genes—in effect, remove or turn off the genes—and observe the effects on organisms or on individual cells. Studies of mutations have always afforded this information, but mutations are random by their nature, which has made systematic study of individual genes difficult (or, in the case of human beings and other complex and long-lived organisms, impossible).

With the recent advent of technology for cloning, or copying, genes during the past decade, it is now becoming realistic to think about selectively turning off or modifying the activity of any given gene. One method is—in principle—remarkably simple: create antisense RNA or DNA molecules that bind specifically with a targeted gene's RNA message, thereby interrupting the precise molecular choreography that expresses a gene as a protein. In this way viruses and bacteria regulate some genes during their life cycles. Today such an approach is practical enough for investigators to apply it to a broad range of problems.

The ability to deactivate specific genes holds great promise for medicine. For example, it may someday be possible to fight viral diseases with antisense RNA and DNA molecules

HAROLD M. WEINTRAUB is a member of the division of basic sciences at the Fred Hutchinson Cancer Research Center in Seattle. He received his Ph.D. from the University of Pennsylvania School of Medicine in 1971 and his M.D. in 1973. After completing his postdoctoral work at the Medical Research Council in Cambridge, England, he spent four years at Princeton University in the department of biochemical sciences. His current research interests are gene regulation and development.

that seek and destroy viral gene products inside a person's cells. Such applications are in their infancy. In the meantime antisense technology is contributing to the birth of a new field, reverse genetics. Classical genetics usually studies the random mutations of all genes in an organism and selects the mutations responsible for specific characteristics; reverse genetics starts with a cloned gene of interest and manipulates it to elicit information about its function.

The traditional genetic approach relies on chemicals or radiation to delete or alter genes randomly. The treated organisms or cells and their progeny can then be observed, and mutated individuals that display characteristics of interest to the experimenter can be studied. The genetic approach has been tremendously successful with microorganisms, some plants and some invertebrate animals. Nevertheless, it is poorly suited to studies of vertebrates. Vertebrates have inconveniently long generation times; they often have small numbers of offspring, which limits how quickly interesting mutants can be produced; and their most intriguing mutations are usually lethal and consequently difficult to propagate and study.

Another shortcoming of any genetic approach is that the observable effect of a mutation may not reveal precisely what the mechanism of the mutation is. For example, a mutation may first be detected as a microorganism's diminished ability to grow on a source of sugar. Is the mutation altering an enzyme that digests the sugar, or is it blocking the cell's uptake of the sugar? Is it perhaps activating enzymes that cause the sugar to be stored instead of digested? Genetics alone cannot provide the answer; genetics can identify the range of genes that influence a process, but additional approaches are often needed to probe exactly what a particular gene does. The new approach involving antisense

technology is one attempt to overcome some of these problems.

To understand how antisense technology works, it is first necessary to review the fundamentals of gene structure and expression. A gene is a coded blueprint for a protein; the code is written in the precisely ordered sequences of four nucleotide bases—adenine (A), thymine (T), guanine (G) and cytosine (C)—that make up molecules of DNA. In addition to the strong linking bonds that these bases can make within DNA strands, A's can form weak bonds with T's in other strands, and G's can form similar bonds with C's.

For this reason, DNA in organisms usually exists as a double helix, or duplex, consisting of two coiled DNA strands. In each duplex, a base on one strand is bound to its complementary base on the other strand; for example, a "sense" sequence that reads A-T-G-C-T-C on one strand pairs with an "antisense" sequence, T-A-C-G-A-G, on the other strand. The high specificity of base pairing is important during DNA replication, when the two complementary strands of each duplex separate: each strand serves as a template for reconstructing its partner, and the result is two identical duplexes.

Base-pairing specificity is also important when genetic information is decoded to make proteins. DNA does not make proteins directly; instead an intermediary molecule of RNA is created for the job. RNA is made of the same bases as DNA except that the base T is replaced by the base uracil (U), which can also pair with A. During transcription, the first stage of reading the genetic code, the sense strand of a gene separates from its antisense partner. Enzymes then assemble an RNA molecule that complements the sequence on the antisense DNA strand. This messenger RNA eventually migrates to cell structures called ribosomes, which read the encoded information and string together the appropriate amino acids to form the encoded proteins.

The antisense strand of DNA in the genes is the template for messenger RNA; the messenger RNA carries the structural code for a protein. But what of the sense DNA strand? Does it produce antisense RNA, and if so, what does this RNA do?

An important discovery about the natural biological function of antisense RNA molecules was made in 1981 by Jun-ichi Tomizawa at the National Institutes of Health (NIH). Tomizawa was studying the replication of a plasmid, or small double-strand ring of bacterial DNA, called ColE1. In this plasmid, DNA replication begins at a specific sequence called the origin. First the primer, a short chain of DNA, opens up the DNA double helix and hybridizes, or pairs, with the origin. The enzyme DNA polymerase then adds A's, T's, C's and G's to the RNA primer, constructing a new DNA strand that is complementary to the origin-containing strand. The number of copies made of the plasmid genetic material depends on the number of available RNA primers inside the cell.

Tomizawa discovered that the availability of RNA primers is controlled not by their total concentration but rather by the ratio of primers to specific inhibitor molecules. He went on to show that these inhibitors are RNA molecules transcribed from the DNA strand complementary to the one that produces the RNA primer. In other words, the inhibitors are the antisense products of the sense DNA strands.

Just as the sense and antisense DNA strands are complementary, so too are the sense RNA primers and the antisense inhibitor molecules. Consequently, the sense RNA and the antisense RNA can hybridize with one another. In this duplexed state, the RNA primer cannot initiate DNA replication, because it cannot pair with the origin of the plasmid.

The function of antisense RNA goes beyond regulation of DNA replication; it also extends to regulation of transcription. In 1983 Nancy E. Kleckner of Harvard University conducted a series of elegant experiments that described how antisense RNA in bacteria controls the synthesis of the enzyme transposase. During transcription, messenger RNA encoding the enzyme is produced from the transposase gene. When the bacteria also transcribe antisense RNA from the sense strand of the transposase gene, the antisense RNA binds specifically with the sense messenger RNA and prevents the ribosome from translating the encoded information into a protein.

Investigators have shown that regulation or inhibition of gene activity with antisense RNA seems to be universal among viruses and bacteria. The mechanism controls many stages of cell metabolism. There is some tentative evidence that antisense RNA may also have a natural role in more complex cells, but this has not yet been proved.

VOCABULARY

Study the meaning of the following words and expressions as used in the text.

1   takes
    - needs
5   to tinker
    - to try to improve, mend or alter
9   to afford
    - to give; to give up naturally
25 thereby
    - by that means
32 broad
    - with wide application
32 range
    - extent
35 to hold great promise
    - to give great reasons to hope; to show signs of future success
36 someday
    - one day in the future
41 infancy
    - (fig.) very early stages
53 to rely on
    - to depend on
54 to alter
    - to change
56 progeny
    - descendants
60 tremendously
    - immensely
63 to suit
    - to be appropriate
67 offspring
    - children
69 to intrigue
    - to fascinate

TEXT BASED EXERCISES

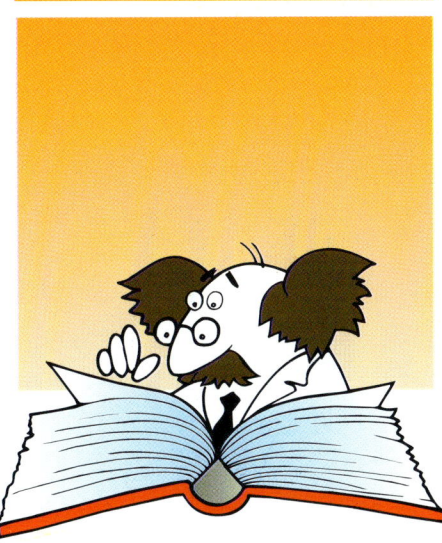

72 a shortcoming
    - a defect
77 to detect
    - to notice
81 uptake
    - intake; act of taking in
110 to coil
    - to move in spirals
121 a template
    - a mould
126 to decode
    - to translate from code
141 to encode
    - to put into code
142 to string
    - to link or join
177 ratio
    - proportion
214 inhibition
    - act of inhibiting; restraining the natural activity

218 tentative
    - proposed or done merely as a suggestion or experiment

1   COMPREHENSION

Write questions to which the following are the answers.

1   About 100,000.
2   It may someday be possible to fight viral diseases with antisense RNA and DNA molecules that seek and destroy viral gene products inside a person's cells.
3   No, such applications are still in their infancy.
4   Classical genetics usually studies the random mutations of all genes in an organism and selects the mutations responsible for specific characteristics; reverse genetics starts with a cloned gene of interest and manipulates it to elicit information about its function.
5   In order to probe exactly what a particular gene does.
6   As a duplex, consisting of two coiled DNA strands.
7   No, an intermediary molecule of RNA is created for the job.
8   The base thymine is replaced by the base uracil.
9   No, it also extends to regulation of transcription.
10 It prevents the ribosome from translating the encoded information into a protein.

2 WORD CHECK

Explain what you understand by the following expressions.

26 molecular choreography
30 life cycles
37 viral diseases
38 antisense RNA and DNA molecules
43 reverse genetics
53 radiation
141 ribosomes
197 transcription

3 ADJECTIVES

Fill in the blanks with the *adjectives* below as used in the text.

✔ systematic
✔ genetic
✔ classical
✔ observable
✔ long-lived
✔ mutated
✔ broad
✔ viral
✔ weak

a .... organisms
b .... diseases
c .... genetics

d .... bonds
e .... study
f .... individuals
g a .... range
h the .... approach
i the .... effect

4 NOUNS FROM VERBS

Find *nouns* in the text related to the verbs below.

Verb	Noun
to experiment	
to generate	
to originate	
to concentrate	
to inhibit	
to produce	
to discover	
to radiate	
to approach	
to express	
to transcribe	
to regulate	

5 OPPOSITES

Give the *opposite* of the following words using expressions found in the text.

✔ possible
✔ to turn on
✔ traditional
✔ systematic
✔ unrealistic
✔ short-lived
✔ death
✔ vertebrates
✔ strong
✔ complex

6 VERBS

Fill in the blanks with the *verbs* below in the form used in the text.

✔ seek
✔ initiate
✔ rely
✔ deactivate
✔ pair
✔ alter
✔ decode
✔ fight
✔ destroy
✔ hold

1 It may someday be possible .... viral diseases with antisense RNA and DNA

molecules that .... and .... viral gene products inside a person's cells.

2 The ability .... specific genes .... great promise for medicine.

3 In this duplexed state, the RNA primer cannot .... DNA replication, because it cannot .... with the origin of the plasmid.

4 The traditional genetic approach .... on chemicals or radiation to delete or .... genes randomly.

5 Base-pairing specificity is also important when genetic information is .... to make proteins.

7

Fill in the blanks with the words below as used in the text.

- ✓ contributing
- ✓ encoding
- ✓ cloning
- ✓ linking
- ✓ turning
- ✓ becoming
- ✓ pairing
- ✓ modifying
- ✓ copying
- ✓ reconstructing

1 In the meantime antisense technology is .... to the birth of a new field, reverse genetics.

2 The high specificity of base .... is important during DNA replication, when the two complementary strands of each duplex separate: each strand serves as a template for .... its partner, and the result is two identical duplexes.

3 In addition to the strong .... bonds that these bases can make within DNA strands, A's can form weak bonds with T's in other strands, and G's can form similar bonds with C's.

4 During transcription, messenger RNA .... the enzyme is produced from the transposase gene.

5 With the recent advent of technology for .... ,or .... ,genes during the past decade, it is now .... realistic to think about selectively .... off or .... the activity of any given gene.

8 PREPOSITIONS

Fill in the blanks with *prepositions* as used in the text.

1 During transcription, messenger RNA encoding the enzyme is produced .... the transposase gene.

2 Molecules that bind .... specific messenger RNA's can selectively turn .... genes.

3 The number .... copies made .... the plasmid genetic material depends .... the number .... available RNA primers .... the cell.

4 Investigators have shown that regulation or inhibition of gene activity .... antisense RNA seems to be universal .... viruses and bacteria.

5 .... this plasmid, DNA replication begins .... a specific sequence called the origin.

6 Tomizawa discovered that the availability of RNA primers is controlled not .... their total concentration but rather .... the ratio .... primers to specific inhibitor molecules.

7 The traditional genetic approach relies .... chemicals or radiation to delate or alter genes randomly.

8 Classical genetics usually studies the random mutations .... all genes an organism and selects the mutations responsible .... specific characteristics.

9 ASKING QUESTIONS WITH PERHAPS

EXTENSION EXERCISES

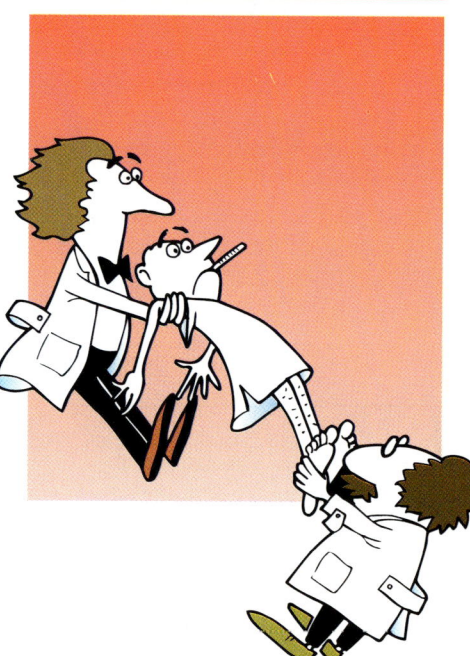

Note the use of the word *perhaps* in the following sentence.

82 Is it *perhaps* activating enzymes that cause the sugar to be stored instead of digested?

Comment on the following sentences. Use the *interrogative* form and the word *perhaps*. Complete the sentences in any suitable form.

e.g. John is very tired.
Is he *perhaps studying* too much?

1 Bill is standing outside the cinema.
2 There are a lot of grey clouds in the sky.
3 Their son failed all his exams but they still expect him to succeed.
4 Doctor Grant hasn't returned home yet.
5 They couldn't come to the party.
6 He won't be here this weekend.
7 She went to bed early.
8 Tony had a car accident.

Notes

WISH + PAST TENSE

Study the following sentence.

If I knew her address, I would visit her.
We can also say:
I wish I knew her address.

We use *wish* to say that we regret that something is *not* as we would like it to be.

N.B. We use *the past* for a present situation after wish.

e.g. I wish I *had* a job at the hospital.

10 GRAMMAR CHECK

Read the sentences below. Make sentences using an appropriate subject and the word *wish* as in the example. Make any changes necessary.

e.g. He smokes too much.
He wishes he didn't smoke so much.

1 I don't know her name.
2 They hate working late.
3 He has to go to the dentist.
4 She can't find a job.
5 They don't like travelling on crowded trains.
6 He doesn't have enough money to buy a new car.

GRAMMAR POINT

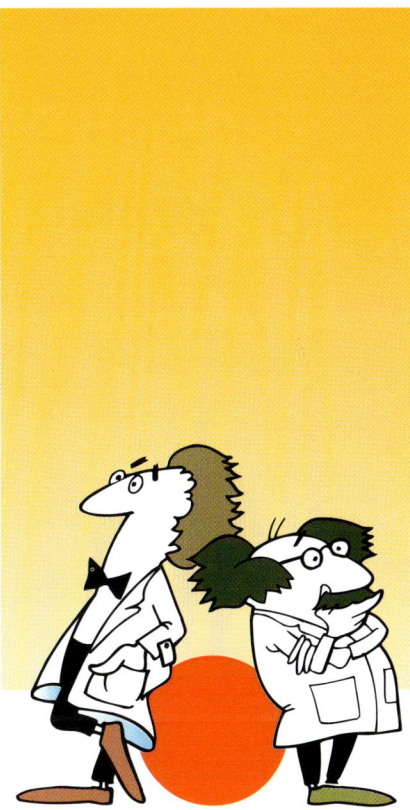

7 I must study tonight.
8 We have to start work very early in the morning.

11 GRAMMAR CHECK

We use *WISH* + *the PAST PERFECT* when we say that we regret something that happened or didn't happen *in the past*.

Read the sentences below. Make sentences in *the Past Perfect* using *wish*. Make any changes necessary.

e.g. I fell asleep in front of the T.V. and missed the end of the film.
I wish I hadn't fallen asleep and missed the end of the film.

1 I had an accident because I was driving too fast.
2 I forgot to post the letter this morning.
3 He didn't go to the doctor when the pain started.
4 I have never studied Russian.
5 We ate too much last night.
6 John didn't know about it.
7 House prices have gone up. I didn't buy my house when I had the chance.
8 I've got a cold. I went out yesterday when it was raining.

12 GRAMMAR CHECK

Translate the following sentences into your native language.

1 We wish we could visit you more often.
2 John wishes he didn't have to go to work today.
3 I wish it would stop snowing.
4 He wishes he could change his job.
5 I wish I knew where they had gone.

WRITING

13 EXPLAINING A PROCESS

Study the diagram below. Explain the processes in your own words. Use the following headings:

1 DNA Duplex.
2 Transcription.
3 RNA Duplex

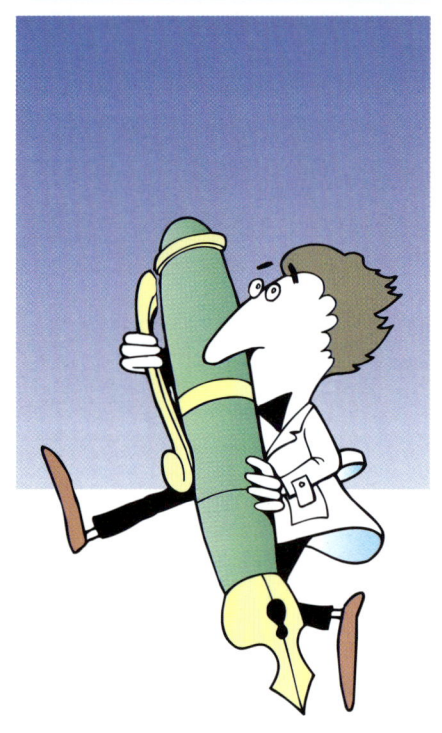

Notes

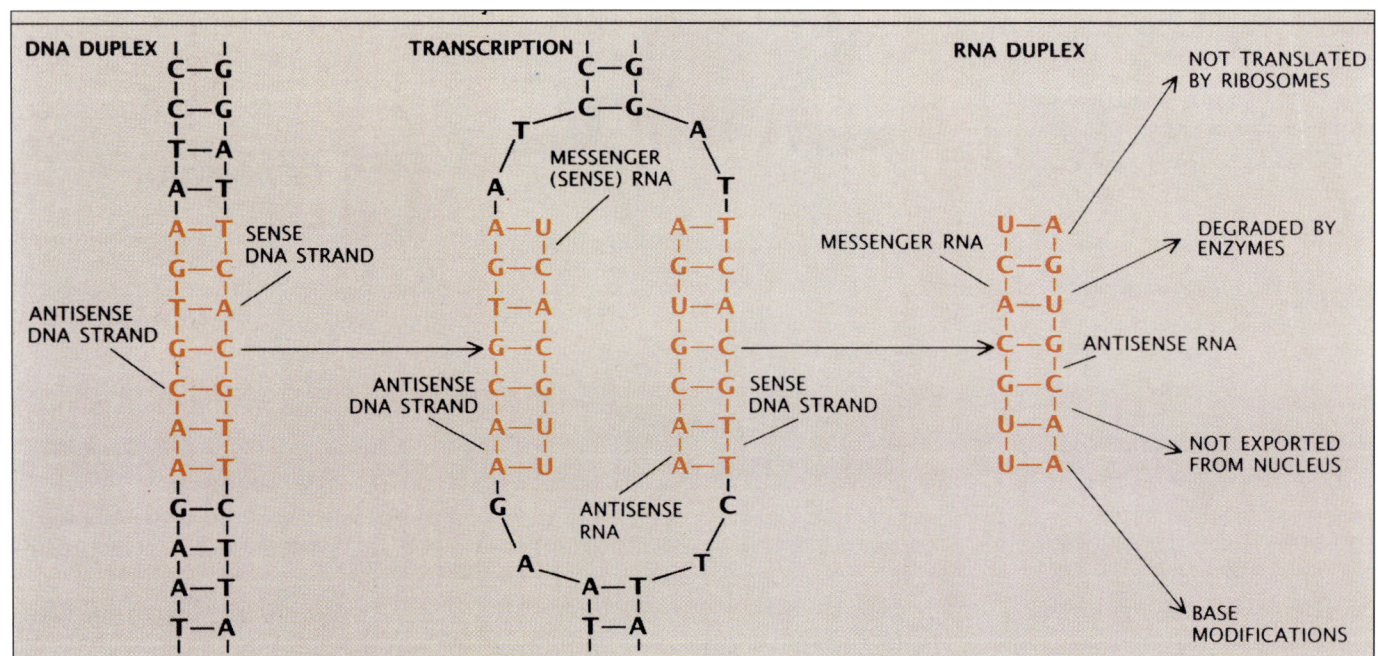

The Human Telomere

Although this specialized DNA cap at each end of the chromosome carries no genes, it is still valuable. Recent evidence indicates that chromosomes need their telomeres to survive

by Robert K. Moyzis

The Nobel laureate Hermann J. Muller proposed more than 50 years ago that the segments at the ends of chromosomes play a criti-
5 cal role in the cell. Before anyone knew that the DNA in chromosomes was double stranded and carried genes, he understood that the terminal material caps chromosomes to prevent their decay.
10 Muller also gave the tips a name: telomere, from the Greek (*telos* means end; *meros*, part).

For decades, little more was learned about the telomere. Then, roughly 10
15 years ago, investigators began to decipher its structure in various species. The composition of the human telomere, however, eluded discovery.

It is a mystery no longer. A few years
20 ago my colleagues and I at Los Alamos National Laboratory developed new research tools that enabled us to clone the human telomere, identify the sequence of its nucleotides (the building
25 blocks of DNA) and learn more about its three-dimensional structure and its function in the cell.

In the course of our experiments, we helped to confirm that the telomere,
30 which carries no genes, is vital to chromosomal survival. This result supports a growing awareness that gene-free regions of chromosomes often play critical roles in the cell, even though they
35 cannot specify the amino acid sequences of the body's proteins. (Proteins are vital to all life processes.) Clearly, investigators who want to understand how chromosomes and individual genes
40 function will have to identify the DNA sequences not only of genes but also of many nongenic regions. They will also have to determine how the various parts of a chromosome interact with
45 one another.

The cloning of the human telomere is already aiding that ambitious effort—by helping to advance the Human Genome Project in the U.S. and similar projects
50 elsewhere. These programs will map the entire human genome (the full complement of chromosomes in the cell), pinpointing the location of every gene. Just as assembling the edges of a jigsaw
55 puzzle simplifies the puzzle's completion, description of the ends of human chromosomes should facilitate completion of chromosomal maps. As the mapping progresses, researchers will un-
60 doubtedly uncover the genetic roots of many diseases and further clarify both how chromosomes direct development and how they ensure that cells operate properly.

ROBERT K. MOYZIS is director of the Center for Human Genome Studies at Los Alamos National Laboratory. He earned his Ph.D. in molecular biology from Johns Hopkins University, teaching there before moving to Los Alamos as genetics group leader in 1984. He accepted his current post in 1989. Moyzis is a member of the committees of the U.S. Department of Energy and the National Institutes of Health that are overseeing American efforts to map and sequence human chromosomes.

Notes

VOCABULARY

8 to cap
- to protect the end of; to put on a cap

9 decay
- decomposition; a gradual weakening

18 to elude
- to escape; to evade

50 elsewhere
- in other places

52 to pinpoint
- to locate with precision

54 edge
- outer extremity; border

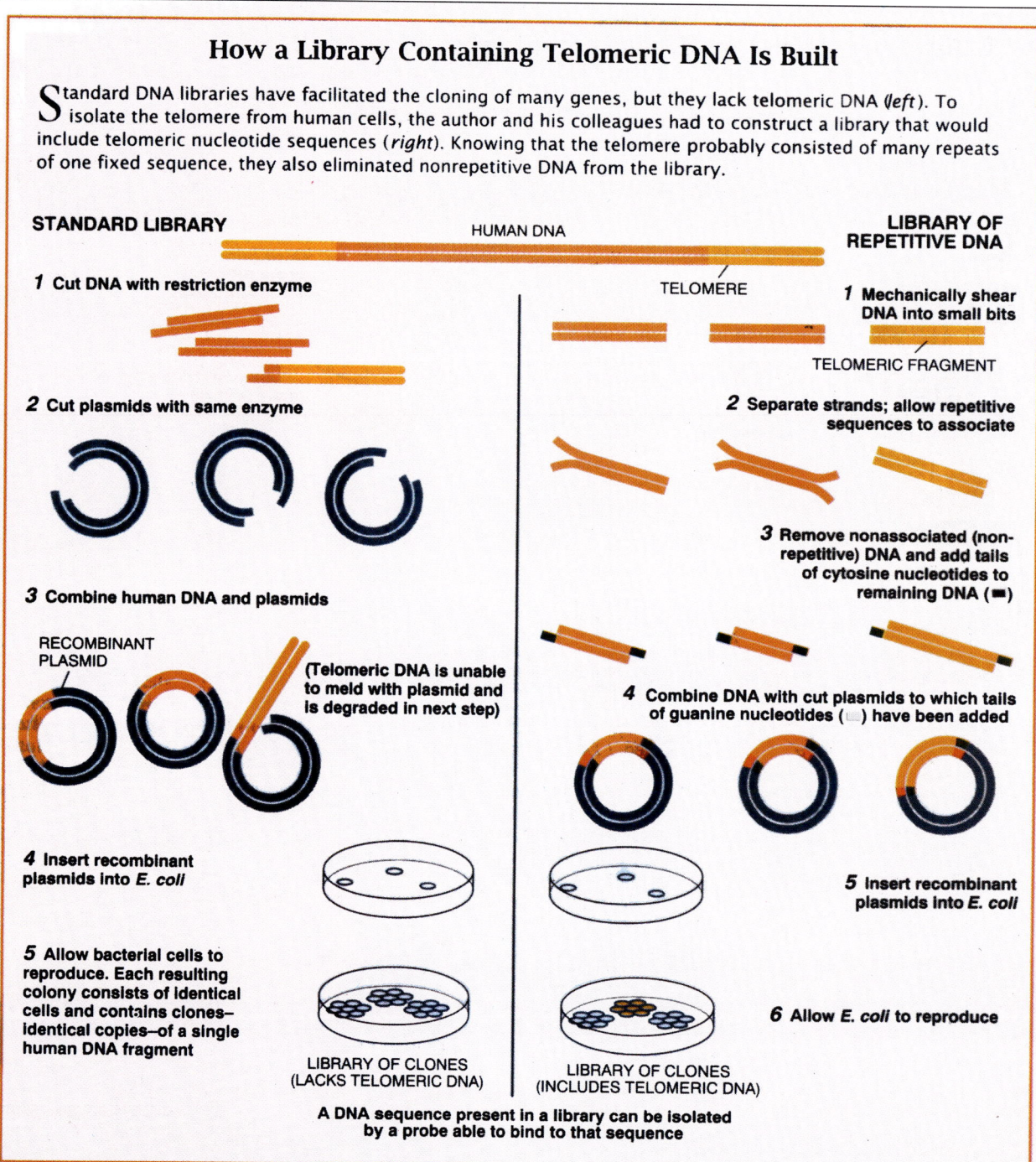

How a Library Containing Telomeric DNA Is Built

Standard DNA libraries have facilitated the cloning of many genes, but they lack telomeric DNA (*left*). To isolate the telomere from human cells, the author and his colleagues had to construct a library that would include telomeric nucleotide sequences (*right*). Knowing that the telomere probably consisted of many repeats of one fixed sequence, they also eliminated nonrepetitive DNA from the library.

STANDARD LIBRARY

HUMAN DNA

LIBRARY OF REPETITIVE DNA

TELOMERE

1 Cut DNA with restriction enzyme

1 Mechanically shear DNA into small bits

TELOMERIC FRAGMENT

2 Cut plasmids with same enzyme

2 Separate strands; allow repetitive sequences to associate

3 Remove nonassociated (nonrepetitive) DNA and add tails of cytosine nucleotides to remaining DNA (▬)

3 Combine human DNA and plasmids

RECOMBINANT PLASMID

(Telomeric DNA is unable to meld with plasmid and is degraded in next step)

4 Combine DNA with cut plasmids to which tails of guanine nucleotides (▭) have been added

4 Insert recombinant plasmids into *E. coli*

5 Insert recombinant plasmids into *E. coli*

5 Allow bacterial cells to reproduce. Each resulting colony consists of identical cells and contains clones—identical copies—of a single human DNA fragment

6 Allow *E. coli* to reproduce

LIBRARY OF CLONES (LACKS TELOMERIC DNA)

LIBRARY OF CLONES (INCLUDES TELOMERIC DNA)

A DNA sequence present in a library can be isolated by a probe able to bind to that sequence

SPEAKING

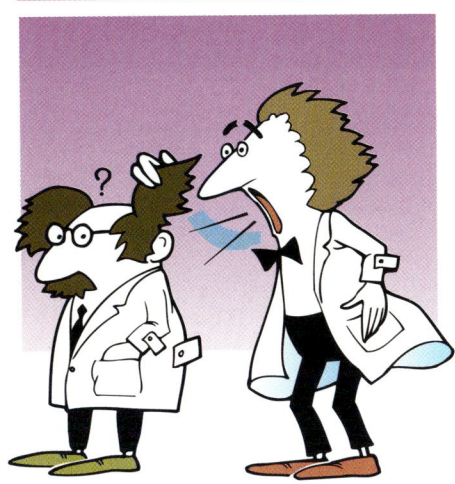

14 TELOMERES

Explain the importance of the human telomere. The words below will help you.

Muller - proposed - more than 50 years ago - the segments - ends of chromosomes - a critical role in the cell.

He - understood - terminal material caps chromosomes - decay.

Muller - name - telomere.

Roughly 10 years ago - investigators - decipher - structure - composition - however - eluded.

Dr. Moyzis and his colleagues - new research tools - clone human telomere - nucleotides - three - dimensional structure.

Course of experiments - confirm - no genes - telomere - vital - chromosome survival.

Supports - gene-free regions of chromosomes - critical roles - even though - cannot - amino acid sequences - body proteins.

Investigators - understand - chromosomes and genes - identify DNA sequence - genes - nongenic regions.

Cloning the human telomere - aiding - Human Genome Project in U.S. - similar projects elsewhere.

These projects - map - entire human genome - pinpointing - location - every gene.

UNDERSTANDING IDIOMATIC ENGLISH

Explain the idiom.

He's got pins
and needles in his feet

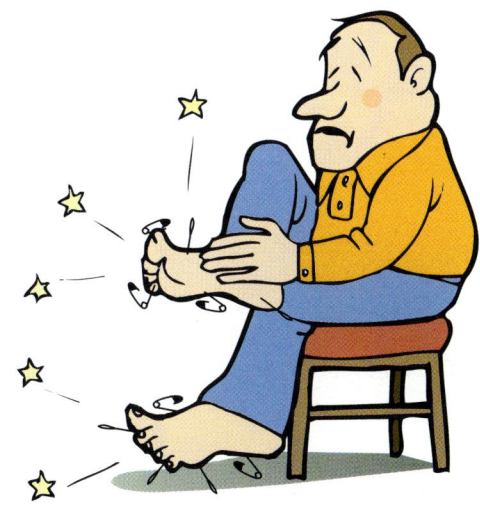

UNIT 22

*Report on smoking raises
new worries*

A Not-So-Happy Anniversary

The Surgeon General's report on smoking raises new worries

Many people look back on Jan. 11, 1964, as a pivotal date in their lives. On that day U.S. Surgeon General Luther Terry warned about the deadly dangers of tobacco in a blockbuster report. Frightened smokers promptly resolved to give up the habit; some scared souls stubbed out cigarettes on the spot. Last week the Federal Government marked the 25th anniversary of that first alarm with a new Surgeon General's report that charts the progress in the war against tobacco. The past quarter-century has seen "a revolution in smoking behavior," declared C. Everett Koop, the current Surgeon General. "In the 1940s and '50s, smoking was chic; now, increasingly, it is shunned." But, he continued, tobacco is still "the single most important preventable cause of death, responsible for 1 out of every 6 deaths in the U.S."

The most disturbing news in the 679-page report was the assertion that smoking has exacted a heavier toll in death and disease than had previously been thought. Among the findings:

▶ Tobacco claims 390,000 lives a year, 90,000 more than earlier estimates. Two-thirds of those deaths result from cardiovascular disease, lung cancer and chronic respiratory ailments like emphysema. The average male smoker is 22 times as likely to die from lung cancer as is a nonsmoker, double the previous risk estimate.

▶ For the first time, the Government has concluded that smoking is a major cause of stroke, accounting for an estimated 26,500 deaths a year. Half of all strokes in people under 65 stem from smoking.

▶ While the incidence of lung cancer has been leveling off for men, it has been rising among women. The report cites the American Cancer Society's estimate that lung cancer has surpassed breast malignancies as the second leading cause of death among women. "Women took up smoking in large numbers about three decades after men did so," explained Koop. "We can envision the catastrophic epidemic of lung cancer that is likely to occur among women in the coming years."

On the bright side, the U.S. has made substantial strides in curtailing cigarette use. Only 29% of adults now light up, down from 40% in 1965. The biggest decline has been among men: 50% smoked in 1965, less than a third today. Nearly half of all living adults who have ever smoked have quit—at least for a while. But the progress has not been spread equally over various groups in the population. Smoking among blacks and blue-collar workers is higher than average. Level of education is the best predictor of tobacco use: the more years of schooling people have, the less likely they are to smoke.

Cigarette use was declining among teenagers, but has now leveled off. Chil-

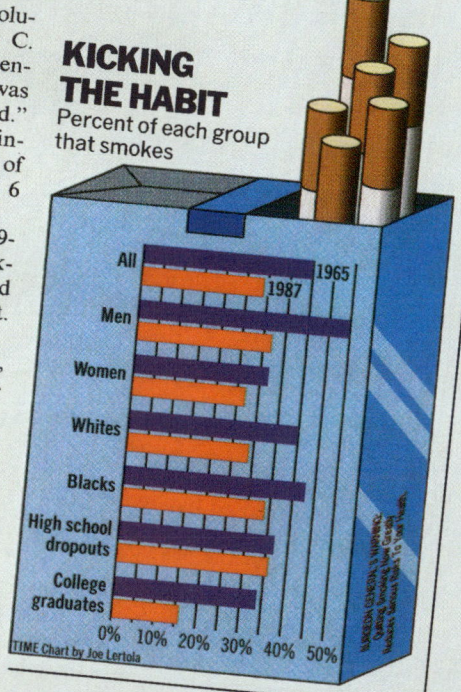

KICKING THE HABIT
Percent of each group that smokes

1965
1987

All
Men
Women
Whites
Blacks
High school dropouts
College graduates

0% 10% 20% 30% 40% 50%

TIME Chart by Joe Lertola

dren, especially girls, are taking up tobacco at a younger age. Among high school seniors who have ever smoked, a quarter took their first puff by the sixth grade and half by the eighth. Restrictions on children's access to cigarettes have weakened; many stores routinely ignore minimum-age-of-purchaser laws.

The tobacco industry, used to harsh reports from the Surgeon General, tried to blunt the latest attack with newspaper ads saying that "enough is enough." Said Brennan Dawson, a spokeswoman for the Tobacco Institute: "The report represents an escalation in the antismoking campaign." Surgeon General Koop certainly hopes so. His stated goal is to make the U.S. a "smoke-free society by the year 2000."

—By Anastasia Toufexis.
Reported by Dick Thompson/Washington

VOCABULARY

Study the meaning of the following words and expressions as used in the text.

2 pivotal
   - as or like a pivot; central; vital

7 a soul
   - (coll.) a person

17 to shun
   - to avoid

23 to assert
   - to declare to be true

24 to exact
   - to demand; to extort

24 a toll
   - (fig.) a loss

31 an ailment
   - an illness; an affliction

32 average
   - ordinary

45 to surpass
   - to exceed

50 to envisage
   - to visualize

54 bright
   - positive

55 a stride
   - a long step

55 to curtail
   - to diminish

75 a puff
   - a short jet of air or smoke

78 a store
   - a large shop

80 harsh
   - hard; severe

82 to blunt (fig.)
   - to make less sensitive or acute

TEXT BASED EXERCISES

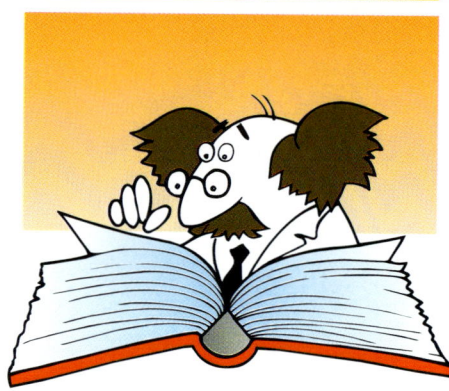

1 WORD CHECK

Explain the following expressions in your own words.

title a not-so-happy anniversary
   4 the deadly dangers of tobacco
   5 a blockbuster report
   8 on the spot
   16 in the 1940's and 50's
   17 chic
   22 disturbing news
   52 the coming years
   61 for a while
   83 enough is enough
   89 a smoke-free society

2 WORD CHECK

Explain the meaning of the following verbs. Give a sentence for each in your own words. Use any suitable tense.

1 to look back
6 to give up
7 to stub out
40 to stem from
42 to level off
47 to take up
56 to light up

3 COMPREHENSION

Correct the following statements.

1 The U.S. Surgeon General Luther Terry issued a short report warning about the dangers of smoking.
2 Smoking behavior has remained the same in the last twenty-five years.
3 Smoking is responsible for 1 out of every 10 deaths in the U.S.
4 Tobacco was previously estimated to have claimed 90,000 lives a year.
5 The average male smoker is twice as likely to die from lung cancer as a nonsmoker.
6 The incidence of lung cancer has been rising among men.
7 Only 40% of adults now smoke in the U.S.
8 Nearly all living adults who have ever smoked have stopped, at least for a while.
9 Race is the best predictor of tobacco use.
10 Cigarette use is now declining among teenagers.

4 NOUNS FROM VERBS

Find *nouns* in the text that are formed from the following verbs.

Verb	Noun
to ail	
to restrict	
to populate	
to attack	
to assert	
to campaign	
to purchase	
to school	
to puff	
to escalate	

5

Fill in the blanks with the words below as used in the text.

✓ estimated	✓ malignancies
✓ estimate	✓ cause
✓ estimates	✓ thirds
✓ cancer	✓ respiratory
✓ time	✓ all
✓ times	✓ incidence
✓ nonsmoker	✓ smoker
✓ rising	✓ cardiovascular
✓ leading	

Tobacco claims 390,000 lives a year, 90,000 more than earlier (1) .... Two (2) .... of those deaths result from (3) .... disease, lung (4) .... and chronic (5) .... ailments like emphysema. The average male (6) .... is 22 (7) .... as likely to die from lung cancer as is a (8) .... , double the previous risk estimate.
For the first (9) .... , the Government has concluded that smoking is a major (10) .... of stroke, accounting for an (11) .... 26,500 deaths a year. Half of (12) .... strokes in people under 65 stem from smoking.
While the (13) .... of lung cancer has been leveling off for men, it has been (14) .... among women. The report cites the American Cancer Society's (15) .... that lung cancer has surpassed breast (16) .... as the second (17) .... cause of death among women.

6 PREPOSITIONS

Fill in the blanks with a *preposition* as used in the text.

1 Last week the Federal Government marked the 25th anniversary .... that first alarm .... a new Surgeon General's report that charts the progress .... the war .... tobacco.

2 "........... the 1940's and '50's, smoking was chic; now, increasingly, it is shunned".

3 Tobacco is still "the single most important preventable cause .... death, responsible .... I .... every 6 deaths .... the U.S.".

4 .... the bright side, the U.S. has made substantial strides .... curtailing cigarette use.

5 Only 29% .... adults now light ...., ... 40% .... 1965.

6 Nearly half .... all living adults who have ever smoked have quit - .... least .... a while.

7 But the progress has not been spread equally .... various groups .... the population.

8 .... high school seniors who have ever smoked, a quarter took their first puff .... the sixth grade and half .... the eighth.

9 The report represents an escalation .... the antismoking campaign.

10 His stated goal is to make the U.S. a "smoke-free society .... the year 2000".

EXTENSION EXERCISES

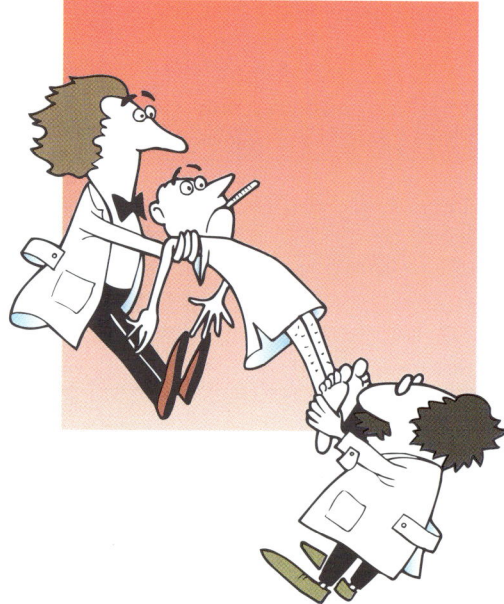

7

Study this sentence.

22 The most disturbing news in the 679-page report was the assertion that smoking has exacted a heavier toll in death and disease *than had previously been thought.*

Change the following sentences. Begin with the words in brackets and complete the sentence with *than had previously been thought.*

e.g. Many people have been influenced by the report. (More people)
More people have been influenced by the report *than had previously been thought.*

1 Tobacco has claimed 390,000 lives a year. (More lives)
2 Many high school students have started smoking. (More high school students)
3 Some people have stopped smoking. (More people)
4 The U.S. has made strides in the antismoking campaign. (More strides)
5 Many men have given up smoking. (More men)
6 A lot of reports have been written. (More reports)
7 Many women have taken up smoking. (More women)
8 Children are smoking at a younger age. (More children)

8 I THINK SO
I DON'T THINK SO
EXPECT/SUPPOSE

Study this sentence.

85 "The report represents an escalation in the antismoking campaign."
Surgeon General Koop certainly *hopes so.*

SO is used in this way after certain verbs e.g. think, expect, hope, suppose, be afraid.
The negative form depends on the verb used.

affirmative	negative
I think so	I don't think so
I expect so	I don't expect so
I hope so	I hope not
I'm afraid so	I'm afraid not
I suppose so	I don't suppose so *or* I suppose not

Answer each of the following questions in the first person singular. Use one of the above expressions as indicated in brackets.

e.g. Is he Italian? (think, affirmative)
I think so.
Is he coming? (expect, negative)
I don't expect so.

1 Is he a good doctor? (think, affirmative)
2 Are they going to London? (suppose, affirmative)
3 Are we going to fail the exam? (hope, negative)
4 Did she get the job? (afraid, negative)
5 Will Jack be late? (expect, affirmative)
6 Does he like skiing? (think, negative)
7 Are they going to the conference? (suppose, negative)
8 Is Mary coming tonight? (expect, negative)
9 Are you going to pass your driving test? (hope, affirmative)
10 Is he in pain? (afraid, affirmative)

9 COMPARATIVES

Study the chart that indicates the percentage of each group that smokes. Make comparative sentences using *more* or *less*. Use the words "*than in*" and the years 1965 and 1987 as in the examples below.

e.g. More men
More men smoked in 1965 *than in* 1987.
Less women
Less women smoked in 1987 *than in* 1965.

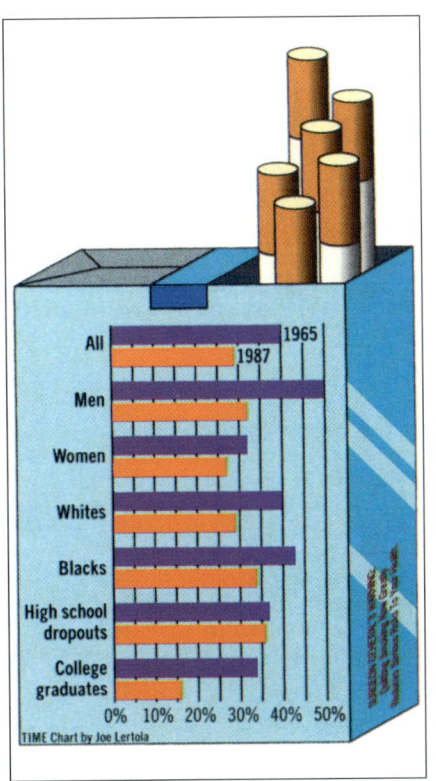

TIME Chart by Joe Lertola

1 More college graduates.
2 More whites.
3 Less men.
4 Less blacks.
5 More high school dropouts.
6 Less college graduates.
7 More women.
8 Less high school dropouts.
9 Less whites.
10 More blacks.

10 COMPARATIVES

Study this sentence.

67 The more years of schooling people have, *the less likely they are* to smoke.

Complete the following sentences in your own words using the expressions *the more likely they are* or *the less likely they are*.

e.g. The more people exercise regularly ....
The more people exercise regularly, *the more likely they are to be fit.*
The more people exercise regularly, *the less likely they are to be unfit.*

a The more people eat ....

b The less alcohol people drink ....

c The less sleep children get ....

d The more the students study ....

e The less people smoke ....

f The more free time people have ....

g The more researchers know about the AIDS virus ....

11

Study this sentence.

8 Last week the Federal Government marked *the 25th anniversary* of that first alarm with a new Surgeon General's report that charts the progress in the war against tobacco.

Now *read aloud* the following expressions.

a Our 29th test.
b The 18th result.
c The 6th attempt.
d His 21st birthday party.
e Your 4th application.
f Their 2nd wedding anniversary.
g The 15th time.
h Her 3rd case.

USED TO/ TO BE USED TO

Be careful not to confuse *USED TO* with *TO BE USED TO*. They are different in both structure and meaning.

Study these examples.

1   *I wasn't used to giving* injections until I started working at the clinic.
2   *I used to give* injections in my previous job. Now I don't.

The meaning is different.

a   *I'm used to* means that something is not new to me. I have often done it and now I am accustomed to it.
b   *I used to* (no verb to be) means that I did something regularly in the past but I don't do it now.

The structure is different.

a   *I used to*

    e.g.   *I used to live* in Manchester.
          used + infinitive with to

In this example *used* is a verb and *to* is part of the following infinitive

b   *I'm used to*

    e.g.   *I'm used to living* in Manchester.
          verb to be + used + to + gerund

In this example *used* is an adjective and *to* is a preposition.

GRAMMAR POINT

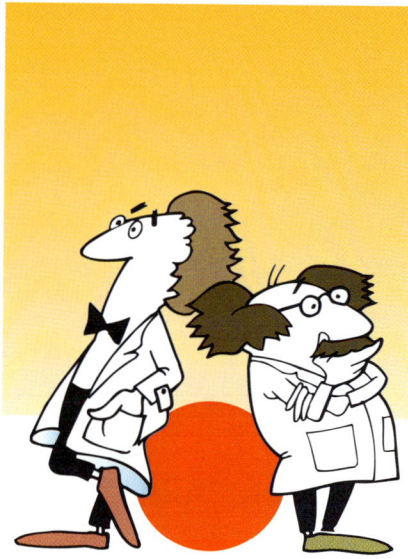

This form can also be followed by a noun or pronoun.

    e.g.   I'm used to the work.
          I'm used to it.

Get may also be used with this form.

    e.g.   You'll soon *get* used to it.

12 GRAMMAR CHECK

Fill in the blanks with a suitable *verb* in the correct form.

When I was a child I used to .... of becoming a doctor. Every night, I used to .... in bed and picture myself in a white coat. I used .... very hard at school. I was used to .... very hard at school. I used to .... hard, so when I went to university it wasn't a problem. I used to .... up at half past six every morning in order to catch the 7.15 bus. I never really got used to .... up so early. I always used to .... at my lectures still half asleep.
Now I am a doctor, I am used to .... irregular hours. Before specializing in surgery, I used to .... in the Casualty Department. I wasn't used to .... on shifts. In the beginning it was difficult but now I'm used to it.

13 GRAMMAR CHECK

Translate the following sentences into your native language.

1   I'm used to reading scientific articles.
2   You used to live in London, didn't you?
3   Jack used to like his job, but now he's bored.
4   He's used to solving difficult problems.
5   They used to work a lot less.

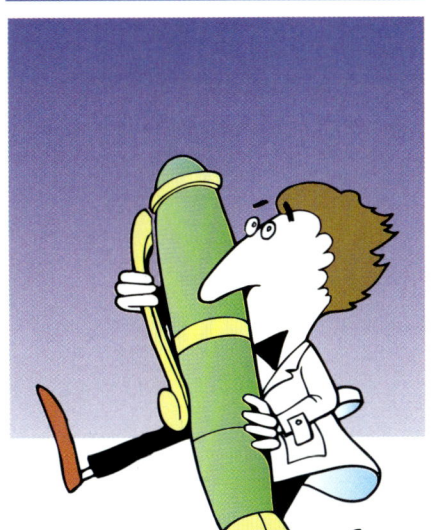

WRITING

14 REPORT ON SMOKING

Write a short summary of the text. The words below will help you.

The past quarter-century - a revolution - smoking behavior.
Chic.
Shunned.
Single - preventable cause - I out of 6 deaths - U.S.

Disturbing news - 679 page report.
390,000 lives a year - 90,000 more - earlier estimates.
Major cause of stroke.
Leveling off for men.
Rising among women.
29% of adults - down from 40% - 1965.
Level of education.
Children - especially girls.

Notes

Study the following article.

A Patch of Hope for Smokers

U.S. doctors will soon begin prescribing a new nicotine device that can help people stay off cigarettes for good

5 Smoking is complex. Just ask the 50 million Americans who continue to do it despite abundant evidence that as a diversion its safety ranks somewhere between bungee jumping and Russian roulette. 10 For the past decade, addiction researchers have struggled to sort through the tangle of biological urges and psychological cravings that stir people to light up, in an attempt to develop better ways to kick the habit. That 15 effort is finally beginning to bear fruit.

Over the next few months, four drug companies will introduce similar versions of a transdermal nicotine patch, a palm-size 20 circular envelope that, when applied to the upper arm or back every 24 hours, releases a steady stream of nicotine into the blood. 25 A study in last week's *Journal of the American Medical Association* found that the patch, when administered with proper counseling, doubled the odds that smokers will successfully quit over a six-30 month period. "It's a major breakthrough in medicine by any measure. It could save thousands of lives," said Dr. Jack Henning-35 field, chief of clinical pharmacology at the U.S. National Institute on Drug Abuse.

The idea of using pure nicotine to help smokers stop was first 40 tried in the mid-1980s with the nicotine-laced chewing gum Nicorette. The drug provides relief from the symptoms of physical withdrawal—anxiety, difficulty 45 concentrating—so that people can focus on the behavioral side of their addiction. But Nicorette has proved disappointing, largely because heavy smokers have trouble getting a sufficient dose to 50 match their craving. In addition, the gum can cause soreness in the mouth and upset stomach. Patches overcome these shortcomings by steadily pumping the drug directly into the bloodstream. After a month 55 of daily use, ex-smokers wean themselves from the nicotine by applying successively smaller patches.

But experts caution that the device will work only when combined with coun-60 seling, which should include advice on setting a "quit date" and on coping with the urges that will persist even with the patch in place. Unfortunately, physicians in the U.S. have a poor record in this regard.

65 Less than half of 2,700 smokers surveyed for a study in last week's *Journal* said their doctors had ever advised them to kick the habit or even to cut down.

Moreover, scientists are only beginning 70 to understand the factors that drive cigarette addiction. A smoker can take a million puffs during a lifetime, and each of those

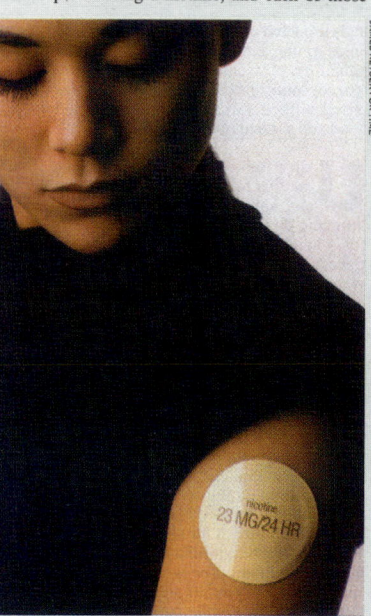

Nicotine is absorbed through the skin

becomes indelibly linked with a particular activity—drinking coffee, talking on the 75 phone, driving. In his recent book, *Smoking: The Artificial Passion*, David Krogh writes, "Addiction and attachment, pharmacology and behavior, personality, culture and genetics all chase each other around 80 like a cat after its own tail when we start to consider the issue of why people smoke."

Inevitably, the new patch will not be able to cure most smokers. According to last week's report, 26% of those wearing 85 the device actually succeeded in abstaining for six months, as opposed to 12% of those using a placebo patch. Still, for smokers the choice seems clear: a 1 in 4 chance of quitting successfully, or the same odds of 90 dying of a tobacco-related disease if they do not.
—By Andrew Purvis

JAMES KEYSER FOR TIME

VOCABULARY

2 **to stay off**
- not to eat, drink, smoke etc. things which, if taken in excess, may be bad for one's health

2 **for good**
- permanently

6 **to rank**
- to classify

10 **a tangle**
- a confused, twisted mass of threads

11 **a craving**
- an intense desire

11 **to stir**
- to set in movement

14 **to bear**
- to produce

40 **to lace**
- to flavour

43 **to withdraw**
- to draw back

50 **soreness**
- state of being painful

52 **steadily**
- in a steady way; regular; constant

54 **to wean**
- (fig.) to cause to break away from an attachment

57 **to caution**
- to warn

67 **to cut down**
- to reduce

SPEAKING

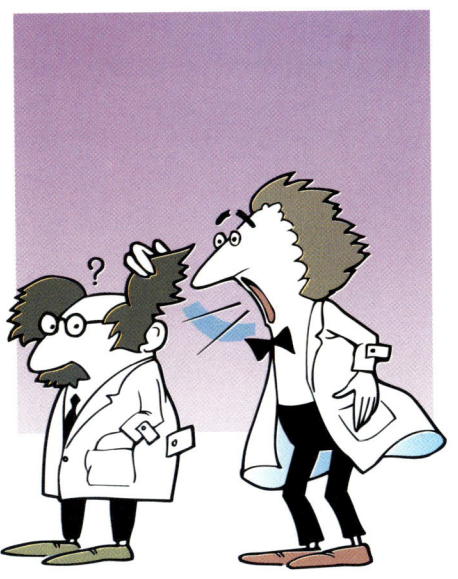

15 TRANSDERMAL NICOTINE PATCH

Explain, in your own words, how the transdermal nicotine patch works and how it will help smokers who are trying to give up the habit.

16 DOCTOR/PATIENT DIALOGUE

Work in pairs.
Coduct the following doctor/patient dialogue.

A heavy smoker comes to ask his doctor how to give up smoking. The doctor should try to give him some practical suggestions.

UNDERSTANDING IDIOMATIC ENGLISH

Explain the idiom.

> He's got eyes in
> the back of his head

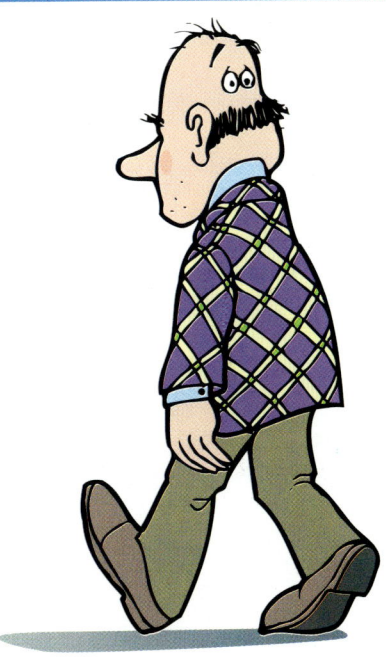

UNIT 23

Training the mind
but neglecting the body

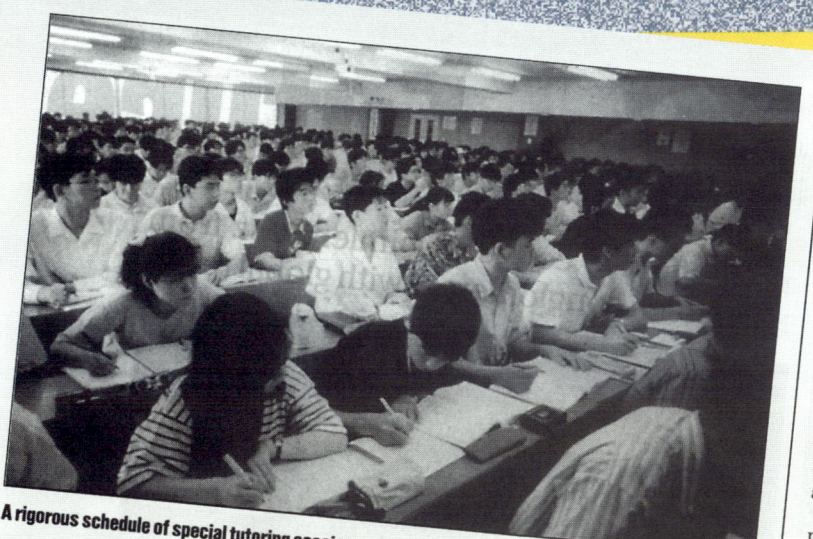

A rigorous schedule of special tutoring sessions: *Cramming for university entrance exams*

JOE McNALLY—SYGMA

The Out-of-Shape Generation

All study, no play is making Japanese kids flabby

Kensuke Suzuki, a 17-year-old Japanese high-school student, hears the same gripes from his classmates every day. "They tell each other how tired they are or complain about a backache," he says. "It's almost like being in an old folks' home." Makoto Hirai, a Tokyo pediatrician for 34 years, notices that his young patients seem to break bones much more often these days. "In the old days when kids ran wild, they did break bones," Dr. Hirai says. "But now the fractures tend to come from just missing a step on the staircase. They don't move their bodies. They don't use their muscles."

The minds of Japanese children benefit from one of the world's most rigorous educational systems, but their bodies are woefully neglected, according to a recently released report by a Japanese professor. Takeo Masaki of Nippon College of Physical Education surveyed 1,231 schools, ranging from nursery schools to high schools, and found pupils yawning in class and complaining about fatigue. Teenagers suffered from stiff shoulders and backaches. Allergies were on the upswing, eyesight was deteriorating. Masaki also found indications that today's youngsters are more passive than those of previous generations. For ex-

ample, 41.3 percent of 193 kindergarten teachers throughout Japan noticed that children tend to fall on their faces, instead of sticking their hands out to protect themselves when confronted with a potential danger.

Textbooks and television: Masaki blames postwar prosperity for the decline in physical fitness. The allergies are probably the result of industrial pollution, changes in diet and food additives, he says. More significant is the lack of exercise. Today's Japanese children are slaves to their studies. The schedule of Nobuo, a 15-year-old from Yokohama, is not atypical: he attends

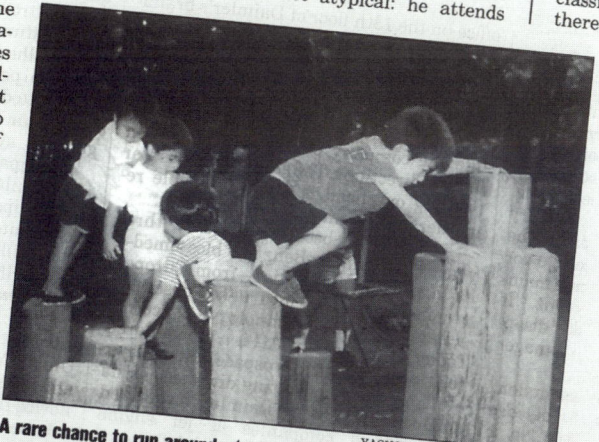

A rare chance to run around: *At Hanegi Playpark in Tokyo*

YASUO KOBAYASHI—NEWSWEEK

school from 8:30 a.m. to 3:30 p.m., joins such afterclass activities as amateur radio until 6 o'clock and then rushes on to a cram school that ends at 9:30. After dinner, there's homework to do—if his mother can keep him awake. "Their days and hours are scheduled between schools and special tutoring sessions. And even when they find a little time to spare, they just stare at a TV screen till the wee hours," Masaki says. That's why they end up yawning the next day in class. He also points out the drastic change in the role of children in Japanese families. "In the old days, children had to help around the house cleaning, washing and carrying things," Masaki says. "It helped to build their back-muscle strength. Now they may study, but they just don't do any of these house chores."

Urban trap: There's literally no room for play in modern Japan. Urban children live in concrete jungles without open space to run around. In Tokyo, there are only 2.5 square meters of park space for every person, compared with 45.7 square meters in Washington and 19.2 square meters in New York. Even in the little outdoor space that's available, kids must abide by a plethora of restrictive rules: No ball playing. No bicycling. No tree climbing. The housing situation contributes to the problem: paper-thin walls mean that kids have to be quiet or the neighbors will complain. So parents buy high-tech toys like Nintendo or rent video movies to keep the noise down. If the youngsters are not glued to the tube, they're stuck to their books. Even in largely rural Shizuoka Prefecture, a recent survey found that only 60 percent of the children played outside an hour a day.

The Education Ministry says that there is a limit to what schools can do to solve the problem. Most elementary and junior high schools offer three hours of physical education a week; administrators say that the classroom curriculum is so demanding that there isn't time for more. Masaki suggests that schools and parents take their children to the country and let them run around for a few days. Some city dwellers have also begun to set up special "playparks" for young children. At Hanegi Playpark in Tokyo on a recent afternoon, children were happily running around, inventing their own games while their mothers presided over a cookout. Unless Japanese youngsters spend a lot more time in playparks and much less time in front of the tube, warns Dr. Hirai, they will come in two varieties: fat, and skinny with a big head. "Give them a slight push," he says, "and both will fall."

HIDEKO TAKAYAMA *in Tokyo*

VOCABULARY

Study the meaning of the following words and expressions as used in the text.

1 flabby
- hanging loose; weak
21 woefully
- miserably
25 to survey
- to inspect and assess
31 stiff
- rigid
33 upswing
- increase
41 to stick out
- to push forward
44 to blame
- to accuse; to find fault with
47 to pollute
- to contaminate; to make dirty
55 to cram
- to study intensively for an examination
55 to rush
- to move rapidly
57 homework
- work to be done by pupils after school hours
61 time to spare
- free time after work is done
62 wee
- small
64 to point out
- to indicate; to call attention to
71 a chore
- a small domestic task
74 concrete
- a mixture of water, sand, stone and cement, used in building
80 a plethora
- a superabundance
80 to abide by
- to do as asked
89 to stick (stuck p.t.)
- to remain attached
103 to dwell (dwellers n.)
- to reside
114 the tube
- (coll.) the television
117 skinny
- very thin

TEXT BASED EXERCISES

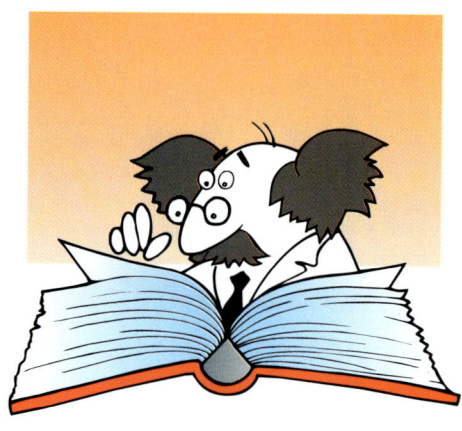

b Animal tissue consisting of highly contractile cells through which movement is effected.
c Part of the body to which an arm is attached.
d A condition of unusually high sensitivity to a substance, contact with which may produce unpleasant physical symptoms.
e Power or range of vision.
f Quality of being strong.
g Exhaustion

1 WORD SEARCH

Find a word in the text which has the following meaning.

a A pain in the back.

2 COMPREHENSION

Answer the following questions.

1 What do Kensuke Suzuki's classmates complain about?
2 What has the Tokyo pediatrician Makoto Hirai noticed about his young patients in recent years?
3 What comparison is made between the minds of Japanese children and their bodies?
4 What did Takeo Masaki of Nippon College of Physical Education find in his survey of 1,231 Japanese schools?
5 What example does Masaki give to show that today's Japanese children are more passive than those of previous generations?
6 What does Masaki blame for the decline in physical fitness?
7 In what way has the role of

children in Japanese families changed?

8 How does the amount of park space per person available in Tokyo compare with that of Washington or New York?

9 What did a recent survey in the largely rural Shizuoka Prefecture find?

10 Why does the Education Ministry say that there is a limit to what schools can do to solve the problem?

3

Some words are formed from two separate words.

e.g. outside (out + side)
playparks (play + parks)
Join a word from column 1 with a word from column 2 to form a single word as used in the text.

Column 1	Column 2
eye	ache
back	swing
out	war
home	door
up	room
post	class
class	sight
stair	work
after	mates
class	case

4 ADJECTIVES

Fill in the blanks with the *adjectives* below as used in the text.

- ✓ rigorous
- ✓ out-of-shape
- ✓ potential
- ✓ stiff
- ✓ restrictive
- ✓ high-tech
- ✓ physical
- ✓ drastic
- ✓ paper-thin
- ✓ industrial

a   .... shoulders
b the .... generation
c a .... schedule
d   .... fitness
e   .... walls
f a .... danger
g   .... pollution
h the .... change
i   .... rules
j   .... toys

5 NOUNS

Fill in the blanks with the following *nouns* as used in the text.

- ✓ allergies
- ✓ fractures
- ✓ strength
- ✓ shoulders
- ✓ backaches
- ✓ diet
- ✓ patients
- ✓ additives
- ✓ bones
- ✓ muscles
- ✓ bodies
- ✓ pediatrician

a Teenagers suffered from stiff (1) .... and (2) ....

b In the old days, children helped around the house. It helped to build their back-muscle (3) ....

c The (4) .... are probably the result of industrial pollution, changes in (5) .... and food (6) ....

d Makoto Hirai, a Tokyo (7) .... for 34 years, notices that his young (8) .... seem to break (9) .... much more often these days.

e Now the (10) .... tend to come from just missing a step on the staircase. They don't move their (11) .... They don't use their (12) ....

EXTENSION EXERCISES

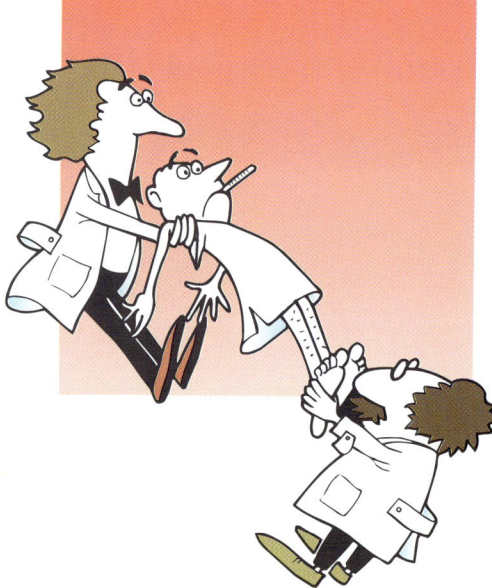

6

Study this sentence.

46 The allergies are *probably* the result of industrial pollution.

Comment on the following statements using the words "*would probably be better*".

e.g. The minds of Japanese children benefit from one of the world's most rigorous educational systems, but their bodies are woefully neglected.

Japanese children *would probably be better* to exercise their bodies as much as their minds.

1 Today's Japanese youngsters are more passive than those of previous generations.
2 Pupils are yawning in school.
3 Children are slaves to their studies.
4 The Education Ministry can't do much to solve the problem.
5 Most elementary and junior high schools offer three hours of physical education a week.
6 Urban children live in concrete jungles without open space to run around.
7 Japanese children study, but they don't do any of the house chores.

7 TELL/SAY

Study this sentence.

5 "They *tell* each other how tired they are or complain about a backache, he *says*."

Put the verbs *tell* or *say* in the blanks below in *a suitable form*.

General rule For most constructions, if you say *who* you are talking to, you should use *tell*.

1 They .... that they are going to be late.

2 He .... me yesterday that he couldn't come.
3 She .... it is going to rain.
4 I want to .... you something important.
5 .... Frank to come at six o'clock.
6 I have been .... you for weeks to phone her.
7 Dick .... that he had seen you on Saturday.
8 They .... lies, but we later discovered the truth.

8 REVISION

Revision - If sentences
Study this sentence.

88 If the youngsters are not glued to the tube, they're stuck to their books.

Complete the following *if* sentences in your own words.

1 If Japanese children study too much ....
2 If you want my advice ....
3 If Japanese children exercised more ....
4 If they had set up more playparks ....
5 If they build houses with paper-thin walls ....
6 If there hadn't been such industrial pollution and changes in diet ....

7   If Japanese parents took their children to the country for a few days ....

8   If the classroom curriculum were less demanding ....

9   IDIOMATIC EXPRESSIONS WITH *MAKE*

Study the following expressions. They are all formed with the verb *TO MAKE*.
Read the following sentences. Replace the part of the sentence *in italics* with one of the idioms below in the correct form.

1   I continued to put off studying for the Histology examination. Then I decided I really had *to begin*.

2   Nurse Jenkins was only a few minutes late for duty. Sister Demptster saw her arrive and started *to scream and shout excitedly*.

3   I've tried to understand Doctor Mason's handwriting but I can't make *it out*.

4   Although Mr. Ridley was still feeling weak after his operation, his doctors told him he should get up. They thought he should try to *do it even if he didn't feel like it*.

5   When Doctor Bradley's wife phoned, he was busy in his surgery and couldn't speak to her. He *remembered* to phone her back later when he had a free moment.

6   It's very difficult in your first year of employment to *have enough money to live on* unless you continue to live with your parents.

7   Doctor Gerald Carter specialized in Cardiology for many years. In fact, he was responsible for several important breakthroughs and *became very well-known*.

8   We are all very busy at the moment so try to *do something to help us*.

9   I've been studying Microsurgery from my text book but I don't seem to be *learning very much*. I think I need to see a few operations to understand what I'm reading.

10 Robert always tended *to exaggerate* when he didn't feel well. Whenever he caught a cold, he was convinced he had pneumonia.

Idiomatic expression	Meaning
to make a start	to begin a task
to make an effort	to do a task, even if you don't feel like it
to make both ends meet	to match expenses to income
to make headway	to move forward satisfactorily
to make oneself useful	to do a task to help someone
to make a mountain out of a molehill	to greatly exaggerate a problem
to make a song and dance	to become unreasonably excited
to make a name for oneself	to earn oneself a reputation in a particular field
not to make head nor tail of	not to understand at all
to make a mental note	to record in one's mind

10   NOUNS FROM VERBS

Give *nouns* formed from the verbs below.

Verb	Noun
to compare	
to notice	
to complain	
to deteriorate	
to protect	
to limit	
to survey	
to warn	
to pollute	
to schedule	

GRAMMAR POINT

VERB+INFINITIVE

a Some common verbs are followed by *the infinitive*

e.g.

✔ agree
✔ appear
✔ attempt
✔ decide
✔ forget
✔ hope
✔ learn
✔ manage
✔ offer
✔ refuse
✔ plan
✔ pretend
✔ promise
✔ seem
✔ tend

If these verbs are followed by another verb, the second verb is in the infinitive form.

e.g. The patient agreed *to undergo* surgery.

b *Not* is used in the negative form.

e.g. We decided *not to wait*.

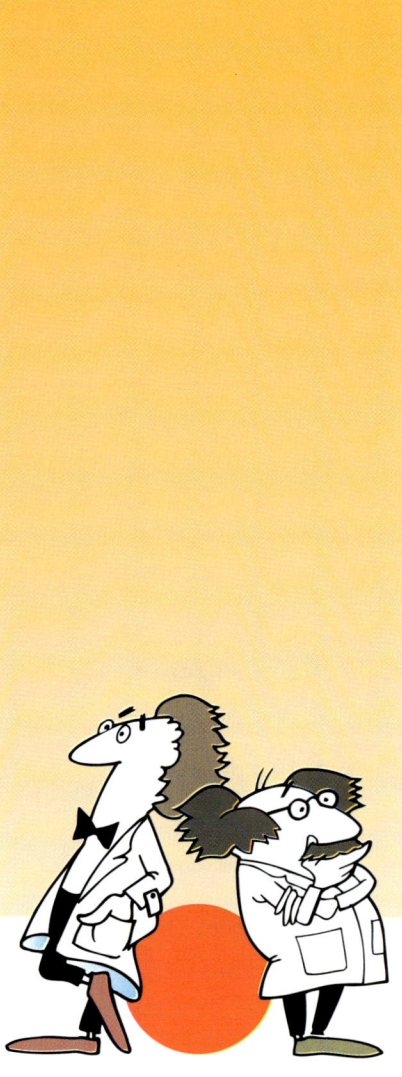

11 GRAMMAR CHECK

Fill in the blanks with a suitable *verb*.

1 David refused .... to the doctor with his complaint.
2 Richard managed .... the examinations because he had studied hard.
3 Doctor Harris decided not .... for a job he had seen advertised in a medical journal.
4 He seems .... put on a lot of weight.
5 Mary pretended not .... afraid.
6 Some patients tend .... to take their medicine and have to be constantly reminded.
7 As John hoped .... a surgeon one day, he would often go and observe operations.
8 Peter offered .... me his lecture notes for the Chemistry course.
9 Mr. Taylor promised .... the doctor's advice about giving up smoking.

WRITING

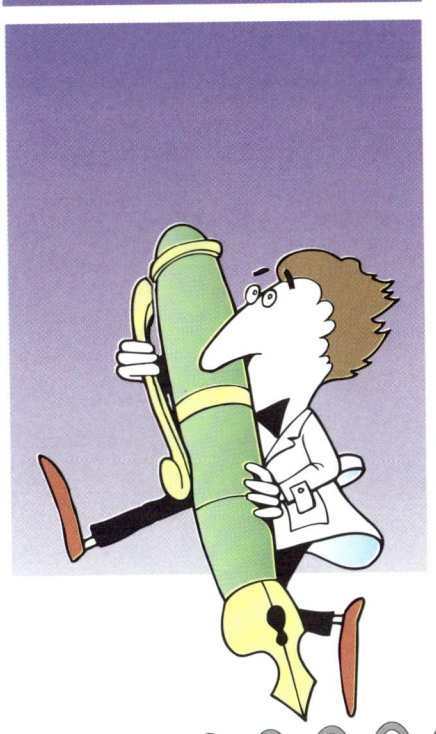

12 MISSING LETTERS

Write the *missing letter*s in the words below.

TIR_D
INSTE_D
BACKAC_E
SC_EDULE
PEDI_TRIC_AN
STREN_TH
YOUN_STERS
GLU_D
OF_EN

YAW_ING
MUS_LES
FATIG_E
SURVE_ED
SLIG_T

13 LETTER WRITING

Write a letter by Takeo Masaki of the Nippon College of Physical Education to the Education Minister. Briefly explain the findings of the survey. Make practical recommendations which would improve the health of Japanese children.

Notes

Study the following article.

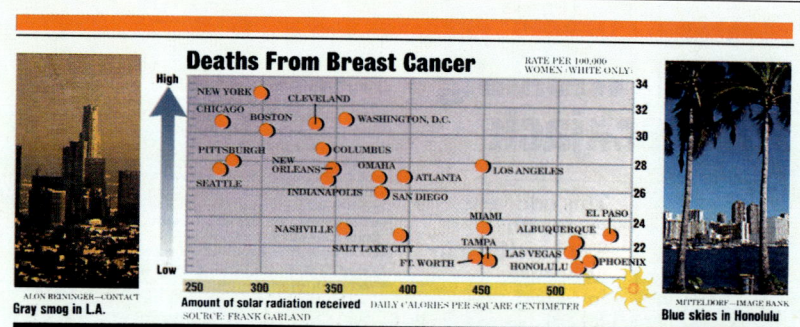

Deaths From Breast Cancer

RATE PER 100,000 WOMEN · WHITE ONLY:

Chart plotting cities by amount of solar radiation received (Daily Calories per Square Centimeter) against breast cancer death rate. Cities shown: NEW YORK, CLEVELAND, CHICAGO, BOSTON, WASHINGTON, D.C., PITTSBURGH, COLUMBUS, NEW ORLEANS, OMAHA, SEATTLE, INDIANAPOLIS, ATLANTA, LOS ANGELES, SAN DIEGO, NASHVILLE, MIAMI, EL PASO, ALBUQUERQUE, SALT LAKE CITY, TAMPA, LAS VEGAS, FT. WORTH, HONOLULU, PHOENIX.

Amount of solar radiation received — DAILY CALORIES PER SQUARE CENTIMETER

SOURCE: FRANK GARLAND

ALON BRININGER—CONTACT
Gray smog in L.A.

MITTELDORF—IMAGE BANK
Blue skies in Honolulu

HEALTH

Can Sunshine Save Your Life?

Vitamin D may help fight colon and breast cancer

Thirty-five years ago, herring fishing was big business in Norway but oncology was fairly slow. Today you could say just the opposite. The annual herring catch has dwindled from more than a million tons to less than 4,000—and the rates of breast and colon cancer have nearly doubled. The increase doesn't surprise epidemiologists Frank and Cedric Garland of the University of California, San Diego. Herring is rich in vitamin D, a nutrient that Norwegians receive only in paltry amounts from the sun. And as the Garland brothers have shown over the past decade, a population's vitamin D intake can be a powerful predictor of two leading malignancies.

Breast and colon cancer are rampant in the industrial world. In the United States, where the average adult gets less than half the recommended daily allowance of vitamin D, nearly a third of all cancers involve the breast or colon. Could a simple vitamin pill help control these common killers? It's still too early to say. "The epidemiologic studies are all there," says Dr. William Harlan, associate director for disease prevention at the National Institutes of Health. "But you need to do an interventional trial before you make clinical recommendations." The NIH is now planning a huge clinical trial that should yield definitive answers over the next decade. And Frank Garland, for one, is optimistic. "I think we'll find that colon and breast cancer are essentially vitamin-deficiency diseases of adulthood," he says.

Medical researchers have long regarded high-fat diets and delayed childbearing as key risk factors for colon and breast cancer. But those factors don't seem to account for the striking geographic patterns these diseases exhibit. The Garlands started puzzling over the patterns in the late 1970s, when a colleague showed them a map of the world color-coded to reflect the prevalence of colon cancer in different countries. The map suggested the disease was virtually unknown at the equator and that its prevalence mounted as the latitude grew higher. One of the few exceptions to this rule was Japan, a country that has traditionally enjoyed low rates of breast and colon cancer despite its northern geography.

Fish oil: What did the lucky populations have in common? They all seemed to be getting plenty of vitamin D, whether from sunshine or (like Japan) from diets rich in fish oil, so the Garlands started exploring the possibility. In a 1980 study, they compared colon-cancer death rates for different regions of the United States. As they'd predicted, the rates were lowest in the sunny South and West and highest in the gray Northeast—even though Northeasterners ate more vegetables, and roughly the same amount of meat, as the other groups.

In subsequent studies, the Garlands and other researchers have put the vitamin D hypothesis to a range of other tests, and it has held up well. In 1985, a team led by Cedric Garland examined the health records of nearly 2,000 Chicago utility workers who recorded everything they ate for 28 days back in the late '50s. Over the next 19 years, the workers who'd consumed at least 150 iu (international units) of vitamin D each day suffered only half as much colon cancer as those who'd consumed lesser amounts (200 iu is the recommended daily allowance for adults). A similar pattern turned up in a study of 101 blood samples drawn from volunteers in Maryland in 1974. The volunteers with the lowest vitamin D levels went on to develop colon cancer at three times the rate of other subjects.

More recently, the Garlands and their San Diego colleague Edward Gorham have concentrated on showing that breast cancer follows the same pattern as colon cancer. In 1990, they analyzed breast-cancer incidence in the Soviet Union and discovered a threefold discrepancy between the northern and southern republics. Back in the United States, a similar study revealed that breast-cancer death rates were more than 1.5 times as high in New York and Boston as in Phoenix or Honolulu (chart). Sunshine isn't the only amenity the South offers and the North lacks, but still other studies suggest it's the crucial one. Gorham has compared communities at similar latitudes and shown that breast and colon cancer are most common in the communities with the most light-blocking air pollution.

No one knows exactly how vitamin D might ward off these diseases. The molecule—which is found in egg yolks, liver and fortified milk as well as in tuna, salmon and other fatty fish—helps the body absorb calcium. Calcium, in turn, can help prevent uncontrolled cell growth. However the vitamin works, its potential benefits are immense. As part of the Women's Health Initiative, the massive NIH research project scheduled to begin in 1992, some 60,000 postmenopausal women will receive either a twice-daily calcium and vitamin D supplement or a placebo for up to nine years. The trial's formal goal is to reduce colon cancer and bone fractures by 25 percent, says Dr. Harlan of the NIH. But investigators will monitor the participants for breast cancer and other conditions as well. If the evidence to date is any indication, they could be in for pleasant surprises.

GEOFFREY COWLEY

80
85
90
95
100
105
110
115
120

VOCABULARY

5 **to dwindle**
- to gradually diminish
12 **paltry**
- very small
40 **to account for**
- to explain
82 **threefold**
- three times as great
82 **discrepancy**
- a difference; a lack of agreement
96 **a yolk**
- the yellow part of eggs

SPEAKING

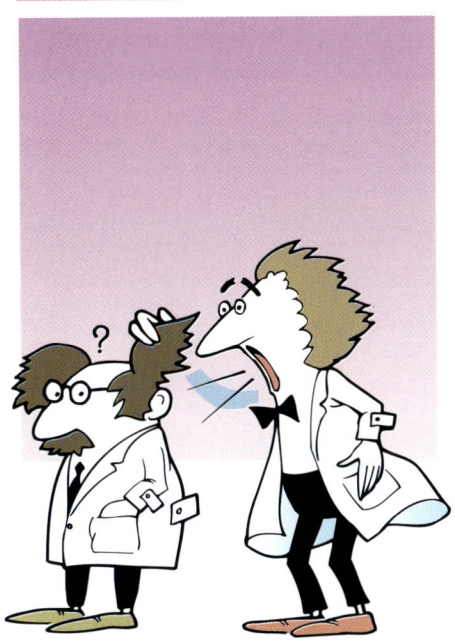

14 FIGHTING COLON AND BREAST CANCER WITH VITAMIN D

Explain, in your own words, the findings that suggest that colon and breast cancer are essentially vitamin-deficiency diseases of adulthood. Make notes before you begin. The following prompts will help you.

Breast and colon cancer are rampant in the industrial world.

Medical researchers have long regarded high-fat diets and delayed childbearing as key risk factors for colon and breast cancer.

The map suggested the disease was virtually unknown at the equator and that its prevalence mounted as the latitude grew higher.

In subsequent studies, the Garlands and other researchers have put the vitamin D hypothesis to a range of other tests, and it has held up well.

In 1990, they analyzed breast-cancer incidence in the Soviet Union and discovered a threefold discrepancy between the northern and southern republics.

No one knows exactly how vitamin D might ward off these diseases.

UNDERSTANDING IDIOMATIC ENGLISH

Explain the idiom.

He has skin like
a rhinoceros

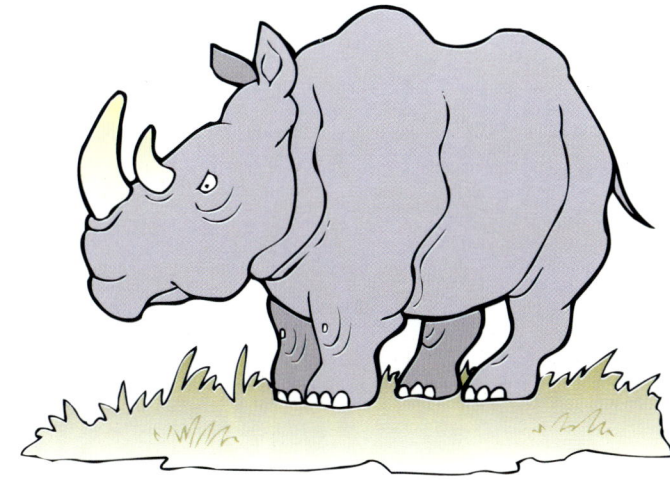

UNIT 24

Fitness pays

Take a Walk—and Live

A new study says even mild exercise can postpone death

Couch potatoes, your last excuse is gone. You knew you should be getting into your running shoes and hitting the pavement. After all, everyone concedes that exercising is one of the best ways to stave off heart attacks and other health problems. But hard physical exertion is downright unpleasant, and you—along with about 50 million other seden-

tary Americans—could be forgiven for putting it off or avoiding it altogether.

No more, though. A study published last week in the *Journal of the American Medical Association* says that even a minimal amount of exercise—a brisk half-hour walk once a day is enough—confers significant protection not only from cardiovascular disease and cancers but also against death from a wide range of other causes. Put plainly, people who exercise just a little bit tend to live longer.

The eight-year, 13,344-subject study, carried out by researchers at the Institute for Aerobics Research in Dallas, is hardly the first to establish a link between moderate exercise and longevity. But it is considered especially significant. For one thing, it includes both men and women, in contrast to earlier, mostly male surveys. For another, it strengthens the evidence that exercise can ward off cancer, a rela-

tionship discovered only in the past few years. And, perhaps most important, it is one of the largest studies ever done that relied on an objective measure of fitness, not just participants' descriptions of how much they exercise.

The researchers measured fitness in a straightforward way: they put people on a treadmill, set them walking, and periodically increased first the incline and then the speed of the treadmill until the walkers could no longer continue. The subjects were grouped into five different fitness levels based on their performance and followed for the next eight years.

At the end of that time, 283 of the participants, all of whom were in good health at the start of the study, had died. And after allowing for various other health-affecting factors, including smoking, age, cholesterol levels, weight, blood pressure and family history of heart disease, they found that deaths were sharply higher in the least-fit category than in the second-most-sedentary group—more than double for men and almost twice as high for women.

In the most-fit groups, which included people in the habit of running up to 40 miles a week, death rates tended to be lower still, but the improvement was not so dramatic. In short, says Carl Caspersen, a physical-activity epidemiologist at the federal Centers for Disease Control in Atlanta: "You don't have to be a marathoner to greatly reduce your mortality. After that first jump in activity, you're not buying that much more reduced risk."

While this and earlier studies agree on the health benefits of regular, moderate exercise, no one is sure of the physiological mechanisms involved. It may be that exercise increases coronary blood flow, decreases clotting or both, which would limit the blood-vessel blockages that cause cardiovascular problems. And some scientists speculate that exercise increases bowel motility, a factor in avoiding colon cancer. Those questions may be answered in part by the next phase of the investigation, which is expected to include more than 40,000 people. Such speculations are literally academic, though. For the average man or woman, the message is clear: get moving.

—By Michael D. Lemonick.
Reported by Andrew Purvis/New York

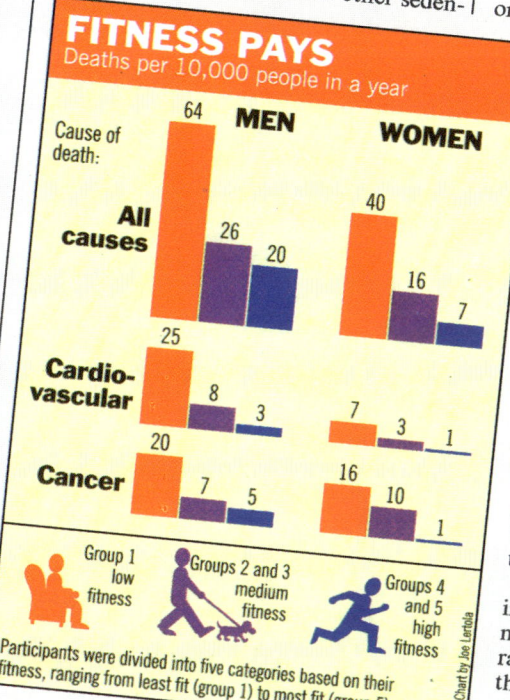

FITNESS PAYS
Deaths per 10,000 people in a year

Cause of death:

MEN   **WOMEN**

All causes — 64 | 26 | 20 — 40 | 16 | 7

Cardiovascular — 25 | 8 | 3 — 7 | 3 | 1

Cancer — 20 | 7 | 5 — 16 | 10 | 1

Group 1 low fitness
Groups 2 and 3 medium fitness
Groups 4 and 5 high fitness

Participants were divided into five categories based on their fitness, ranging from least fit (group 1) to most fit (group 5).

TIME Chart by Joe Lertola

TEXT BASED EXERCISES

VOCABULARY

Study the meaning of the following words and expressions as used in the text.

chart to pay
- to be profitable or advantageous
1 a couch
- a sofa
5 to stave off
- to avert temporarily
7 exertion
- vigorous activity
7 downright
- thoroughly
8 to put off
- to postpone
9 altogether
- entirely
13 brisk
- quick-moving
18 plainly
- clearly; simply
24 a link
- a connection; that which connects two parts
39 straightforward
- trustworthy; honest
62 twice
- two times
82 a blockage
- an obstruction

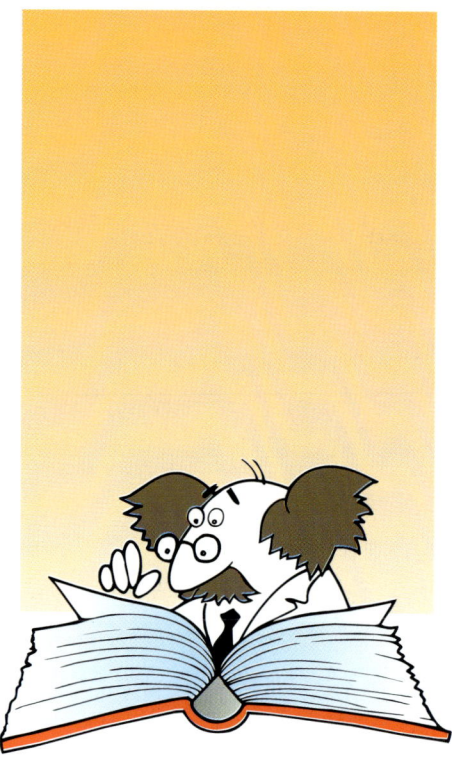

1 WORD CHECK

Explain the meaning of the words and expressions below.

2 getting into
3 hitting the pavement
5 ways
22 carried out
27 thing
35 an objective measure
46 performance
87 in part

2 RECONSTRUCTION

Rearrange the words below in order to make complete sentences.

1 Hard - downright - physical - unpleasant - exertion - is.
2 A brisk - a day - half-hour - once - walk - enough - is.
3 It - ward off - strengthens - exercise - cancer - the evidence - can - that.
4 The researchers - straightforward - fitness - way - measured - in - a.
5 The - levels - subjects - five - different - fitness - grouped - were - into.
6 You - your mortality - don't - a marathoner - reduce - to - greatly - have to be.
7 Some scientists - increases - exercise - bowel motility - avoiding - speculate - a factor - colon cancer - that - in.
8 People - exercise - just a little - to live - bit - tend - longer - who.

3 NOUNS FROM VERBS

Find *nouns* in the text that are formed from the following verbs.

to range	to participate
to link	to benefit
to exert	to block
to incline	to investigate
to perform	to speculate

4 NOUNS

Fill in the blanks with the *nouns* below as used in the text.

- ✔ walk
- ✔ study
- ✔ category
- ✔ measure
- ✔ disease
- ✔ mechanisms
- ✔ protection
- ✔ factors
- ✔ groups
- ✔ blood flow

a cardiovascular ....
b the physiological ....
c significant ....
d the eight-year ....
e coronary ....
f the least-fit ....
g the most-fit ....
h a half-hour ....
i health-affecting ....
j an objective ....

5 ADVERBS

Fill in the blanks with the following *adverbs* as used in the text.

- ✔ especially
- ✔ only
- ✔ literally
- ✔ sharply
- ✔ hardly
- ✔ greatly
- ✔ mostly
- ✔ plainly
- ✔ periodically

a The eight-year, 13,344-subject study, carried out by researchers at the Institute for Aerobic Research in Dallas, is .... the first to establish a link between moderate exercise and longevity. But it is considered .... significant. For one thing, it includes both men and women, in contrast to earlier, ... male surveys. For another, it strengthens the evidence that exercise can ward off cancer, a relationship discovered .... in the past few years.

b After allowing for various other health-affecting factors, including smoking, age, cholesterol levels, weight, blood pressure and family history of heart disease, they found that deaths were .... higher in the least-fit category than they were in the second most sedentary group.

c They put people on a treadmill, set them walking and .... increased first the incline and then the speed of the treadmill until the walkers could no longer continue.

d You don't have to be a marathoner to .... reduce your mortality.

e Put .... , people who exercise just a little bit tend to live longer.

f Such speculations are .... academic, though.

6 PREPOSITIONS

Fill in the blanks with *prepositions* as used in the text.

1 The subjects were grouped .... five different fitness levels based .... their performance and followed .... the next eight years.

2 .... the end .... that time, 283 .... the participants, all .... whom were .... good health .... the start .... the study, had died.

3 You knew you should be getting .... your running shoes and hitting the pavement.

4 The researchers measured fitness .... a straightforward way: they put people .... a treadmill, set them walking, and periodically increased first the

incline and then the speed .... the treadmill until the walkers could no longer continue.

5 Some scientists speculate that exercise increases bowel motility, a factor .... avoiding colon cancer.

6 Those questions may be answered .... part .... the next phase .... the investigation.

7 Hard physical exertion is downright unpleasant and you could be forgiven .... putting it .... or avoiding it altogether.

8 In the most-fit group, which included people .... the habit .... running .... to 40 miles a week, death rates tended to be lower still, but the improvement was not so dramatic.

9 It is one .... the largest studies ever done that relied .... an objective measure .... fitness, not just participants' descriptions .... how much they exercise.

10 It strengthens the evidence that exercise can ward .... cancer, a relationship discovered only .... the past few years.

7

Fill in the blanks with the following words.

✔ sedentary
✔ health
✔ pressure
✔ habit
✔ various
✔ participants
✔ allowing
✔ history
✔ including
✔ included
✔ improvement
✔ dramatic
✔ twice
✔ weight
✔ still

At the end of that time, 283 of the (1) .... , all of whom were in good (2) .... at the start of the study, had died. And after (3) .... for (4) .... other health-affecting factors, (5) .... smoking, age, cholesterol levels, (6) .... , blood (7) .... and family (8) .... of heart disease, they found that deaths were sharply higher in the least-fit category than they were in the second most (9) .... group – more than double for men and almost (10) .... as high for women. In the most-fit groups, which (11) .... people in the (12) .... of running up to 40 miles a week, death rates tended to be lower (13) .... but the (14) .... was not so (15) ....

Notes

8 THE VERB *TEND*

When the verb TEND is followed by another verb, the infinitive + to is used with the second verb (see Unit 23).

Study these sentences.

18 Put plainly, people who exercise just a little bit *tend to live* longer.

63 In the most-fit groups, which included people in the habit of running up to 40 miles a week, death rates *tended to be* lower still, but the improvement was not so dramatic.

Complete the following sentences in your own words using the verb *TEND* in any suitable verbal form.

1 People who sit on couches too much, glued to the T.V. ....

2 Every time I tell John he should study more ....

3 Last summer, I went to England to practise my English but ....

4 When Tom sits behind his driving wheel ....

5 It has been reported in the newspapers that many teenagers ....

6 If I watch a horror film late at night ....

7 Last year, the number of deaths from smoking related diseases ....

EXTENSION EXERCISES

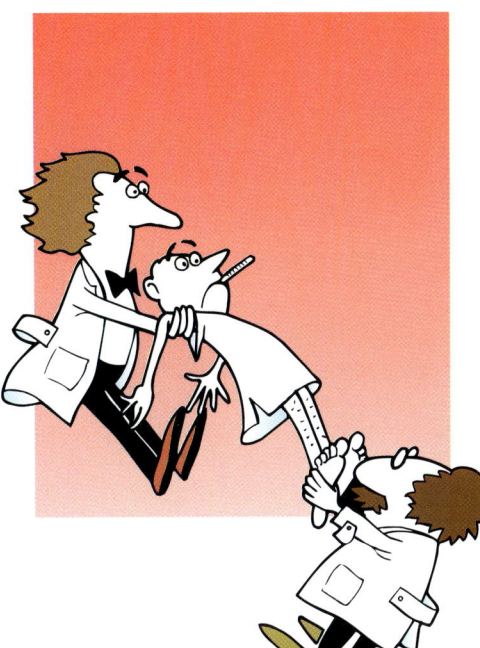

8 Whenever I ask Jane about her health ....

9 Paul likes to tell a story but ....

10 Never arrive on time for an appointment with George because ....

9 THERE WERE + NUMBER

13,400 people took part in the study. If you had been one of the subjects, you could say, "*There were 13,400 of us.*"

Make sentences beginning with "There were". Use the number and the pronoun in brackets to form the sentences.

e.g. 25 (them)
There were 25 of them.

a	10	(us)
b	55	(them)
c	4	(us)
d	16	(you)
e	30	(them)
f	100	(you)
g	260	(us)
h	15,000	(them)

Notes

10 REVISION OF IDIOMS

Fill in the missing words in the following idiomatic expressions.

1 You look as if you've seen a .... You're very pale.
2 When you have very little money it's often hard to make .... meet.
3 Harry likes to play practical jokes on his colleagues. Yesterday he got a .... of his own medicine when they played one on him.
4 She made a song and .... about the situation.
5 Instead of writing down the message, he made a .... note.
6 You should always look before you ....
7 They are getting too .... for their boots.
8 There is really nothing to worry about. Don't make a .... out of a molehill.
9 He's got pins and .... in his feet.
10 His patients loved him for his .... manner.
11 He's got a .... in the cupboard.
12 The .... is worse than the disease.
13 Her new car cost her an .... and a ....
14 She's got .... in the back of her head.
15 As he was feeling very generous, he offered to .... the bill.

11 PHRASAL VERBS WITH *MAKE*

Study the meanings of the verbs below. They are all formed with the verb *TO MAKE*.

Phrasal verb	Meaning
to make out (1)	to understand the nature of
to make out (2)	to discover the meaning of
to make out (3)	to write a cheque
to make for	to move towards; to escape
to make up	to prepare by mixing various ingredients
to make up for	to compensate
to make up to	to increase to a particular level
to make up one's mind	to come to a decision
to make up a story	to invent it
to make application to	to write; to apply

Complete the following sentences. Add the missing part of the phrasal verb.

1 I've been offered two jobs but I can't make .... my mind which to accept.
2 Patients often complain that they can't make .... the doctor's handwriting on their prescriptions.
3 Gordon hadn't studied all term. As there were only two weeks until the examination, he was forced to study night and day to make .... lost time.
4 I think I'll make an application .... the Bristol General Hospital. I'm interested in the post of anaesthetist I saw advertised yesterday.
5 The liquid was too concentrate. It had to be made .... a litre by adding water.
6 The doctor didn't believe Mr. Green's explanation of how the accident happened. He thought that the patient had made .... the whole story.
7 When the fire bell rang, everyone made .... the fire escape.
8 Patient: "Can I pay my hospital bill by cheque?" Clerk: "Certainly. You should make it .... to the Maxwell clinic."
9 Robert is behaving very strangely. I can't make him ....
10 The medicine is made .... by mixing the contents of these two bottles.

GRAMMAR POINT

VERB + GERUND

Some common verbs are followed by *the gerund*.

e.g.

- ✔ admit
- ✔ avoid
- ✔ consider
- ✔ delay
- ✔ dislike
- ✔ dread
- ✔ enjoy
- ✔ finish
- ✔ keep
- ✔ mind
- ✔ postpone
- ✔ risk
- ✔ suggest
- ✔ remember
- ✔ stop

e.g. Would you *mind helping* me?
Most people *dread going* to the dentist.

12 GRAMMAR CHECK

Fill in the blanks with a suitable verb in the correct form.

1 I suggested .... on holiday in July this year.
2 Would you mind .... this note to Doctor Baxter?

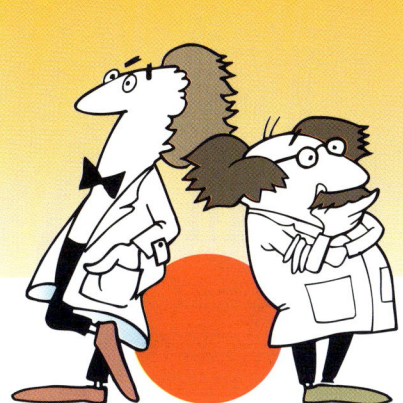

3 Most students dread .... examinations.
4 She considered .... for the job and then changed her mind.
5 Mr. Green admitted not .... the doctor's instructions.
6 Without the necessary vaccination, you'll risk .... the disease.
7 The lectures were so boring that after a while the students stopped ....
8 The doctors postponed .... any decision about the patient's treatment until they had examined the results of his tests.
9 I remember .... the letter on my desk, but now I can't find it.
10 John enjoys .... detective stories.

13 GRAMMAR CHECK

Translate the following sentences into your native language.

1 He considered going abroad.
2 She avoided meeting him.
3 He admitted telling lies.
4 Would you mind opening the window?
5 They suggested trying a different method.
6 John risked losing his job.
7 He remembered having been shown the report.
8 We enjoyed working on the new project.

Notes

WRITING

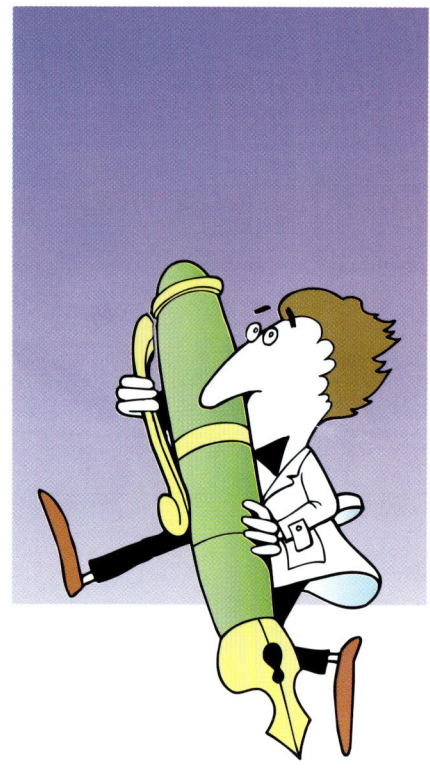

14 FITNESS QUESTIONNAIRE

HOW FIT ARE YOU?

Answer the following questions.

1 Do you consider yourself fit?

| YES | NO |

2 Do you exercise regularly?

| YES | NO |

3 How many times a week do you take part in regular exercise?

....

4 How many kilometres do you walk per day?

....

5 Do you take the lift rather than use the stairs?

| ALWAYS |
| SOMETIMES |
| NEVER |

6 How many press-ups can you do in one minute?

....

7 How many sit-ups can you do in one minute?

....

8 How many hours of TV do you watch per week?

....

9 Do you smoke?

| YES | NO |

10 If you answered yes to question 1, do you still consider yourself fit?

| YES | NO |

15 HEALTH BENEFITS

Explain, in your own words, the health benefits to be gained from regular, moderate exercise.

Notes

SPEAKING

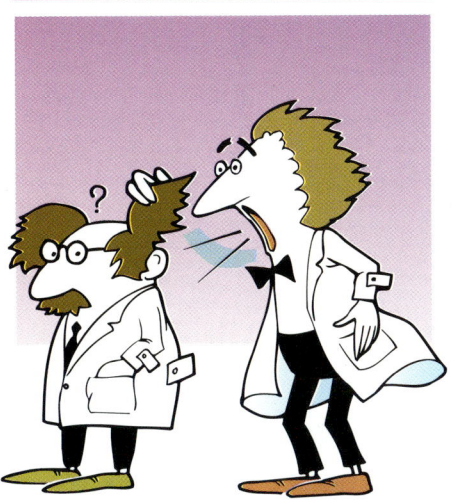

16 AN OBJECTIVE MEASUREMENT OF FITNESS

Explain how the study published in the *Journal of the American Medical Association* was carried out. The words below will help you.

Researchers - straightforward way - treadmill - increased the incline - the speed - grouped - five different fitness levels - performance - followed - eight years.

At the end of that time - 283 had died - allowing for health-affecting factors - deaths sharply higher - least-fit category - most sedentary group.

In the most fit groups - included people - running up to 40 miles a week - death rates lower still - improvement not so dramatic.

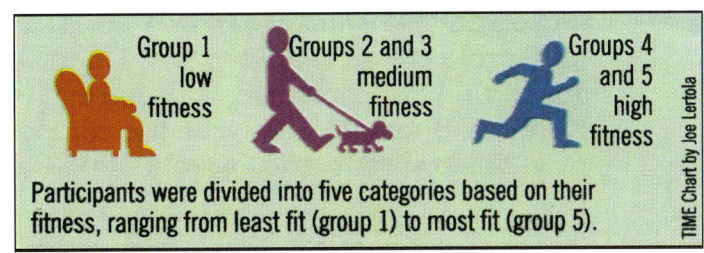

Participants were divided into five categories based on their fitness, ranging from least fit (group 1) to most fit (group 5).

UNDERSTANDING IDIOMATIC ENGLISH

Explain the idiom.

She has a big mouth!

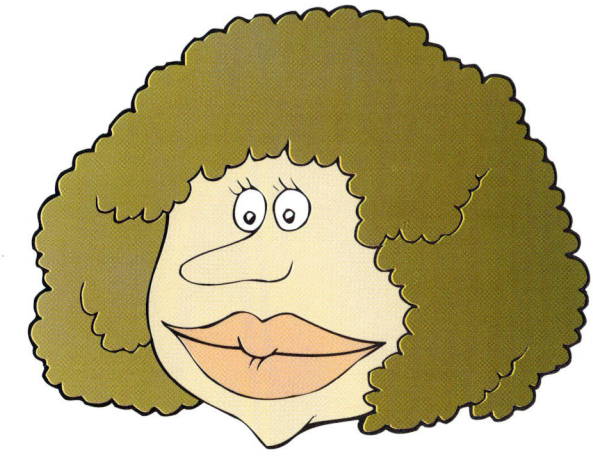

UNIT 25

Telephoning for specialist information

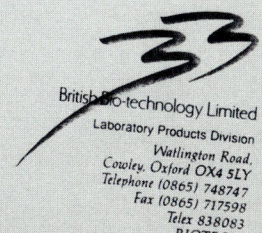

VOCABULARY

Study the meaning of the following words and expressions as used in the text.

6   a kit
    - equipment; a collection of tools or other articles
22 whole
    - complete; total
24 to look into
    - to investigate

1   MIXED VERBAL FORMS

Fill in the blanks with the verbs below in the form used in the text.

✓ be
✓ sound
✓ assume
✓ use
✓ hear
✓ provide
✓ supply
✓ give
✓ see
✓ synthesise
✓ like
✓ believe
✓ think
✓ amplify
✓ look into

TEXT BASED EXERCISES

"Good morning! I .... some advice about Molecular Biology Products. I .... that you supply 3' and 5' Labelling Kits. .... they for labelling oligonucleotide probes to a high specific activity?... I .... so, and I .... that optimised protocols .... ? ... Good! Now I .... how good your Designer Genes and Designer Probes are, but can you .... probes and genes to my own specifications? ... You can? I .... that your new TaqCheck kit is an amplification reaction control kit ... and it .... a guide to the number of DNA copies .... ? ... Yes, it does .... useful. Can you supply custom primers too? ... Wonderful!
Well, yes I could certainly .... the advice of one of your Molecular Biologists. Excellent! You .... me a whole new perspective!"
BRITISH BIO-TECHNOLOGY: the company for Molecular Biologists to be ....

Notes

EXTENSION EXERCISES

2 NOUNS FROM VERBS

Give *nouns* related to the verbs below.

Verb	Noun
to advise	
to guide	
to think	
to specify	
to supply	
to activate	
to amplify	
to copy	
to believe	
to synthesise	

3 UNCOUNTABLE NOUNS

ADVICE is *an uncountable noun* in English.

N.B. 1 Uncountable nouns are things that you *cannot count.*
2 They take a *singular verb.*
3 *Do not* use A/AN with these nouns.

Make sentences *in your own words* with each of the following nouns.

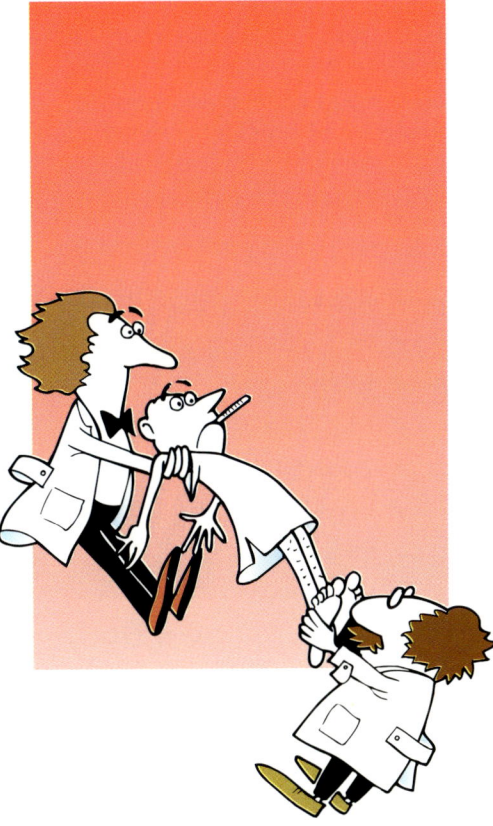

Use the words given as the subject of the sentence. N.B. *Not all* of the nouns take a singular verb.

a Information.
b Accomodation.
c News.
d People.
e Behaviour.
f Scissors.
g Advice.
h Hair.
i Furniture.
j Police.

4 NEGATIVE/ AFFIRMATIVE INTERROGATIVES

Line 6 begins with a question using the words *aren't they.* "*Aren't they* for labelling oligonucleotide probes to a high specific activity?"

The negative interrogative is used when the speaker expects an affirmative answer.

Read the sentences below. Ask questions using the negative interrogative at the beginning of your sentences. Remember to read this type of interrogative with the appropriate intonation.

e.g. He's the man who told us the news.
      Isn't he the man who told us the news?

1 The meeting is tomorrow.
2 He should have left by now.
3 It was a rather difficult operation.
4 Doctor Baxter would like some advice.
5 We met them on holiday last year.
6 These are the articles you were telling me about.
7 This is the patient who attends the clinic for treatment.
8 She will apply for a job as soon as she graduates.
9 They have forgotten something.
10 I could do it for you.

5

Study this sentence.

17 Yes, it does *sound* useful.

Comment on the sentences below in your own words. Use *don't* or *doesn't* and one of the following words.

✓ look
✓ sound
✓ smell
✓ taste
✓ feel

e.g. He's ill.
 He *doesn't look* ill.

1 The water is cold.
2 The bread is stale.
3 They are very tired.
4 This is a dry wine.
5 This milk is off.
6 These blankets are warm.
7 This is a true story.
8 They are old.
9 The coffee's hot.
10 That's John's voice.
11 Her perfume's French.
12 He feels sad.
13 Her hands are soft.
14 I burnt the cake.
15 This is a silk blouse.

6

In the text, the words *GOOD, WONDERFUL* and *EXCELLENT* are used to express an opinion. *Reply* to the statements below with an expression *of your own choice.* Choose from the following:

✓ REALLY!
✓ GOOD!
✓ FINE!
✓ EXCELLENT!
✓ WONDERFUL!
✓ WHAT A PITY!
✓ OH, DEAR!
✓ I'M SORRY!
✓ CONGRATULATIONS!

a Bob can't come tonight.
b I got the job.
c Barbara has broken her leg.
d They'll help us.
e I've passed my examination.
f My wife's mother is coming to stay with us for a week.
g He's got the flu.
h I'll telephone you later.
i My brother failed his driving test.
j I had to pay a fine for parking my car in a no parking area.

7 REVISION PHRASAL VERBS

Fill in the missing parts of the phrasal verbs in the blanks below.

1 The biggest problem is keeping them .... doing too much.
2 I'm looking .... to the holidays.
3 Less fat builds ...., but the artery still narrows.
4 Half of all strokes in people under 65 stem .... smoking.
5 If you can't remember his telephone number, look it .... in the telephone directory.
6 It is now becoming realistic to think .... selectively turning .... or modifying the activity of any given gene.
7 Look .... these reports until you find Mr. Mason's.
8 Surgeons cut .... the fetus, whose abdominal organs have spilled .... the chest.
9 Type I diabetes is brought .... by an insufficient supply of insulin.
10 While the incidence of lung cancer has been leveling .... for men, it has been rising among women.

GRAMMAR POINT

8 COMMENT TAGS

a These are formed with auxiliary verbs, just like question tags (see Unit 15). However, there are two important differences.
1 After an *affirmative* statement a *positive tag* is used.
2 After a *negative* statement a *negative tag* is used.

b A comment tag can be added to an affirmative statement to indicate that the speaker notes the fact just mentioned.

e.g. Optimised protocols are supplied, are they?
They synthesised the probes, did they?

c Comment tags can also be spoken in answer to an affirmative or negative statement.

e.g. A. I'm working in surgery now.
B. Are you?

A. He didn't get the job.
B. Didn't he?

d The main use of these tags is to express the speaker's reaction to a statement. By the tone of his voice, he can indicate surprise, anger, disbelief etc.

e A comment tag can be used

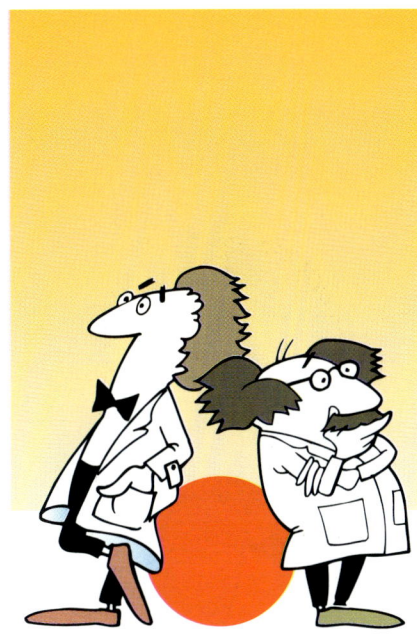

after a question has been asked and the answer received. The order is not inverted.

e.g. Can you synthesise probes and genes to my own specifications?
You can?

9 GRAMMAR CHECK

Use comment tags to reply to the following statements as in the example. Remember to read the comment tag with the appropriate intonation.

e.g. A. John's ill.
B. Is he?

A. Mark isn't coming.
B. Isn't he?

1 He's heard about the product.
2 They'd like some advice.
3 Tom didn't telephone.
4 It's an amplification reaction control kit.
5 I've passed my exam.
6 She hasn't arrived yet.
7 They could use our advice.
8 The new drug was tested.
9 He doesn't need any help.
10 The doctors were happy with the results.

10 GRAMMAR CHECK

Ask questions using the words below as in the example. Begin the first question with the word in brackets. Remember to read the comment tag with the appropriate intonation.

e.g. (would) to London?
Would you like to go to London for the week-end?
You would?

1 (will) see him?
2 (have) told?
3 (could) try?
4 (do) like?
5 (are) tomorrow?
6 (does) at the hospital?
7 (were) last night?
8 (has) already left?
9 (did) telephone?
10 (is) ready?

11 ANAGRAMS

Rearrange the letters below to form words used in the telephone conversation.

EDAICV	TCAOIENR
RAEDH	EUDIG
TSKI	LSUUEF
VEELBIE	GHHTTUO
SBROEP	LEHOW
LORTCON	LESDPPIU
PFCCIISE	GTSSOOLIIB
NOW	EIPOCS

WRITING

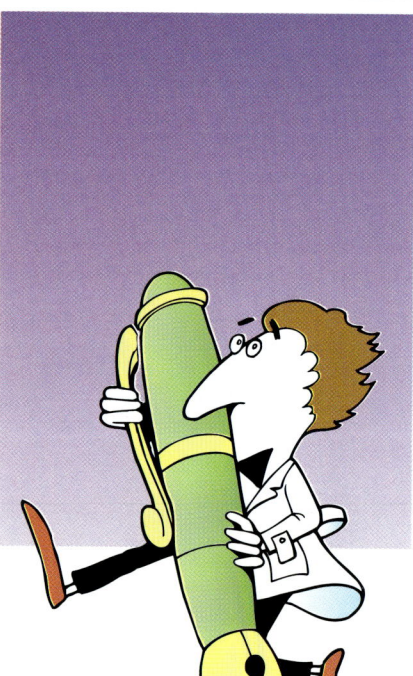

12 WRITING QUESTIONS

Write questions based on the telephone conversation.

e.g. He'd like some advice about Molecular Biology Products, wouldn't he?

Optimised protocols are supplied, aren't they?

Notes

SPEAKING

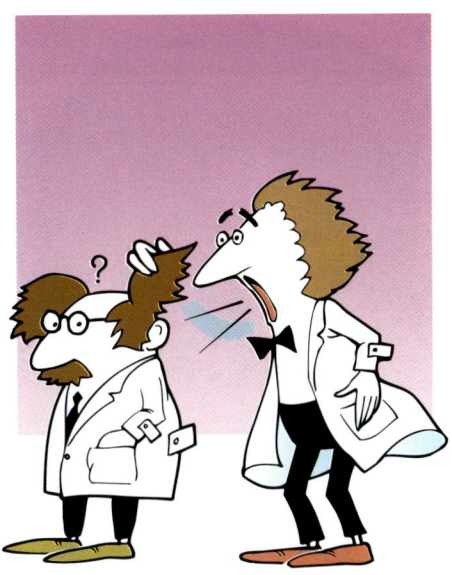

13 TELEPHONING

Conduct the following telephone conversations.

Work in pairs.

a You have read British-Bio Technology's advertisement in a magazine for Molecular Biology Products. Conduct a telephone conversation with a representative of the Technical Service Department asking for more information.

b *Doctor/patient*
You are on call at your home. In the middle of the night a patient telephones to say his wife is unwell. Ask questions to ascertain if a home visit is necessary.

c You are going to attend a three-day conference in London. Unfortunately, you will have to miss the first day. Phone your hotel and advise them of this change.

UNDERSTANDING IDIOMATIC ENGLISH

Explain the idiom.

He had to sit down as his feet were killing him

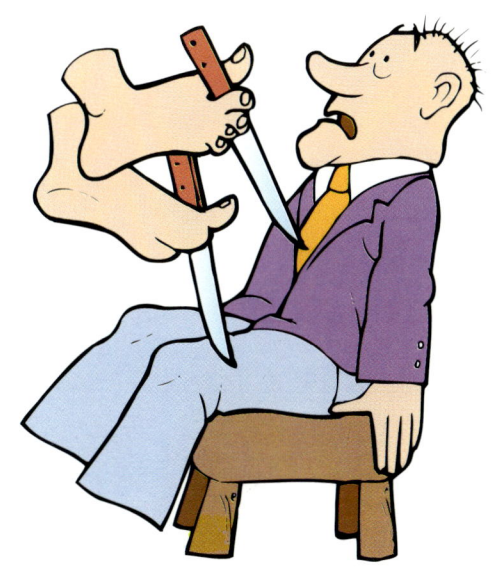

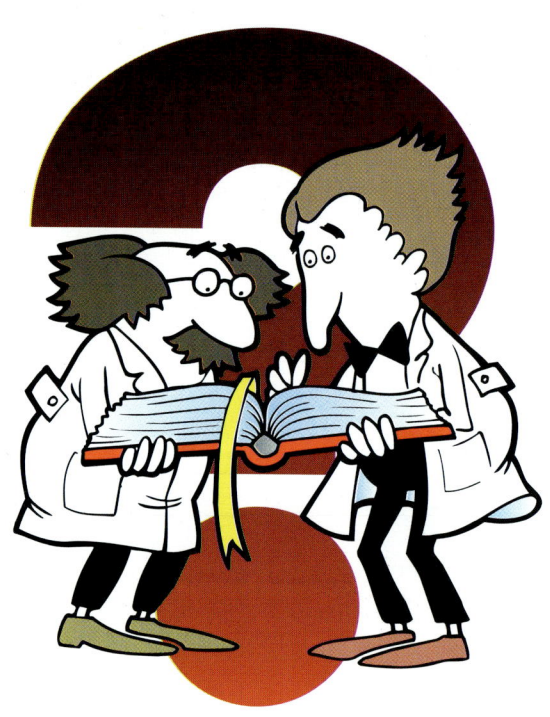

MEMORY TESTS

● *Try* these memory tests after completing each unit.

● *A revision test* follows every fifth unit.

● *Try* to answer the tests from memory.

● *Consult* the text of the unit if you cannot remember the relative word or expression.

● *Write down* your score at the end of each test.

UNIT 1

1. A cut. ....
2. A photograph of an organ or bone. ....
3. The main nerve cord of all vertebrates. ....
4. Used to close a wound. ....
5. To protect with soft material. ....
6. The opposite of minor. ....
7. Anaesthesia that is not local. ....
8. A noun from remove. ....
9. A hospital department that receives patients who live at home but attend for treatment. ....
10. An adjective that refers to pain lasting a long time. ....
11. A pain-killing drug. ....
12. To stand on. ....
13. To clean by a rush of water. ....
14. The opposite of a failure. ....
15. An adjective meaning small. ....

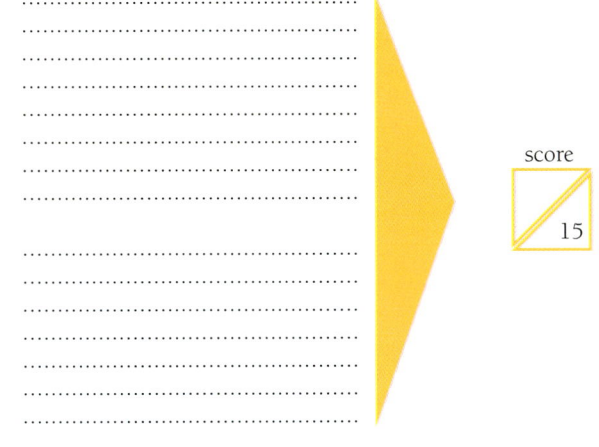

score

15

UNIT 2

1. A verb meaning to lead a project. ....
2. To want to avoid. ....
3. An approach based on rules. ....
4. An expression meaning close behind. ....
5. To compel by force. ....
6. The opposite of useful. ....
7. To financially support a project. ....
8. To put their data into a common fund. ....
9. Living and active. ....
10. The opposite of pessimistic. ....
11. To make a preliminary sketch. ....
12. A feature by which one can recognize a locality. ....
13. Completely new. ....
14. To violently move the foot forward. ....
15. A little push with the elbow. ....

score

15

Answers 1. to head – 2. to shy away from – 3. a rule-based approach – 4. close on its heels – 5. to enforce – 6. useless – 7. to fund – 8. to pool – 9. alive and well – 10. optimistic – 11. to draft – 12. a landmark – 13. brand new – 14. to kick – 15. a nudge

Answers 1. an incision – 2. an X-ray – 3. the spinal cord – 4. a stitch – 5. to cushion – 6. major – 7. general – 8. removal – 9. outpatient department – 10. chronic – 11. an analgesic – 12. to step on – 13. to flush – 14. a success – 15. tiny

MEMORY TESTS

UNIT 3

1. A first public appearance.
2. To cure.
3. The opposite of permanently.
4. Six.
5. An adjective meaning taking up a lot of space.
6. Dangerous.
7. One who has just arrived.
8. A verb meaning to introduce into.
9. The cutting part of a tool.
10. Not able to do something.
11. A disadvantage.
12. Amazing.
13. A ticket showing a price.
14. These may become narrowed.
15. The past participle of to drive.

score

15

UNIT 4

1. An illness.
2. A place or point of union.
3. The past participle of to bend.
4. The opposite of external.
5. A verb meaning to make able or possible.
6. A noun from replace.
7. The opposite of fortunate.
8. Paralysis of the lower part of the body and both legs.
9. A noun from deform.
10. To conquer.
11. The opposite of lower.
12. To throw out of balance.
13. A doctor who performs surgery.
14. A verb meaning to make flat.
15. The opposite of backwards.

score

15

UNIT 5

1. A noun from true.
2. An organic substance that acts as a catalyst in chemical changes.
3. A thing causing obstruction.
4. A noun from divide.
5. A prize given for merit.
6. A carrier of hereditary characteristics.
7. An adjective from molecule.
8. Worthy of notice.
9. A noun from discover.
10. One of the sections of a book.
11. An adjective from pride.
12. Prominent, remarkable.
13. A noun from achieve.
14. Every year.
15. An adjective from biology.

score

15

REVISION – UNITS 1-5

1. One who suffers.
2. A cardiac arrest.
3. A mark left by a wound.
4. Vessels that carry blood away from the heart to all parts of the body.
5. A mechanical gadget.
6. A sticking plaster.
7. A verb used to describe the continuous movement of blood.
8. Part of the body joining head to shoulders.
9. A disposable pump that can handle most of the heart's workload.
10. One who maps chromosomes.
11. Posterior part of the foot.
12. An adjective from cardiology.
13. The opposite of comfort.
14. A room where patients recover after an operation.
15. The protrusion of an organ through an aperture in its containing wall.

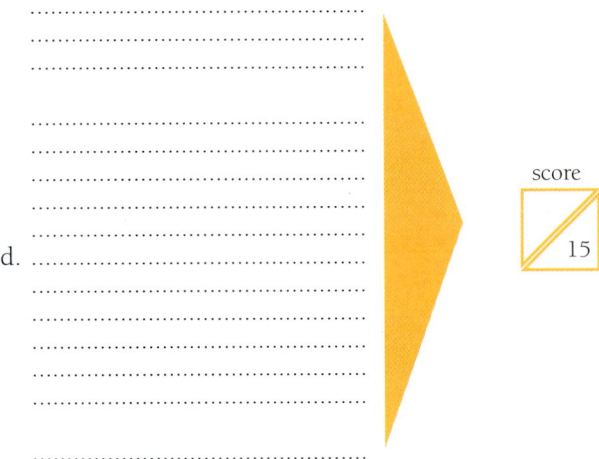

score

15

Answers 1. a sufferer – 2. a heart attack – 3. a scar – 4. arteries – 5. a device – 6. a Band Aid – 7. to flow – 8. neck – 9. a Hemopump – 10. a mapper – 11. heel – 12. cardiac – 13. discomfort – 14. recovery room – 15. a hernia

Answers 1. truth – 2. an enzyme – 3. an obstacle – 4. division – 5. an award – 6. a chromosome – 7. molecular – 8. remarkable – 9. discovery – 10. a chapter – 11. proud – 12. outstanding – 13. achievement – 14. yearly – 15. biological

MEMORY TESTS

UNIT 6

1. The part of the cell that contains the chromosome.
2. A verb meaning to decode.
3. The opposite of low.
4. An aim.
5. The structural unit of which living organisms are built.
6. A deficiency of poor quality red corpuscles in blood.
7. The opposite of far.
8. A genealogical table.
9. One hundred years.
10. An adverb meaning "in the past".
11. An adverb used for emphasis which means really or certainly.
12. A figurative use of a word meaning the origins or basic causes.
13. A condition of unusually high sensitivity to a substance, contact with which may produce unpleasant physical symptoms.
14. To set in motion.
15. A group of similar or related things meant to be used as a whole.

score
15

UNIT 7

1. A noun from develop.
2. A segment of the DNA that contains the instructions for a complete protein.
3. A word meaning probable.
4. What do the letters RFLP stand for?
5. A verb meaning to receive as hereditary characteristics.
6. A glass cylinder used in testing chemical reactions in the laboratory.
7. An adverb meaning principally.
8. The process by which cells divide.
9. A verb meaning to cut into pieces.
10. The slight differences in each pair of chromosomes that can be used as signposts to help locate genes.
11. A verb meaning to produce.
12. A noun from generate.
13. A small piece of paper or other material for fixing to an object and inscribing with a name.
14. A verb meaning to join or stick.
15. An adjective from electricity.

score
15

Answers 1. development – 2. a gene – 3. likely – 4. restriction-fragment-length-polymorphisms – 5. to inherit – 6. a test tube – 7. primarily – 8. cell division – 9. to chop up – 10. markers – 11. to yield – 12. generation – 13. a label – 14. to attach – 15. electric

Answers 1. nucleus – 2. to decipher – 3. high – 4. a goal – 5. a cell – 6. anemia – 7. near – 8. a family tree – 9. a century – 10. ago – 11. indeed – 12. roots – 13. an allergy – 14. to launch – 15. a set

UNIT 8

1. A noun from dense.
2. A risk.
3. An unpleasant effect of a drug.
4. A noun from thick.
5. Each other.
6. A noun from deteriorate.
7. Near.
8. The past participle of to know.
9. An adjective meaning only one.
10. A noun from mobile.
11. To happen.
12. The comparative of fast.
13. The opposite of to hide.
14. The lower part of the large intestine.
15. A noun meaning that which has been made larger.

score

15

UNIT 9

1. A noun from effect.
2. Combinations of various symptoms of a disease.
3. A tendency; general direction of development.
4. A catalogue of words.
5. An adjective meaning suitable.
6. An example or portion showing the qualities and characteristics of a group.
7. An adjective meaning to be in hospital.
8. Not able to be controlled.
9. Terrifying.
10. Rigid.
11. The opposite of practically.
12. Supply the next word: first, second.
13. To classify again.
14. An adjective from clinic.
15. A system of grading by size, quality or degree.

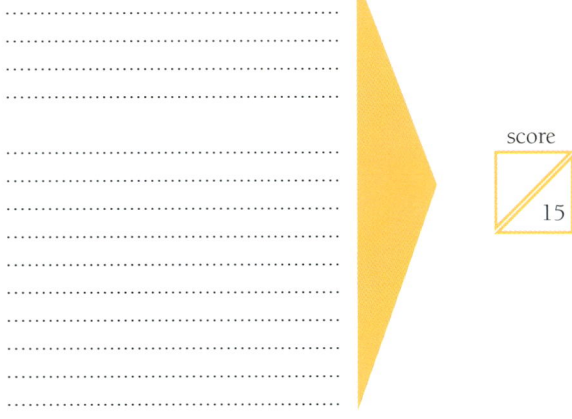

score

15

Answers 1. effectiveness – 2. a syndrome – 3. trend – 4. a list – 5. appropriate – 6. a sample – 7. hospitalized – 8. uncontrollable – 9. frightening – 10. stiff – 11. theoretically – 12. third – 13. reclassify – 14. clinical – 15. a scale

Answers 1. density – 2. a hazard – 3. a side effect – 4. thickness – 5. one another – 6. deterioration – 7. close – 8. known – 9. single – 10. mobility – 11. to occur – 12. faster – 13. to reveal – 14. colon – 15. enlargement

UNIT 10

1. A noun from to be born.
2. One less than a triplet.
3. Another word for difficulty.
4. Understanding; discernment.
5. A state of being cleaned.
6. Something partially similar or corresponding.
7. An adjective from prepare.
8. A period of ten years.
9. A plural noun from capable.
10. An adjective meaning single, singular or unrivalled.
11. An answer to a problem.
12. A verb meaning to acquire or obtain by effort.
13. An adverb meaning perhaps.
14. Unexpected.
15. A degree of being big or small.

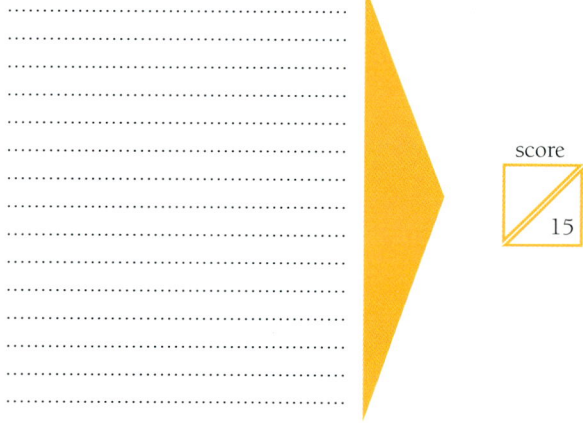

score

15

REVISION – UNITS 6-10

1. The transmission from parents to children of physical and mental characteristics.
2. An adjective that means of the lungs.
3. A chemical messenger secreted by endocrine glands directly into the blood stream.
4. A drug that gives relief from pain.
5. An adjective meaning produced by synthesis.
6. A process by which genes are copied.
7. An adjective meaning without fat..
8. A compound containing two or more amino acids linked together.
9. An adjective that means without feeling.
10. A chemical that chops up the DNA chain into shorter pieces.
11. An adjective that means of the liver.
12. A very small opening.
13. A remedy for all disorders.
14. Two words used together meaning immediately.
15. A noun from weigh.

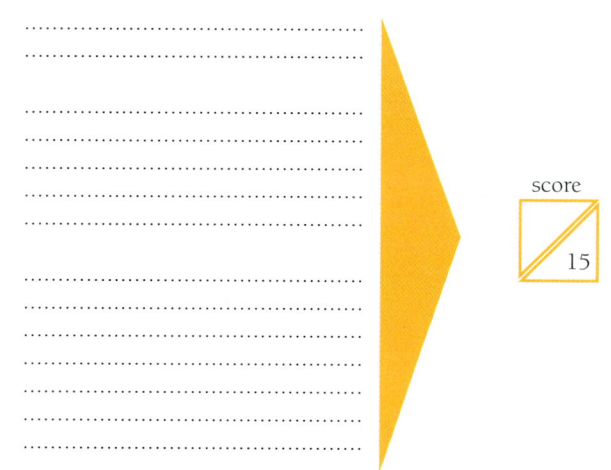

score

15

Answers 1. heredity – 2. pulmonary – 3. a hormone – 4. an analgesic – 5. synthetic – 6. cloning – 7. lean – 8. a protein – 9. numb – 10. a restriction enzyme – 11. hepatic – 12. a pore – 13. a panacea – 14. right away – 15. weigh

Answers 1. birth – 2. a twin – 3. trouble – 4. insight – 5. purification – 6. an analogue – 7. preparative – 8. a decade – 9. capabilities – 10. unique – 11. a solution – 12. to gain – 13. maybe – 14. unpredictable – 15. size

UNIT 11

1. The superlative of tiny.
2. The opposite of to block.
3. The fluid surrounding a fetus.
4. Another word for uterus.
5. You find these on each hand.
6. The opposite of known.
7. The muscular separation between the thorax and abdomen.
8. An adjective from defect.
9. A large organ which secretes bile and purifies the blood.
10. An adjective from technique.
11. A noun from block.
12. Found within the skull.
13. A pair of excretory organs.
14. A soft organ to the left of the stomach.
15. A verb meaning to make bigger.

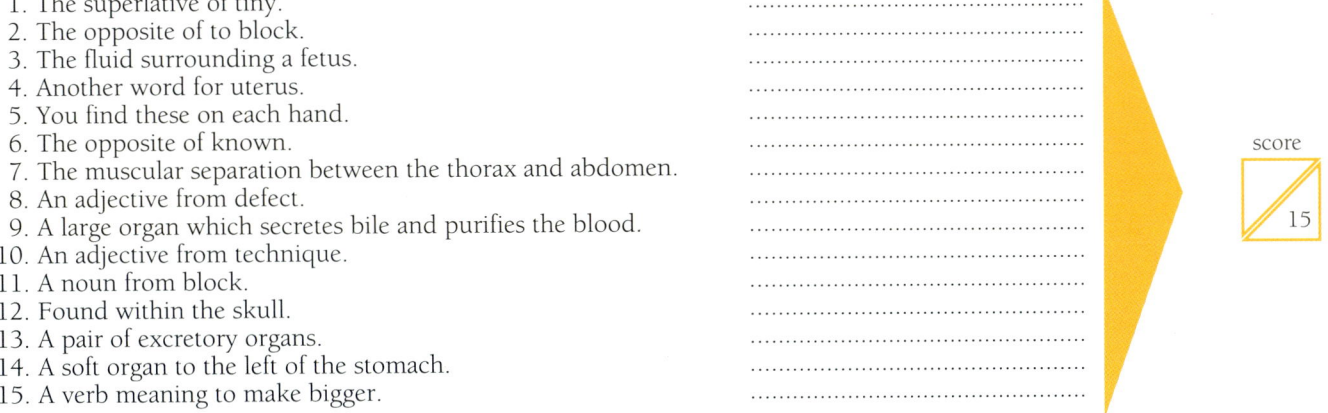

score
/ 15

UNIT 12

1. An adjective meaning strange.
2. A doctor who studies the functions of the nervous system and its related diseases.
3. An ailment or disease.
4. A noun meaning work that must be done.
5. A verb meaning to observe.
6. An adjective meaning giving information.
7. A deficiency or imperfection.
8. The opposite of forwards.
9. A provisional explanation of observed facts.
10. A verb meaning to baffle.
11. A noun meaning a sequence of objects arranged in order.
12. Two words meaning that the upper part has become the lower.
13. A noun from possible.
14. Half of a sphere.
15. An adjective meaning incorrect, not right.

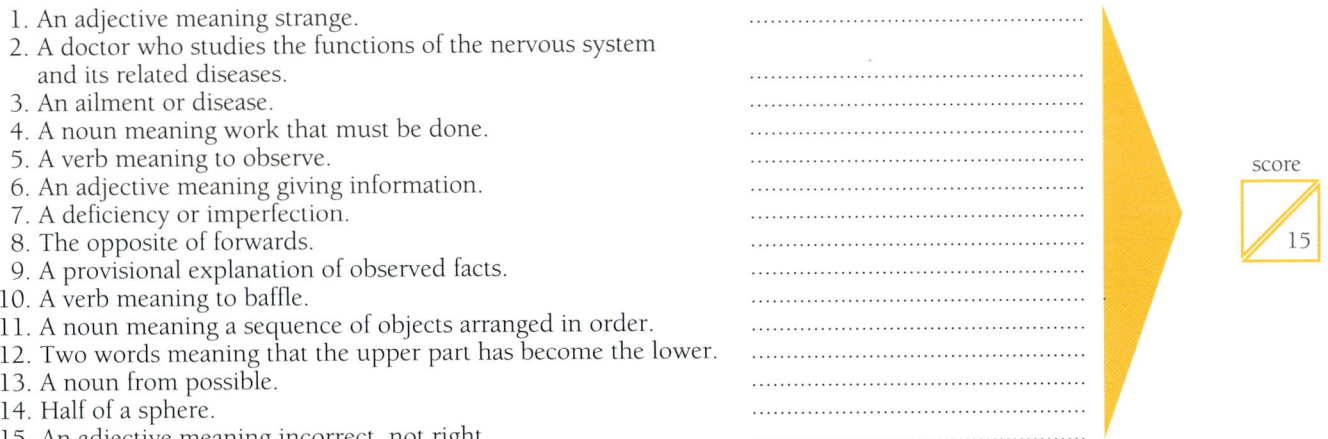

score
/ 15

Answers 1. curious – 2. a neurologist – 3. a disorder – 4. a task – 5. to notice – 6. informative – 7. a defect – 8. backwards – 9. a hypothesis – 10. to puzzle – 11. a series – 12. upside-down – 13. a possibility – 14. a hemisphere – 15. wrong

Answers 1. tiniest – 2. to unblock – 3. amniotic fluid – 4. womb – 5. fingers – 6. unknown – 7. the diaphragm – 8. defective – 9. the liver – 10. technical – 11. blockage – 12. the brain – 13. kidneys – 14. the spleen – 15. to enlarge

MEMORY TESTS

UNIT 13

1. A track formed by constant walking.
2. An adverb from simple.
3. The part of blood that thickens and separates from the serum.
4. An adjective meaning related to the arteries supplying blood to the heart.
5. A sudden involuntary muscular contraction.
6. A verb followed by a preposition that means to start or to cause.
7. Material used to cover an inner surface.
8. A scientist who studies the chemistry of living things.
9. A noun from able.
10. A verb followed by a preposition meaning to break into smaller pieces.
11. A structure by means of which two bones fit together.
12. A verb followed by a preposition that means to produce.
13. A verb from congregation.
14. A verb followed by a preposition that means to accumulate.
15. A disease characterized by excessive production of sugar.

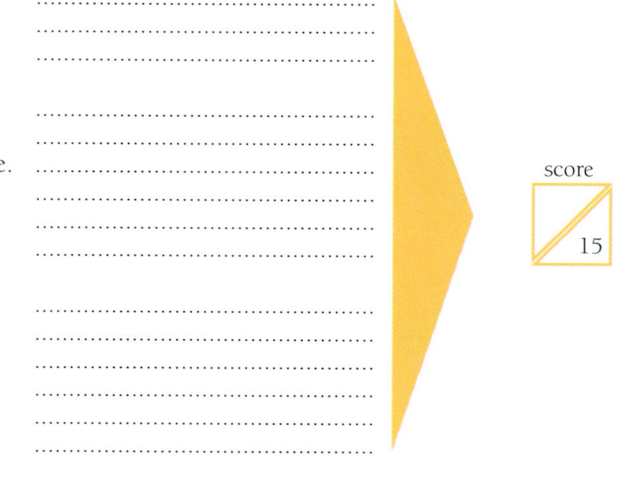

score

15

UNIT 14

1. An adjective meaning not normal.
2. The opposite of to succeed.
3. To inject again.
4. An adjective meaning you can wear it.
5. The opposite of comfort.
6. A verb meaning to take a photograph.
7. A noun from trace.
8. Without motion.
9. An adjective meaning approximate, not complete.
10. A verb meaning to extract a liquid.
11. A noun from accurate.
12. A substance used for colouring.
13. The opposite of strong.
14. An adverb meaning unable to be reversed.
15. A noun from interpret.

score

15

Answers 1. abnormal – 2. to fail – 3. to reinject – 4. wearable – 5. discomfort – 6. to snap – 7. a tracer/tracings – 8. motionless – 9. rough – 10. to draw – 11. accuracy – 12. a dye – 13. weak – 14. irreversibly – 15. interpretation.

Answers 1. a path – 2. simply – 3. a clot – 4. coronary – 5. a spasm – 6. to set off – 7. a lining – 8. a biochemist – 9. ability – 10. to break down – 11. a joint – 12. to turn out – 13. to congregate – 14. to build up/to pile up – 15. diabetes

264

UNIT 15

1. A white substance present in human tissues. ....
2. That which provides proof or strong probability. ....
3. A noun meaning frequency of occurrence. ....
4. A verb meaning to make weak. ....
5. A cooking utensil in which food is cooked under steam pressure. ....
6. An adjective meaning conducive to good health. ....
7. An annoyance. ....
8. An adjective from stress. ....
9. An adjective meaning not patient. ....
10. The past tense of to teach. ....
11. An idea. ....
12. The opposite of detected. ....
13. A noun from hostile. ....
14. One who suffers through no fault of his own. ....
15. A series of questions, especially in a written form. ....

score
/ 15

REVISION – UNITS 11-15

1. An adjective meaning a type of material that does not let water pass. ....
2. To say or write the letters of a word in the correct order. ....
3. What do the letters LDL's refer to? ....
4. One who remains alive after experiencing some danger. ....
5. A specialist in obstetrics. ....
6. A layer of nerve fibres sensitive to light forming the lining of the eyeball. ....
7. The arguments for and against. ....
8. Therapies that save lives. ....
9. A strong band of fibrous tissue connecting bone to bone. ....
10. A test that provides tracings of the heart's electrical activity. ....
11. A test in which a catheter is threaded through a vein in the groin or arm into the heart. A dye is injected that produces X-ray images of the coronary arteries. ....
12. An adjective from abdomen. ....
13. The period of time when one is a child. ....
14. An adjective from neurology. ....
15. A test that reveals how much blood the heart's left chamber holds and pumps. ....

score
/ 15

Answers 1. waterproof – 2. to spell – 3. low-density lipoproteins – 4. a survivor – 5. an obstetrician – 6. the retina – 7. the pros and cons – 8. lifesaving therapies – 9. a ligament – 10. an electrocardiogram – 11. an angiography – 12. abdominal – 13. childhood – 14. neurological – 15. a Stress-Gated Blood-Pool Scan

Answers 1. cholesterol – 2. evidence – 3. incidence – 4. to weaken – 5. a pressure cooker – 6. healthy – 7. an aggravation – 8. stressful – 9. impatient – 10. taught – 11. a notion – 12. undetected – 13. hostility – 14. a victim – 15. a questionnaire

MEMORY TESTS

UNIT 16

1. A disease characterized by intermittent attacks of difficult breathing.
2. A verb meaning to order a treatment.
3. A noun meaning a state of being extremely fat.
4. A noun from limit.
5. A step taken in advance to avoid an accident.
6. Two words that mean for example.
7. A noun from require.
8. A choice.
9. An adjective meaning not dangerous.
10. A noun from consult.
11. An area of study.
12. A noun from adapt.
13. An adjective meaning excellent.
14. An adjective meaning suffering from some disease.
15. An invalid's chair on wheels.

score

15

UNIT 17

1. A person suffering from diabetes.
2. A supply kept for future need.
3. A verb meaning to make normal.
4. A state of being complicated.
5. A noun from fail.
6. A noun from survive.
7. A verb meaning to work too much.
8. A noun from react.
9. A verb meaning to begin; to set in motion.
10. A course of remedial treatment.
11. To colour with a dye.
12. A noun from dehydrate.
13. The past of to mean.
14. Something produced in the process of manufacturing another article.
15. A noun from isolate.

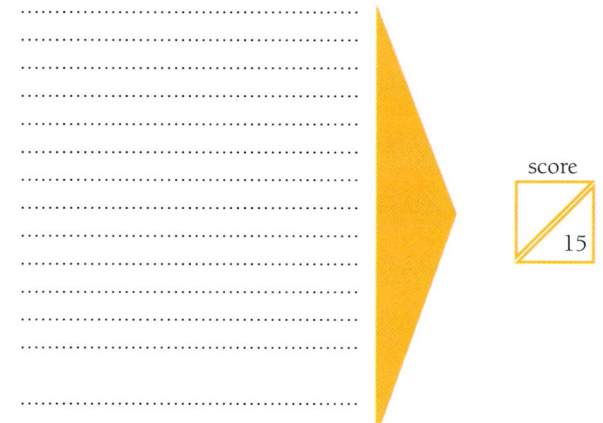

score

15

Answers 1. a diabetic – 2. a store – 3. to normalize – 4. a complication – 5. failure – 6. survival – 7. to overwork – 8. a reaction – 9. to initiate – 10. a cure – 11. to stain – 12. dehydration – 13. meant – 14. a by-product – 15. isolation

Answers 1. asthma – 2. to prescribe – 3. obesity – 4. a limitation – 5. a precaution – 6. such as – 7. a requirement – 8. an option – 9. safe – 10. consultation – 11. a field – 12. an adaptation – 13. superb – 14. sick – 15. a wheelchair

UNIT 18

1. An adjective meaning deadly.
2. A fluid secreted into the mouth to soften and partially digest food.
3. A noun from protect.
4. A noisy, violent expulsion of air from the lungs.
5. An adjective meaning ceaseless; without end.
6. Drops of salty liquid secreted by a gland near the eye.
7. An adjective meaning to cause damage.
8. An object used for attack or defence.
9. A wild, uncultivated land with dense undergrowth; an equatorial forest.
10. An obstruction or obstacle preventing access; an impediment.
11. A convulsive and loud ejection of air through the nostrils because of irritation of the nose.
12. A verb meaning to recognize differences; to discriminate.
13. To insert an instrument into a wound to ascertain its depth; to investigate.
14. A noun from know.
15. An adjective used with the word therapies and meaning likely to succeed in the future.

score
15

UNIT 19

1. An adjective meaning able to resist infection.
2. You insert a key into this.
3. One who defends.
4. An adjective meaning complete or total.
5. A noun from extend.
6. An unnatural enlargement of a part of the body.
7. A noun from explode.
8. A condition of illness with high temperature.
9. An adverb meaning happening at the same time.
10. One who fights.
11. Buildings in which goods are manufactured.
12. Proteins capable of recognizing and binding to viruses.
13. An adverb that means lasting only a moment or a short time.
14. Redness and swelling with heat and pain.
15. An adjective meaning porous.

score
15

Answers 1. immune – 2. a lock – 3. a defender – 4. entire – 5. extension – 6. a swelling – 7. explosion – 8. fever – 9. simultaneously – 10. a fighter – 11. factories – 12. antibodies – 13. momentarily – 14. inflammation – 15. permeable

Answers 1. lethal – 2. saliva – 3. protection – 4. a cough – 5. unending – 6. tears – 7. harmful – 8. a weapon – 9. a jungle – 10. a barrier – 11. a sneeze – 12. to differentiate – 13. to probe – 14. knowledge – 15. promising

MEMORY TESTS

UNIT 20

1. The opposite of effective.
2. Another word for influenza.
3. A noun from grow.
4. A system of related organs.
5. An adjective meaning to cause trouble.
6. An apoplectic attack, especially one causing partial paralysis.
7. A verb meaning to make stronger.
8. An adjective from explode.
9. An allergic catarrh of nose and throat, caused by inhaling pollen, dust or other irritants.
10. An adjective meaning inactive; sleeping.
11. An instrument or apparatus; an implement used by workmen.
12. A soft, fatty substance in the cavities of bones.
13. An adjective from immunology.
14. To examine carefully and thoroughly.
15. A mistake.

score / 15

REVISION – UNITS 16-20

1. The faculty of mentally retaining impressions of past experiences.
2. A verb meaning to deal successfully with a difficulty.
3. A two-word expression meaning as and when desired.
4. To stay in good condition by exercising.
5. A plural noun meaning probability or chance in favour of one side in a contest.
6. To educate or instruct by systematic practice.
7. A noun from expect.
8. A substance that dilates blood vessels and makes it easier for cells to pass through the capillary walls.
9. What do the letters MHC stand for?
10. An attack in reply to enemy advance.
11. An infectious disease characterized by the presence of tubercles in tissues.
12. To die of hunger.
13. A preparation of a virus used for inoculation.
14. A noun from progress.
15. These cells probably work by sending out chemical signals that slow or stop an immune reaction after an invader has been defeated.

score / 15

Answers 1. memory – 2. to cope – 3. at will – 4. to keep fit – 5. odds – 6. to train – 7. expectation – 8. histamine – 9. major histocompatibility complex – 10. a counterattack – 11. tuberculosis – 12. to starve – 13. a vaccine – 14. progression – 15. suppressor T cells.

Answers 1. ineffective – 2. flu – 3. growth – 4. a tract – 5. troublesome – 6. a stroke – 7. to strengthen – 8. explosive – 9. hay fever – 10. dormant – 11. a tool – 12. bone-marrow – 13. immunological – 14. to scrutinize – 15. an error.

UNIT 21

1. A system of special symbols for transmitting messages.
2. One who carries a message.
3. The formation of a compound from elements or simpler compounds.
4. The period of being an infant.
5. Another word for cloning genes.
6. To translate from a code.
7. A noun from regulate.
8. A verb meaning to change; to make or become different.
9. A noun from active.
10. To construct again.
11. A proportion; a numerical relation.
12. A phrasal verb meaning to stop the action or flow of.
13. The act of transcribing.
14. A verb meaning to control or handle.
15. A noun from available.

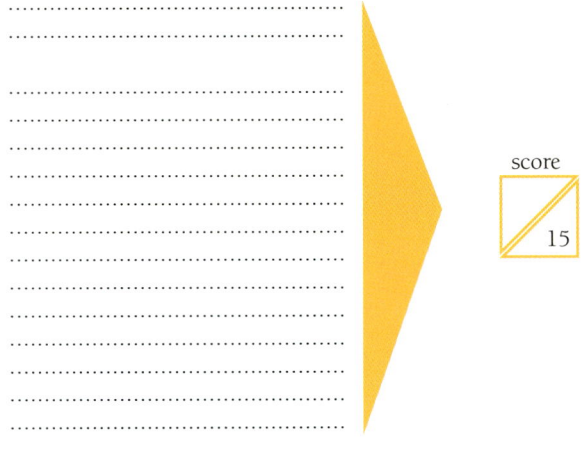

score

15

UNIT 22

1. A person who smokes.
2. The opposite of an increase.
3. A period of 25 years.
4. A sound that gives warning of an approaching danger.
5. An adjective from prevent.
6. To give information of an approaching danger; to advise a person to be prudent.
7. Rules imposed by authority.
8. An adjective from respire.
9. A person who does not smoke.
10. To exceed; to go beyond.
11. A phrasal verb meaning to start a habit or pastime.
12. An adjective from catastrophy.
13. An expression that means for a short time.
14. An adjective meaning likely to be fatal; cancerous.
15. An abbreviation for the word advertisements.

score

15

Answers 1. a smoker – 2. a decline – 3. a quarter-century – 4. an alarm – 5. preventable – 6. to warn – 7. laws – 8. respiratory – 9. a nonsmoker – 10. to surpass – 11. to take up – 12. catastrophic – 13. for a while – 14. malignant – 15 ads

Answers 1. a code – 2. a messenger – 3. synthesis – 4. infancy – 5. copying/reproducing – 6. to decode – 7. regulation – 8. to alter – 9. activity – 10. to reconstruct – 11. a ratio – 12. to turn off – 13. transcription – 14. to manipulate – 15. availability

UNIT 23

1. An increase.
2. One who attends the same class.
3. A pain in the back.
4. An institution for old people.
5. These are added to food.
6. A noun from strong.
7. The opposite of inside.
8. One who administrates.
9. School work to be done by pupils at home.
10. The opposite of oldsters.
11. A past participle meaning glued.
12. The opposite of to improve.
13. Tiredness.
14. The opposite of indoor.
15. Not typical.

score
15

UNIT 24

1. The opposite of pleasant.
2. A noun from exert.
3. One who takes part.
4. A phrasal verb meaning to postpone.
5. A noun from improve.
6. An adjective meaning habitually sitting for long periods.
7. A phrasal verb meaning to perform or conduct an experiment or study.
8. A machine on which fitness is measured by walking.
9. Another word for the colon.
10. An adverb meaning at regular intervals.
11. A noun from speculate.
12. A stage or period in a developing process.
13. A noun from perform.
14. A noun meaning that which connects two parts, a connection.
15. A test or questionnaire carried out on a representative sample for the purpose of inspection and assessment.

score
15

Answers 1. unpleasant – 2. exertion – 3. a participant – 4. to put off – 5. improvement – 6. sedentary – 7. to carry out – 8. a treadmill – 9. the bowel – 10. periodically – 11. speculation – 12. a phase – 13. performance – 14. a link – 15. a survey

Answers 1. an upswing – 2. a classmate – 3. a backache – 4. an old folks' home – 5. additives – 6. strength – 7. outside – 8. an administrator – 9. homework – 10. youngsters – 11. stuck – 12. to deteriorate – 13. fatigue – 14. outdoor – 15. atypical

UNIT 25

1. An adjective from specify. ....
2. A set of tools or equipment. ....
3. The opposite of useless. ....
4. The past of to hear. ....
5. A detailed statement of work to be done or a list of orders. ....
6. An adjective meaning complete. ....
7. A phrasal verb meaning to investigate. ....
8. An opinion on a question of action. ....
9. The past of to think. ....
10. Marvellous. ....
11. A verb meaning to supply or furnish. ....
12. An adverb meaning also. ....
13. To take for granted; to accept as true without proof. ....
14. An adjective meaning belonging to oneself. ....
15. A perception of the relative importance of facts and ideas. ....

score
15

REVISION – UNITS 21-25

1. A technology that turns off or modifies the activity of a gene. ....
2. A noun from assert. ....
3. An action or practice that has become automatic through repetition. ....
4. To move in spirals. ....
5. Granules present in all cells on which proteins are synthesized. ....
6. To study intensively for an examination. ....
7. A noun from replicate. ....
8. A verb meaning to contaminate; to make dirty. ....
9. A book from which a particular branch of knowledge can be studied. ....
10. An adjective meaning very thin. ....
11. The opposite of activate. ....
12. A state of being fit. ....
13. A phrasal verb meaning to stop or renounce. ....
14. Anxieties; preoccupations. ....
15. This approach to genetics starts with a cloned gene of interest and manipulates it to elicit information about its function. ....

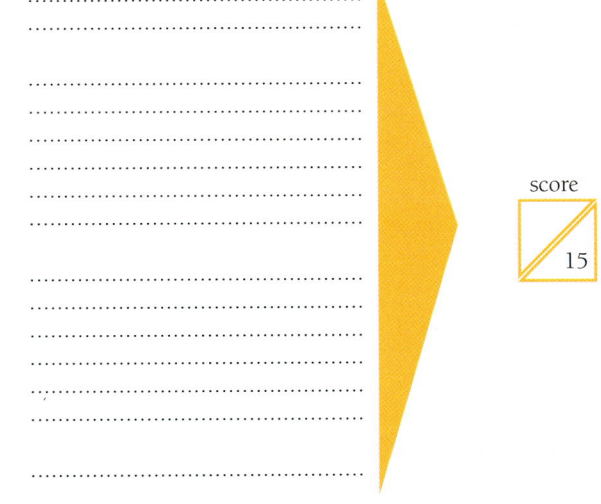

score
15

Answers 1. antisense – 2. assertion – 3. a habit – 4. to coil – 5. ribosomes – 6. to cram – 7. replication – 8. to pollute – 9. a textbook – 10. skinny – 11. deactivate – 12. fitness – 13. to give up – 14. worries – 15. reverse genetics

Answers 1. specific – 2. a kit – 3. useful – 4. heard – 5. specifications – 6. whole – 7. to look into – 8. advice – 9. thought – 10. wonderful – 11. to provide – 12. too – 13. to assume – 14. own – 15. a perspective

VOCABULARY

The following are the words and expressions that appear in the vocabulary lists at the beginning of each chapter. The number indicates the unit where the meaning of the word is given.

A

to abide by	23
to abound	18
to account for	23
to ache	9
an adage	12
adulthood	17
to affect	4
to afford	8, 21
an aggravation	15
to aid	19
to ail	3
an ailment	22
alien	18
alive and well (inf.)	2
all but	14
altogether	24
aptly	12
apt to be	8
armpit	20
to arrange	7
aside	11
to assert	22
as well as	4
to attach	19
to attenuate	20
at will	18
average	22
an award	5
awestruck	18
awry	18

B

a badge	19
a band	7
a band aid	1
to back up	15
to baffle	12
to be in pain	1
to bear	22
to bend	4
to benefit	16
to bind	17

to blame	23
a blister	9
a blockage	24
to bloom	18
a blotch	20
blown (fig.)	1
a blueprint	7
to blunt (fig.)	22
a bond	10
to boost	18
bowel	18
brand new	2
to break through	18
breezed (coll.)	1
bright	22
to bring on	20
to bring about	12
brisk	24
broad	21
a bruise	20
a bubble	20
a bug (coll.)	20
to bulge	13
bulky	3
to bump into	19
a burden (fig.)	15
to burrow	19
a bystander	11
by the turn of	17

C

a cable	3
to call off	19
carnage	19
a catch	19
to caution	22
to chop up	7
a chore	23
to cite	6
to claim	20
to clamp	13
to clarify	17
to clog	14
a clot	13
to cluster	17
a coat	20
to coil	21
to coin	10
to come of age	12
compliance	16
concrete	23
to confine	16
to cope	15

a core	17
to corrode	18
a couch	18
to counter	8
to couple	19
to cram	23
cramp	9
a craving	22
to cripple	4
to cure	18
current	14
to curtail	22
to cushion	1
to cut down	22

D

to damage	14
dead	20
a deadline	15
debatable	10
to decipher	6
to decode	21
a defect	21
to defy	18
to delineate	12
to deploy	19
to detect	14
devastating	17
a device	1
to devise	18
to disable	4
discrepancy	23
a disease	4
dismal	20
to display	19
a dividend	16
dizzy	9
downright	24
to draft	2
a draft call	19
to drain	11
to draw	14
a drawback	3
dual	19
duly	8
a dwarf	8
to dwell	23
to dwindle	23
a dye	14

E

to ease	15
elderly	16

to elicit	20	to gobble up	18	**L**	
elusive	14	to grade	16	to lace	22
to emaciate	8	a grant	2	laid-back	15
to employ	16	a grasp	19	a landmark	2
to enable	4	a gripe (sl.)	15	latter	10
to encounter	18	groin	3	to launch	18
to endanger	11	a groove	19	layout	12
endowed	18			to lead	8
ends (fig.)	2	**H**		to leak out	19
to engulf	19	half a dozen	3	lean	8
to enhance	8	a hallmark (fig.)	17	leery	2
entire	4	to halt	17	likelihood	12
to envisage	22	to handle	15	likely	7
to exacerbate	17	to hang onto (in.)	2	to liken	19
to exact	22	to harden	13	to link	3
excrutiating	1	to harm	15	a link	24
exertion	24	harmful	18	to loathe	2
to expedite	20	harsh	22	to lodge	1
to extubate	16	hay fever	20	a log	15
to eye	11	haywire (coll.)	18	to look into	25
eyelids	20	a hazard	8	to loom (fig.)	11
		to heal	3	a lot	10
F		a heel	2		
to fail	1	to hold at bay	18	**M**	
fairly	10	hollow	1	to make up	17
far	2	homework	23	malady	14
faulty	12	to hone	18	malignancy	18
to fight off	18	hordes	18	to map	6
to finger	15	a host	18	marrow	20
to fire (coll.)	19	to house	17	to match	18
to fit	19	a hunt	6	maybe	10
a fixture	10	a hurdle (fig.)	11	to mean	20
flabby	23	to hurt	9	to meet up with	19
to flatten	4			mere	6
a flood (fig.)	19	**I**		to miss	14
to flourish	18	to impair	12	missing	20
to flush	1	to imprison	15	mistakenly	14
folks	8	infancy (fig.)	21	a mold	20
for good	22	ingenuity	12	to mystify	20
formidable	6	an inhaler	20		
fragile	20	to initiate	17	**N**	
a fuel	17	insides	19	to neglect	12
		in the offing (fig.)	11	to nestle	19
G		to intrigue	21	a newcomer	3
to gain	8	an islet	17	nitty-gritty (inf.)	19
to gather	13	an itch	9	nomenclature	10
to gear up	19			norm	13
gel	7	**J**		notoriously	5
a giveaway	20	jarring	13	a nudge	2
to give rise to	17			numb	9
a glance	16	**K**			
a glob	13	to keep fit	16		
a goal	6	a kick	2		

VOCABULARY

O

to occur	4
odds	19
offspring	21
an onset	17
an onslaught	15
outcome	12
to outline	16
outset	12
outstanding	5
to outweigh	8
to overcome	4

P

to pack	10
pale	20
paltry	23
a panacea	8
a patch	11
to pave the way for	11
to pay	24
to pile up	13
pivotal	22
plagued	11
plainly	24
plenty	17
a plethora	23
a plight	4
to point out	23
a poll	19
pollen	20
to pollute	23
to pool	2
poor	20
a pore	10
to pose	16
pouchy	8
to pound	9
to pour forth	8
a practice	16
pregnant	16
to prescribe	16
a pressure-cooker	15
pretty	6
a prey	18
to prime	19
prior	16
to probe	18
progeny	21
the pros and cons	14
to prove	20
proven	18
to pry loose	18

a puff	22
pulpy	1
purplish	13
to put off	24
to puzzle	12

Q

a quarry	19
a quest	8
to quit (coll.)	15
a quota	15

R

rampart	20
random	12
to range	10
to rank	22
to recur	18
relentless	19
to rely on	21
remarkable	5
renowned	16
to retain	10
to revamp (sl.)	15
ridden	19
right away	10
to review	19
risky	3
root	17
rough	14
to rout	18
to rove	19
a row	12
rude	18
to ruffle	19
to run into	19
to rush	23

S

to scale-up	10
a scalpel	18
to scar	13
scary	9
to scatter	17
a scavenger	19
to scoop up	13
a score	9
to screen	14
to seek out	19
a segment	6
to set the stage	15
settings	9
shooting	9

a shortcoming	21
a shot (coll.)	18
to show up	7
to shun	22
to shy away from	2
to sicken	9
a siege	18
a sign	17
a site	4
skill	18
skinny	23
to slacken	8
a slab	7
slender	3
a slice	17
slight	7
a snap (coll.)	6
to snap	14
so far	3
so far as	20
soil	18
somehow	12
sore	9
soreness	22
to sort	9
a soul	22
to spare	17
speed	17
speedy	20
to spell	12
spherical	17
to spin	3
to splice	20
to split	7
to spread	18
to spur	18
to stab	9
a stack	9
stage	4
to stand to reason	8
a stare	6
to starve	17
to stave off	24
to stay off	22
steadily	22
to stem from	17
to stick	23
to stick out	23
sticky	18
stiff (coll.)	11
stiff	23
still	6
to sting	9

274

Common medical abbreviations

a.c. before meals (L.*, *ante cibum*)
ACTH adrenocorticotropic hormone
ad Latin preposition, to, up to
a.d. alternating days (L., *alternis diebus*)
alt. dieb. every other day (L., *alternis diebus*)
alt. hor. every other hour (L., *alternis horis*)
alt. noct. every other night (L., *alternis noctibus*)
AM, a.m. before noon (L., *ante meridiem*)
amt amount
anat anatomy, anatomic
anes anesthesia
ant anterior
appl applicable, application, appliance
approx approximate
av average

bact bacterium (-ia)
BCC basal cell carcinoma
BF bone fragment
bib drink (L., *bibe*)
b.i.d. twice a day (L., *bis in die*)
biol biologic, biology
BMR basal metabolic rate
BP blood pressure
BS blood sugar
BSA body surface area
BUN blood urea nitrogen
Bx biopsy

C centigrade
C one hundred (L., *centum*)
c with (L., *cum*)

(*) L.– latin

C-1 to **C-7** cervical vertebrae 1 to 7
CA cardiac arrest
CA chronologic age
Ca calcium
Ca carcinoma
cal calorie
caps capsules
cav cavity
CBC complete blood count
CC chief complaint
cc cubic centimetre
cent centigrade
CHD childhood disease
CHF congestive heart failure
chr chronic
cm centimetre
c.m. tomorrow morning (L., *cras mane*)
c/min cycles per minute
cm/s centimetres per second
CNS central nervous system
CO carbon monoxide
CO cardiac output
CO$_2$ carbon dioxide
COD condition on discharge
comp compound
conc concentrated
cond condition
cpd compound
c.p.s. cycles per second
Cs conscious, consciousness
CSF cerebrospinal fluid
Cu copper (L., *cuprum*)
cu cubic
CV cardiovascular
CVA cerebrovascular accident
CY calendar year

d dose (L., *dosis*)
D-1 to **D-12** dorsal vertebrae 1 to 12
dbl double

deg degree
dev develop, development
Dg diagnosis
diag diagnosis
dil dilute (L., *dilue*)
dis disease
disc discontinue
disch discharge
DOA dead on arrival
DOB date of birth
doz dozen
Dr. doctor
d.t.d. give of such a dose (L., *datur talis dosis*)
DTR deep tendon reflexes
DTs delirium tremens
DU duodenal ulcer
D/W dextrose and water
Dx diagnosis

EBL estimated blood loss
ECG electrocardiogram
ECT electric convulsive therapy
ed effective dose
EDTA ethylenediamine tetraacetic acid
EEG electroencephalogram
EENT ears, eyes, nose, and throat
e.g. for example (L., *exempli gratia*)
EKG electrokardiogram (German)
emerg emergency
ENT ears, nose, and throat
epith epithelial
equiv equivalent
esp especially
est estimate, estimation
et Latin conjunction, and
et al. and others (L., *et alii*)
etc. and so on, and so forth, and others (L., *et cetera*)
EUA examination under anaesthesia

F Fahrenheit
F female
FB foreign body
FBS fasting blood sugar
FD fatal dose
ff following
FH family history
fl fluid
frac fracture
frag fragment
freq frequent, frequency
FSH follicle-stimulating hormone
ft foot
FUO fever of undetermined origin
Fx fracture

g gram
gal gallon
GB gallbladder
GH general hospital
GI gastrointestinal
glob globulin
gm gram
GP general practitioner
gt drop (L., *gutta*)
gtt drops (L., *guttae*)
GU genitourinary
G/W glucose and water

H, h, hr hour (L., *hora*)
H₂O water
Hb, hgb hemoglobin
HBD has been drinking
HBP high blood pressure
h.d. at hour of lying down at bedtime
    (L., *hora decubitus*)
hosp hospital
HPI history of present illness
HR heart rate
h.s. hour of sleep (L., *hora somni*)
ht height
HVD hypertensive vascular disease
Hx history

IA incurred accidentally

ibid. in the same place (L., *ibidem*)
ICT inflammation of connective tissue
ICU intensive care unit
id the same (L., *idem*)
i.e. that is (L., *id est*)
IH infectious hepatitis
in inch
in d. daily (L., *in dies*)
inj injection, injury
inoc inoculate
inop inoperable, inoperative
int internal
i.q. the same as (L., *idem quod*)
IV intravenous

K potassium (L., *kalium*)
kc kilocycle
kg, kgm kilogram
kilo kilogram
kV kilovolt

L-1 to L-5 lumbar vertebrae 1 to 5
L & W living and well
lab laboratory
lb pound (L., *libra*)
LBP low back pain
LD lethal dose
lig ligament
LN lymph node
LSH lutein-stimulating hormone
lt left
lymphs lymphocytes

m murmur
m metre
m. dict. as directed (L., *modo dictu*)
M male
M. mix (L., *misce*)
MA mental age
mcg microgram
Mc megacycle
MDR minimum daily requirement
MED minimal effective dose
med medical, medicine
mEq milliequivalent

mg, mgm milligram
micro microscopic
min minute
min minimum
mm millimetre
mo month
MS multiple sclerosis
msec millisecond
MSH melanocyte-stimulating
    hormone

narc narcotic, narcotism
NDF no disease found
neg negative
N₂O nitrous oxide
non. rep. do not repeat
norm normal
NP neuropsychiatry
NPC no previous complaint
NPH no previous history
NPN nonprotein nitrogen
n.p.o. nothing by mouth (L., *nil per
    os*)
NR normal record
n.r. not to be repeated (L., *non
    repetatur*)
NS not significant
NSA no significant abnormality
NTP normal temperature and pressure
N/V nausea and/or vomiting

OB obstetrics
OB-GYN obstetrics and gynecology
o.d. every day (L., *omni die*)
o.d. right eye
O/E on examination
o.h. every hour (L., *omni hora*)
o.m. every morning (L., *omni mane*)
o.n. every night (L., *omni nocte*)
op operation
OPC outpatient clinic
OPD outpatient department
Ophth ophthalmology
opp opposite, opposed
OPS outpatient section, or service

ABBREVIATIONS

OR operating room (U.S.)
org organism, organic
o.s. left eye
OT occupational therapy
OT operating theatre (U.K.)
oz ounce

P pulse
P̄ after (L., *post*)
PATH pituitary adrenotropic hormone
path pathology
PBI protein-bound iodine
p.c. after meal (L., *post cibum*)
PCN penicillin
Ped pediatrics
pen penetrating
perf perforating
PH past history
PI present illness
p.m. after noon (L., *post meridien*)
PM after death (L., *post mortem*)
PMH past medical history
PO postoperative
p.o. by mouth (L., *per os*)
POD 1, 2, etc. postoperative day, first, second, etc.
pos positive
postop postoperative
pp postpartum
PPLO pleuropneumonia-like organism
ppt precipitate
prep preparation, prepare (for surgery)
p.r.n. as required, as the occasion arises (L., *pro re nata*)
prog prognosis
PT physical therapy, physiotherapy
pt patient
pulm pulmonary, pulmonic

q. every (L., *quaque*)
q.d. every day (L., *quaque die*)
q.h. every hour (L., *quaque hora*)
q.2h every second hour (L., *quaque secunda hora*)
q.i.d. four times a day (L., *quater in die*)
q.l. as much as pleased (L., *quantum libet*)
q.n. every night (L., *quaque nocte*)
q.p. at will (L., *quantum placeat*)
q.q.h. every 4 hours (L., *quaque quarta hora*)
q.s. a sufficient quantity
qt quart
q.v. as much as liked (L., *quantum vis*)

RA rheumatoid arthritis
RBC red blood cells
reg regular
req requires, required
Rh Rh factor in blood (L., *Rhesus*)
RHD rheumatic heart disease
RNA ribonucleic acid
RQ respiratory quotient
rt right

s without (L., *sine*)
sec second, secondary
SG skin graft
SI seriously ill
Sig. write on label
SIL seriously ill list
sol solution
spec specimen
sp. fl. spinal fluid
S/S signs and symptoms
stat immediately (L., *statim*)
std standard
surg surgeon, surgery
Sx symptom
sym symmetric
symp symptom
sys system

T temperature
T-1 to T-12 thoracic vertebrae 1 to 12
T & A tonsils and adenoids; tonsillectomy and adenoidectomy

tab tablet
TAT tetanus antitoxin
TB, TBC tuberculosis
tbsp tablespoon
TC treatment completed
t.i.d. three times a day (L., *ter in die*)
TPR temperature, pulse, respiration
TSH thyroid-stimulating hormone
tsp teaspoon

U, u unit
UCHD usual childhood diseases
UGA under general anaesthesia
ung ointment (L., *unguentum*)
unk unknown
URI upper respiratory tract infection
ut. dict. as directed

V, v volt
VD venereal disease
VDH valvular disease of the heart
VIT vitamin
viz that is, namely (L., *videlicet*)
vol volume
v.s. see above (L., *vide supra*)
vs versus

WBC white blood cells
w-d well-developed
Wd ward
WF white female
wh white
WM white male
w-n well-nourished
wnd wound
WNL within normal limits
wt weight

x times: 4 x, four times

yd yard
YOB year of birth
yr year

z unknown quantity

Irregular verbs

Verbs with all 3 forms the same

Infinitive	Simple past	Past participle
burst	burst	burst
cost	cost	cost
cut	cut	cut
hit	hit	hit
hurt	hurt	hurt
let	let	let
put	put	put
set	set	set
shed	shed	shed
shut	shut	shut
slit	slit	slit
split	split	split
spread	spread	spread
thrust	thrust	thrust

Verbs with 2 forms the same

Infinitive	Simple past	Past participle
beat	beat	beaten
become	became	become
bend	bent	bent
bind	bound	bound
bleed	bled	bled
breed	bred	bred
bring	brought	brought
build	built	built
burn	burnt	burnt
buy	bought	bought
catch	caught	caught
come	came	come
cling	clung	clung
deal	dealt	dealt
dig	dug	dug
dream	dreamt	dreamt
feed	fed	fed
feel	felt	felt
fight	fought	fought
find	found	found
get	got	got
have	had	had
hear	heard	heard
hold	held	held
keep	kept	kept
kneel	knelt	knelt
lay	laid	laid
lead	led	led
learn	learnt	learnt
leave	left	left
lend	lent	lent
lose	lost	lost
make	made	made
mean	meant	meant
meet	met	met
pay	paid	paid
read [ri:d]	read [red]	read [red]
run	ran	run
say	said	said
seek	sought	sought
sell	sold	sold
send	sent	sent
shine	shone	shone
shoot	shot	shot
sit	sat	sat
sleep	slept	slept
slide	slid	slid
sling	slung	slung
smell	smelt	smelt
spend	spent	spent
stand	stood	stood
stick	stuck	stuck
strike	struck	struck
string	strung	strung
sweep	swept	swept
swing	swung	swung
teach	taught	taught
tell	told	told
think	thought	thought
understand	understood	understood
win	won	won

Verbs with all 3 forms different

Infinitive	Simple past	Past participle
be	was/were	been
begin	began	begun
bite	bit	bitten
blow	blew	blown
break	broke	broken
choose	chose	chosen
do	did	done
draw	drew	drawn
drink	drank	drunk
drive	drove	driven
eat	ate	eaten
fall	fell	fallen
fly	flew	flown
forget	forgot	forgotten
freeze	froze	frozen
give	gave	given
go	went	gone
grow	grew	grown
hide	hid	hidden
know	knew	known
lie	lay	lain
ride	rode	ridden
ring	rang	rung
rise	rose	risen
see	saw	seen
shake	shook	shaken
shrink	shrank	shrunk
sing	sang	sung
sink	sank	sunk
speak	spoke	spoken
steal	stole	stolen
swim	swam	swum
take	took	taken
tear	tore	torn
throw	threw	thrown
wear	wore	worn
write	wrote	written

ANSWER BOOK

Check-Up can be used by students following a course or studying by themselves.

*In exercises where the student is asked to explain 'in your own words',
the answers given are possible explanations.*

CONTENTS

Unit

UNIT 1

TEXT BASED EXERCISES

1

title Loops of thread used to close a wound.

5 Analgesics.

20 A technique performed on patients who live at home but attend the hospital for treatment etc.

26 The initial tests carried out in order to test the effectiveness of the procedure.

29 A laminectomy.

45 A flexible instrument introduced into a wound or cavity for purposes of exploration.

57 A room in an outpatient department where the patient rests after a minor operation.

71 Fibrous tissue that is formed directly from granulation tissue by the activity of fibroblasts (a scar-mark left by a wound, burn or sore).

73 Pain that lasts for a long time or occurs frequently.

2

1 Lower back pain.

2 Bed rest, exercise and pain-killers.

3 A ruptured spinal disk pressing on nerve roots.

4 A laminectomy is a major operation that requires general anesthesia, the dissection of muscle and removal of bone. A percutaneous automated diskectomy is an outpatient procedure performed under local anesthesia through a tiny incision in the back.

5 It costs approximately one-third the cost of conventional surgery.

6 An operation in which damaged tissue is removed typically from knee joints, through a hollow tube.

7 Until the tip of the instrument rests against the disk.

8 The procedure usually takes less than an hour and requires no stitches.

9 They do too much too soon because they feel so much better.

10 Reoperation is much more difficult because of the scar tissue and adhesions that often form around the nerve roots causing chronic pain and loss of flexibility.

11 It works only for a contained rupture.

12 They require a second operation because X rays failed to reveal that the tissue had already burst out of the disk and lodged against a nerve.

3

1	traumatic	6	are back
2	local anesthesia	7	works
3	an incision	8	failed to reveal
4	performed	9	only partial relief
5	guillotine – like blade	10	surgeon

4

1 procedure / stitches

2 operation / surgery / tissue / joints

3 cases / treatments / relief

4 technique / X ray / incision / instrument

5 probe

5

1	under	6	into / of / on
2	in	7	around
3	on	8	for / through
4	into	9	of / against
5	down	10	of / by

EXTENSION EXERCISES

6

a a heart-shaped object

b a non-narcotic analgesic

c a labour-saving device

d a pain-killer
e a life-threatening disease
f a pump-like action
g a long-term effect
h calcium-rich foods

7

lower	→	upper / higher
lucky	→	unlucky
majority	→	minority
usual	→	unusual
comfort	→	discomfort
advantage	→	disadvantage
partial	→	complete
enthusiastic	→	unenthusiastic
reduce	→	increase
success	→	failure

8

reconstruction   reformation
redevelopment   reorientation
reinvestigation   reproduction
republication   reorganization
redistribution   reinsertion

9

remake   rejoin
reconsider   remould
reconstruct   redouble
reissue   retrace

10

1 C   4 B
2 E   5 D
3 A

GRAMMAR POINT

11

1 I'll answer it.
2 I'll look for them.
3 I'll teach him.
4 I'll explain it.
5 I'll visit her.
6 I'll make it.
7 I'll help him.
8 I'll tell them.

12

1 No, they're going to be cardiologists.
2 No, he's going to pass it.
3 No, I'm (we're) going to play football.
4 No, she's going to marry George.
5 No, they're going to be on time.
6 No, I'm going to read a book.
7 No, he's going to bring (or come with) his brother.
8 No, they're going to buy (or get) a new one.

IDIOM

Meaning

The cure is more
painful or harmful
than the disease itself

e.g. A. You're getting very fat. Why don't you go on a
        diet?
     B. No, thanks! The cure would be worse than the
        disease.

UNIT 2

TEXT BASED EXERCISES

1

5 Largely, to a large extent.

9 Willingly.

36 An approach that sets down rules.

37 Following closely behind.

64 Provided NIH provides some money.

75 His own purposes.

89 An approach that does not set down any rules.

94 That which has taken a long time to find.

103 Extensive sequencing.

116 First of all.

2

1	B	6	C
2	A	7	B
3	B	8	A
4	A	9	A
5	C	10	C

3

Around the world investigators / are working on / pieces of the same puzzle.

A DOE committee / has drafted / some guidelines.

Watson / has just set up / a sequencing subcommittee.

Still others / argue / that they should be able to hang onto the data until they are done, period.

We are very loathe to / impose / rules on anyone unless we are forced to.

David Patterson of the Eleanor Roosevelt Institute for Cancer Research / is getting / a complete set of these YAC clones.

He thinks that rules are clearly in order and that the NIH / ought to get on with / drafting them.

4

a pieces

b a common set

c a vast amount

d the entire group

e lots of groups

f some

5

1 issues

2 venture

3 debate

4 experiment

5 approach

6 guidelines

7 role / role / interest

8 view / sequence

6

a intensely

b publicly

c essentially

d highly

e truly

f clearly

g perfectly / promptly

7

informal   contracts

intense   unacceptable

cooperation   researchers

confront   reagents

subcommittee

EXTENSION EXERCISES

8

1 ought to be available
2 ought to take
3 ought to have
4 ought to be able
5 ought to be made

9

a shouldn't have drafted any
b shouldn't have called
c shouldn't be getting
d shouldn't become
e shouldn't suggest
f shouldn't develop (or shouldn't be developing)
g shouldn't have pooled

10

1 armful
2 spoonful
3 cupful
4 plateful
5 mouthful
6 fistful
7 bowlful
8 glassful

11

1 run out of sugar
2 run down
3 run over
4 running them down
5 I ran into another car
6 running him over
7 run over them
8 I ran into (or across) him
9 run down
10 run up against any difficulties

GRAMMAR POINT

12

1 is taking
2 is coming
3 is not giving
4 is having
5 is starting
6 are meeting
7 am going
8 am having
9 are you doing / I am studying
10 is expecting

13

1 When are their findings being published?
2 When are they drafting the guidelines?
3 When is he meeting the major groups?
4 When are we sending out our DNA probes?
5 When is the debate taking place?
6 When is the project starting?
7 When is the issue being discussed?

IDIOM

Meaning

A bedside manner is the pleasant, reassuring calmness shown by a doctor when speaking to a patient. The patient may or may not be in bed

UNIT 3

TEXT BASED EXERCISES

1

a   A heart attack
b   A transplant
c   An astonishing device
d   A transplanted heart
e   A Hemopump
f   Coronary-care units
g   Flow of blood
h   Whirling blades
i   Narrowed arteries
j   Price tag

2

1   FALSE (temporarily)
2   TRUE
3   TRUE
4   FALSE (within days)
5   FALSE (it is small)
6   TRUE
7   TRUE
8   FALSE (they feared)
9   FALSE (it may be too large)
10 FALSE (it's a bargain)

EXTENSION EXERCISES

3

risk
bleeding / blood

insertion
occurrence
treatment
device
saving
test
improvement
tolerance / toleration
invention
beat / beating

4

1   measures
2   increases
3   receives
4   rebuild
5   reconverts
6   emulsifies
7   absorb
8   open / close / contracts
9   contain
10 support

5

bound
bled
dealt
fought
froze
grew
hurt
knelt
led
stuck

6

1   in
2   over

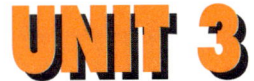

3 away / back
4 up
5 out of
6 up to
7 in for
8 for
9 out

10 mitral valve
11 left ventricle
12 pericardium

GRAMMAR POINT

7

1 I'll be
2 you see / is looking for
3 will be / doesn't pass
4 I'll phone / tell / am getting
5 come / I'll try
6 goes
7 is meeting (or meets)
8 return / you'll feel
9 will you know / they'll tell / decide
10 starts (or is starting or will start)

IDIOM

Meaning

From the bottom of one's heart means sincerely, with genuinely felt emotion

WRITING

8

1 pulmonary arteries
2 superior vena cava
3 right auricle
4 tricuspid valve
5 inferior vena cava
6 right ventricle
7 aorta
8 pulmonary veins
9 left auricle

Notes

UNIT 4

TEXT BASED EXERCISES

1

1 A crippling orthopaedic disease characterized by a spinal deformity with a flattening of the normal lumbar lordosis and an increasing thoracic kyphosis.

2 When left untreated and allowed to progress.

3 A surgeon who deals with bone deformities.

10 An ugly posture with the patient bent forward.

11 Due to the severely flexed position, the patient has difficulty in seeing straight ahead with the field of vision limited to the area around the feet.

17 The surgical cutting of the bone by which the spine is hyperextended in the lumbar region.

23 Complications of the functions of the nervous system.

24 Paralysis of the lower part of the body and both legs.

36 An operation in which a defective hip bone is removed and replaced.

40 The bones surrounding and protecting the thorax.

2

1 What is one of the most crippling diseases seen by the orthopaedic surgeon when allowed to run its own course?

2 What are the characteristics of the spinal deformity?

3 What eventually happens as the disease progresses?

4 Apart from being functionally disabling, what other effect can this disease have on the patient?

5 What is a spinal osteotomy?

6 When the operation is successful, what difference does it make to the patient's field of vision?

7 Have many surgeons attempted the operation since Smith-Peterson and colleagues published their paper?

8 What percentage of patients suffered neurological complications?

9 What is the main indication for the operative correction of the severely flexed posture in a patient with ankylosing spondylitis?

10 Are all regions of the spine and hips affected?

11 How can severe flexion contracture of the hips often be corrected?

12 When is a spinal osteotomy indicated?

13 How is a thoracic deformity best overcome?

14 When could a lumbar osteotomy possibly unbalance the patient and still not enable him to see straight ahead?

15 What should one favour when the decision to perform a lumbar or cervical spinal osteotomy is not clear?

3

1	run	11	entire
2	one	12	by
3	crippling	13	stage
4	surgeon	14	bent
5	spinal	15	at
6	flattening	16	only
7	increasing	17	functionally
8	neck	18	but
9	forwards	19	also
10	junction	20	psychologically

4

hip replacement
serious complications
thoracic cage
lumbar osteotomy
spinal column
bent forward
ugly posture
straight ahead

5

contribution
complications
deformity
extension
correction

decision
creation
replacement
indication
modification

6

a closure
b kyphosis
c patients
d complications
e rate

f posture
g deformity
h junction
i spine

EXTENSION EXERCISES

7

backward
inferior
backwards
external
outward
externally

outwards
anterior
downward
lower
downwards
outer

8

a crippling disease
a deformed position
a life-threatening illness
a weakened immune system
a severely damaged spine
disturbing news
a functionally disabling posture
health-affecting factors
a smoking related disease
a widely used technique

9

1 I'm afraid that
2 I'm not made that way
3 I was a dab hand
4 be a blind bit of use
5 touch and go
6 been off my food

6 been off my food
7 glad to see the back of it
8 dog tired
9 be cruel to be kind
10 he was dead right

GRAMMAR POINT

10

1 but some are more bent than others.
2 but some are more unfortunate than others.
3 but some were more serious than others.
4 but some could be more life-threatening than others.
5 but some are more expensive than others.
6 but some have been more successful than others.
7 but some have been more damaged than others.
8 but some are more painful than others.

11

more serious / most serious
better / best
younger / youngest
less / least

worse / worst
slower / slowest
more / most
more difficult / most difficult

IDIOM

Meaning

She had a sudden
good idea

UNIT 5

TEXT BASED EXERCISES

1

pain killers
cell biology
chromosome ends
cell division
research group
award ceremony
outpatient department
blood flow
heart transplant
emergency room

2

1 The discovery was made by Dr. Elizabeth Blackburn and her research group.

2 Dr. Blackburn has identified a key enzyme that is necessary for chromosomes to make copies of themselves before cell division.

3 She accomplished this by studying chromosome ends.

4 Their biological properties make these ends notoriously difficult to study.

5 Dr. Blackburn overcame all obstacles.

6 Dr. Blackburn is professor of molecular and cell biology at the University of California.

7 Dr. Blackburn has received the 1990 Award for Molecular Biology from the National Academy of Sciences.

8 Monsanto Company is proud to be the sponsor of this award.

9 This award is given yearly by the Academy to an outstanding scientist.

10 We join with the Academy in congratulating Dr. Blackburn for her remarkable achievement

EXTENSION EXERCISES

3

a The task was relatively easy.
b The field is intensely competitive.
c The results were radically different.
d It is a functionally disabling disease.
e It is a highly reliable test.
f It was an exceptionally difficult problem.
g It is a psychologically disturbing condition.
h It is an extremely quick procedure.

4

neurologist
immunologist
psychologist
paediatrician
surgeon
cardiologist
radiologist
pathologist
physiotherapist
psychiatrist

5

a hourly
b daily
c weekly
d monthly

6

1 going on holiday
2 reading his book

3 working with the research group
4 dancing
5 trying again
6 staying at home
7 emigrating
8 helping
9 making you wait
10 finding it
11 handling most of the heart's workload
12 performing the operation
13 coming with me
14 having been told to stay in bed, he decided to get up
15 waiting

7

1 nucleus
2 man's chromosome count
3 the chromosomal material
4 the centrosome
5 a spindle of ray-like fibres of protoplasm
6 chromatids
7 the cell cytoplasm
8 nuclear membranes

8

1 daughter
2 around
3 material
4 once
5 stage
6 mitotic
7 again
8 full-grown
9 species
10 generation
11 pass
12 hereditary

GRAMMAR POINT

9

A neurologist is a specialist who deals with the structure and functions of the nervous system.

An aspirin is a tablet that can be found in all chemist shops.

These are the results of the tests that were carried out yesterday.

A dermatologist is a specialist who deals with the skin and its diseases.

Rabies is a disease that humans can catch from infected dogs.

A cardiologist is a specialist who deals with the heart and its diseases.

The Lancet is a medical magazine that informs the medical profession of new techniques and breakthroughs.

A paediatrician is a specialist who deals with children's diseases.

An electrocardiogram is a test that records the action currents in the heart.

A psychiatrist is a specialist who treats mental and nervous disorders.

N.B. Who is normally used when the subject of the sentence is a person.

IDIOM

Meaning

To say something
or to do something very
stupid or careless

TEXT BASED EXERCISES

9 TRUE
10 FALSE (it will have a great impact)

1

15 The number of years since Watson and Crick first discerned the structure of DNA.

18 The small part of the human genome that scientists have managed to decipher.

22 The time period in which scientists hope to reach the goal of the genome project.

28 Gene therapy.

35 Beta-thalassemia major.

45 Waiting for someone to get sick and then cutting and druging them.

53 A genetic marker.

73 The cell's ability to read and decipher the genetic code.

74 The scientists' efforts to read and decipher the genetic code.

81 The proportion of premature coronary heart disease that was thought to have come from inherited abnormalities ten years ago.

84 The proportion of premature coronary heart disease that is now thought to come from inherited abnormalities.

95 The root causes of many disorders.

2

1 FALSE (don't know)
2 FALSE (largely)
3 FALSE (estimated cost)
4 TRUE
5 TRUE
6 TRUE
7 FALSE (will radically change)
8 FALSE (not all family members were affected)

3

a estimated
b complete
c complex
d high
e formidable
f controversial
g preventive
h affected
i genetic
j inherited

4

1 discerned / have managed
2 sequencing / should accelerate
3 using / inserting
4 is convinced / mapping / will radically change
5 working / concluded / had indeed found / was located
6 could benefit
7 are caused / would require / being contemplated

5

in	by	of	of	in
from	on	by	to	of
of	of	of	of	with
from	in	of		

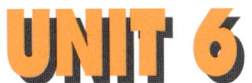

EXTENSION EXERCISES

6

a   to a large extent
b   extremely
c   in fact
d   correctly
e   greatly; fundamentally
f   at last
g   at an earlier time
h   evidently; seemingly; clearly

7

map / mapping
proposal / proposition
project / projection
cause
prediction
conviction
stare
prevention
support
suggestion

estimate / estimation
sample
explanation
confirmation
conclusion
progress / progression
location
cure
predisposition
acceleration

8

1   sticking plaster
2   drops
3   plaster
4   crutches
5   wheelchair
6   tablets
7   bandage
8   stretcher
9   sling
10 syringe

GRAMMAR POINT

9

1   was / started
2   have just heard / has been admitted (was is better when the time is mentioned)
3   left / arrived
4   did you work / worked
5   have you been
6   have just checked
7   was / had / did
8   met
9   have applied (applied is possible but refers to a completed past action rather than one considered up to the time of speaking) / has been
10 have just seen
11 have looked / haven't found
12 telephoned
13 have you finished
14 were
15 liked

IDIOM

Meaning

To do something knowing it
will cause pain to another.
The person inflicting the pain
suffers remorse for the action
he considers necessary

UNIT 7

TEXT BASED EXERCISES

1

a Body in nucleus that contains the genetic code.

b Deoxyribonucleic acid, the master chemical that controls the development and functioning of organisms.

c One of the organic compounds forming the basic constituents of living matter.

d Maps showing the location of genes on a chromosome.

e Differences between the shorter pieces of DNA that form a valuable series of markers along the chromosome.

f A defect in the genetic code.

g A small transparent tube used for chemical experiments.

h The propagation of DNA from a single ancestor.

2

1 Genetic information is present on the 46 chromosomes. This information controls the development and functioning of the organism.

2 The chromosomes are principally made up of DNA.

3 The sequence of the nitrogenous bases.

4 The closer two genes are to each other on a chromosome, the more likely they are to stay linked and be inherited together.

5 They use a large set of chemicals known as restriction enzymes.

6 Researchers have studied the differences between RFLPs and how frequently certain RFLPs are inherited together in several generations of large families and thus how close to one another the RFLPs are on the DNA chain.

7 RFLPs form a valuable series of markers along the chromosomes and make it possible, in many cases, to track down the location of the genetic defect that causes a disease.

8 A radioactive label.

9 In order to break the chain wherever that base occurs.

10 Not immediately, after a time.

3

1 sequence / bases / order
2 segment / chain / instructions
3 member / pair
4 pairs / pieces
5 set
6 series / markers
7 process / copies
8 label / strand
9 reactions
10 pattern / bands

4

blueprint
telltale
signposts
radioactive
breakpoints

5

a crucial
b complementary
c large / shorter
d close / approximate
e valuable
f electric
g distinctive
h complete

296

EXTENSION EXERCISES

6

1 e	3 a	5 g	7 d
2 f	4 h	6 c	8 b

7

1 I have my own business.
2 My wife has her own car.
3 My son has his own key.
4 She has her own ideas.
5 They have their own methods.
6 We have our own house.
7 My grandmother has her own teeth.
8 Does he have his own bank account?
9 They have their own rules.
10 The house has its own garden.

8

1 his own
2 her own
3 my own
4 our own
5 their own
6 your own
7 his own
8 my own

9

1 round
2 off
3 up for
4 up
5 across

6 up against
7 off
8 round
9 up
10 out

GRAMMAR POINT

10

1 Gastric juices are secreted by glands in the stomach wall.

2 Bile is stored by the gall bladder.

3 The amount of sugar that passes into the general circulation is regulated by the liver.

4 The actions of the body are controlled and co-ordinated by the nervous system.

5 Many of the elements needed for growth are provided by mineral salts.

6 The DNA was separated into four test tubes.

7 A large set of chemicals is used to chop up the DNA chain into smaller pieces.

8 Their approximate location on a chromosome can be determined.

9 A chemical is added that destroys one of the four bases.

IDIOM

Meaning

To gain experience of what best to do, and how to do it, in a new environment, a new job etc.

e.g. A. Have you settled into your new job yet?
      B. I'm still finding my feet.

TEXT BASED EXERCISES

1

1 A source that will provide what is needed to stay young.

6 A laboratory-produced version.

11 A course of treatment lasting six months.

19 A remedy that will prevent aging.

22 People who are no longer young but are in good health.

24 Treatment using injections of growth hormones.

26 Defects of the endocrine system.

60 Possible unpleasant effects.

69 The frequency of occurrence of leukemia.

88 Safer and more reliable ways to good health.

2

1 FALSE
2 FALSE
3 FALSE (can slow)
4 TRUE
5 FALSE
6 TRUE
7 FALSE
8 FALSE
9 TRUE
10 FALSE
11 FALSE
12 TRUE

3

body mass
endocrine deficiencies
body composition
heart failure
colon cancer
muscle loss
fat buildup
side effects
cancer connection

4

1 colon cancer
2 body mass
3 side effects / heart failure
4 muscle loss / fat buildup
  endocrine deficiencies
5 body composition
6 cancer connection

5

The six-month regimen / seemed to / undo 10 to 20 years of skin, bone and muscle deterioration.

It / would / cost about $ 14,000 a year at current prices.

A second reason for caution is that the observed effects / don't necessarily / represent improved health.

It stood to reason that aging patients / might / benefit from the treatment.

The treatment / may not / enhance "muscle strength, mobility or the quality of life".

The treatment / might even / pose hazards.

There is also a / possible / cancer connection.

The hormonal drug megestrol acetate / could / help emaciated cancer patients gain weight.

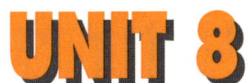
EXTENSION EXERCISES

6

1 come and go
2 come as you are
3 he came alive
4 come unstuck / come what may / come true / come, come / to come up roses / come to think of it
5 come out of his shell

7

to make or become strong or stronger

to make or become weak or weaker

to make or become light or lighter

to make or become loose or looser

to make or become flat or flatter

to make or become quick or quicker

to make or become wide or wider

to make or become long or longer

to make or become short or shorter

GRAMMAR POINT

8

hasn't	haven't
don't	doesn't
wasn't	weren't
didn't	hadn't

shan't	won't
shouldn't	wouldn't
can't	couldn't
mustn't	needn't

9

1   The others won't.
2   The others couldn't.
3   The others don't.
4   The others wouldn't.
5   The others weren't.
6   The others are.
7   The others do.
8   The others couldn't.
9   The others mustn't.
10 The others have.

IDIOM

Meaning

> To get a dose (or taste) of one's own medicine means to receive treatment of the same kind as one has given someone else

e.g. A. Tom is always playing practical jokes on people.
     B. It's about time he got a dose of his own medicine.

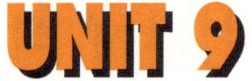

UNIT 9

TEXT BASED EXERCISES

1

1 Where were the three studies conducted?

2 Have children's pain descriptors been found to be similar or different from adult pain words?

3 Why is the development of a measure of pain quality important?

4 What was the age range of the children who took part?

5 How were the three groups of words classified that the children were asked to sort?

6 What was the criterion set for a word to be included on a pain quality word list?

7 How many words met the 50% criterion when the data from the 2 student samples were combined?

8 What trend was observed that was also found in previous research?

9 What assumption does this age-related trend support?

10 Which words were selected more frequently by girls?

11 How many words exhibited no selection bias?

12 Which 9 words were reclassified consistently by less than 70% of the children?

2

1 important assessment parameter

2 clinical specialists

3 sorting procedure

4 additional research

5 age-related trend / general assumption

6 hospitalized children

7 pediatric pain syndromes / analgesic therapies

3

a aching

b hurting

c pinlike

d stabbing

e pinching

f scratching

g stinging

4

1 a

2 a

3 b

4 c

5 b

6 a

7 c

8 b

5

a are recognized / are theoretically organized / have been used / have been found / have not been organized

b was reviewed / were identified / was printed / were asked / knew / used / knew / would not use / not known / repeated / had / was not included

c were organized / had organized / categorized / believed / determined / produced

EXTENSION EXERCISES

6

```
  8  more, further
  8  necessary, required
 30  make, draw up
 50  one by one, separately
 64  fixed
 74  unhappy
114  chosen
```

7

a seeing and believing
b testing and retesting
c including and excluding
d reporting and reviewing
e seeking and finding
f constructing and identifying
g organizing and categorizing
h selecting and rejecting
i examining and comparing
j determining and producing

8

assessment   assumption
organization   combination
practice   observation
development   research / researcher
review   description

GRAMMAR POINT

9

1 She had fallen when skiing.
2 He had received good news.
3 I had left the water running.
4 He had worked hard all day.
5 He hadn't got the job.
6 He had lost it.
7 She had forgotten to post it.
8 He hadn't set his alarm.

10

a She had just got up.
b They had just had something to drink.
c He had just gone out.
d He had just argued with his boss.
e We had just had an emergency case.
f His car had just broken down.

IDIOM

Meaning

To be applauded warmly
and vigorously

UNIT 10

TEXT BASED EXERCISES

1

4   Assistance.

6   An opportunity to test one's ability.

12 For 30 years.

15 Understanding.

21 The size of the opening.

26 Obtainable.

2

5   The challenge is usual and not uncommon.

19 Being new it is worth trying.

22 Pure.

30 The solution offered by the product is easy in comparison to the difficulty of the problem.

15 The special problems need specialist help.

21 It is of high precision.

24 This cartridge system is successful and well-liked.

31 Used to highlight the easy way to solve the problem.

3

experience
phase
size
resolution
purification
analysis
system
dimensions
work
capabilities

4

1   is
2   synthesized
3   offer
4   purifying
5   learned / gained / associated
6   put / to work / reverse
7   selective
8   packed
9   preparative
10 to separate / related

5

1   from
2   into / of / with
3   of / in
4   with / for
5   in
6   for / for / with
7   in
8   of
9   without
10 over / about

EXTENSION EXERCISES

6

a   unpopular
b   unavailable
c   indirect
d   unpredictable
e   impossible
f   unrelated
g   to unpack
h   to disassociate

7

N.B. It is also possible to begin the sentences with "not only".

1   There are columns not only for analytical work but also for preparative work.

2   I have not only studied many new expressions but also learned some phrasal verbs and idiomatic expressions.

3   I have passed not only the Biology exam but also the Anatomy exam.

4   It can help you not only to separate two closely related peptides but also to see the unpredictable triplet.

5   This medium is ideal not only for high resolution peptide purification but also for analysis.

6   They have not only the same mother and father but also the same date of birth.

7   The research group has not only studied chromosome ends but also identified a key enzyme.

8   Not only those with rare genetic disorders could benefit but also those who suffer from diabetes.

9   The treatment is not only very long but also very expensive.

10 The new procedure not only takes less than an hour but also requires no stitches.

3   How long have they been working at the hospital? They have been working at the hospital since May.

4   How long have you been waiting for them to telephone? I've been waiting for them to telephone since this morning

5   How long has she been trying to find a job? She has been trying to find a job since she left school.

6   How long has Dr. Fielding been talking to the patient? He's been talking to the patient for ten minutes.

7   How long has the patient been taking these tablets? He has been taking these tablets for a year.

8   How long has Linda been putting off going to see her doctor? She has been putting off going to see her doctor for a month.

9   How long have we been standing in the queue? We have been standing in the queue for 20 minutes.

10 How long has Mrs. Oliver been learning to drive? She has been learning to drive since September.

GRAMMAR POINT

9

| 1 | for | 3 | for | 5 | for | 7 | for |
| 2 | since | 4 | since | 6 | since | 8 | since |

10

1   How long has he been trying to give up smoking? He has been trying to give up smoking for many years.

2   How long has Jack been looking for a parking space? He's been looking for a parking space for half an hour.

IDIOM

Meaning

To be something that (finally) solves a problem

e.g. A. I've tried several remedies and nothing has helped.
     B. Why don't you try Wonder Drugs' new product? It will do the trick.

UNIT 11

TEXT BASED EXERCISES

1

3 A malfunctioning diaphragm.

8 The fluid surrounding the fetus.

10 The organs situated in the abdomen.

45 A technique that uses very high frequency sound to assemble an image of the shape and movement of parts of the body.

59 Operating on a fetus that is still in its mother's uterus.

62 A doctor skilled in obstetrics.

64 Derived lipids including sterols and certain hormones.

64 Lungs that have not fully developed.

67 Metabolisms that are not normal.

101 A machine that is used to provide artificial respiration.

2

1 Doctors open up the uterus and lift aside the fetus's left arm.

2 Surgeons cut into the fetus, whose abdominal organs have spilled into the chest.

3 Surgeons move the abdominal organs into their proper place, giving the lungs room to develop.

4 They close the diaphragm with a Gore-Tex patch and fill the chest cavity with a saline solution.

5 They enlarge the fetus's abdomen, so its organs fit, with more Gore-Tex.

6 The stomach, intestines, spleen and part of the liver can spill into the chest, leaving the lungs with no room to grow.

7 For years obstetricians have given transfusions to anemic fetuses, steroids to those with underdeveloped lungs and other medications to those with abnormal metabolisms.

8 Last year Harrison and his team operated on a 24-week fetus with the defect.

9 He spent three weeks on a respirator.

10 Only the UCSF team know how to perform it.

EXTENSION EXERCISES

3

1 Bile, produced in the livier, emulsifies fat.

2 Villi, finger-like projections, extend inward from the intestinal wall.

3 That's when the diaphragm, separating (that separates) the abdomen and chest, should close.

4 Now, at least for those fetuses in which the hernia has been detected by ultrasound, there is hope.

5 People with acromegaly, a condition caused by excess growth hormone, are at increased risk of colon cancer.

6 The pituitary gland, called the master gland, is located at the base of the brain.

7 Geneticist James Gusella discovered a particular piece of DNA, called a genetic marker, that seemed to be present in people suffering from Huntington's disease.

8 Lower back pain, as prevalent as the common cold, is the price human beings pay for walking upright.

4

careless

harmless

helpless

painless

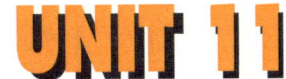
powerless
thoughtless
useless
colourless

5

a a two-inch incision
b a three-month contract
c a fifty-minute operation
d a twenty-year search
e a six-month regimen
f a five-year waiting list
g a sixty-second reaction
h a ten-day therapy

6

1 took
2 operated
3 died
4 opened / pushed
5 led
6 was
7 closed / filled
8 emphasized / understood
9 gave
10 spent

7

a done without your help
b can do without
c done in
d done up
e do with
f did well / did badly / what to do with himself / for

GRAMMAR POINT

8

1 so
2 so
3 such
4 such
5 so
6 such

9

1 It was such a long investigation that I thought they wouldn't find a solution.
2 He was such a healthy-looking man that nobody believed he was ill.
3 It was such a horrible medicine that the patient stopped taking it.
4 It was such an expensive treatment that few patients could afford it.
5 It is such a painless procedure that patients are soon able to return home.
6 It was such a small incision that it didn't leave a scar.

IDIOM

Meaning

> To be very expensive

TEXT BASED EXERCISES

1

1 strange

3 about

6 suitably named

43 additional

51 in a way still unknown

54 ingenious

92 pertinent

97 for example

122 proposed, suggested, advanced

128 considered

2

1 A curious neurological disorder.

2 Towards the beginning of this century.

3 A lesion in the left parietal lobe.

4 She could read the left sides of words well but made gross errors with right halves.

5 In particular with words spelled backwards and with words in which the letters were arranged in a vertical string.

6 She still had difficulty with their second halves.

7 They concluded that the centre of a word must somehow occupy a fixed point in the recognition and production systems for written words.

8 Most people would say that more words begin with 'r' than have 'r' as the third letter because we address words by their initial letter and, in reading, words are usually fixated just to the right of their beginning.

9 Some of the patients copied all the objects, not just those on the same side as the lesion. Patients with right-sided lesions, tended to miss out those parts of each object that lay on the opposite side of the lesion.

10 Whereas in the past it concerned itself with where a function is carried out, it is now investigating how it is carried out.

3

1	disorder	9	suggest
2	noticed	10	positioned
3	suffering	11	earlier
4	difficulty	12	mentioned
5	stimuli	13	however
6	side	14	explanation
7	fail	15	forward
8	puzzling	16	well-known

4

a backwards

b vertical

c the same

d the beginning

e left-hand side

f uncommon

g faulty

h non-dominant

5

1	caused	7	were shown
2	found	8	had
3	could read	9	tended
4	made	10	lay
5	would read	11	spelled
6	should not have been	12	were arranged

6

1 from / in / on / on / of / by / on
2 of / of / in
3 out / of / on
4 at / from / of / on / in
5 in / of
6 in / by
7 in
8 in / with / of

7

a fully
b potentially
c similarly / vertically
d perfectly
e amazingly / exactly / incidentally
f usually

EXTENSION EXERCISES

8

1 put forward
2 putting across
3 put off
4 put in for
5 put her off
6 puts away
7 put forward
8 put in
9 put away
10 put forward

9

a stimulate
b spell
c recognize
d produce
e centre
f represent
g draw
h find

GRAMMAR POINT

10

1 She'll have read the report by tomorrow morning.
2 They'll have spent the money on the project by next year.
3 Will John have left by six o'clock?
4 The laboratory will have completed the tests by tonight.
5 The doctor won't have finished his rounds by midday.
6 They'll have announced the results of the competition by June.
7 He'll have returned the book he borrowed by Wednesday.

11

1 will have been working
2 will have been typing
3 will have been studying
4 will have been operating
5 will have been living
6 will have been following
7 will have been saving up

IDIOM

Meaning

> To be clumsy and awkward

e.g. A. Why isn't John dancing?
  B. He says he can't. He's got two left feet.

UNIT 13

TEXT BASED EXERCISES

1

title The build up of factors that lead to a heart attack.

11 Stop the flow of blood.

20 The blood has difficulty in passing through coronary arteries that have slowly narrowed over time.

20 The arteries supplying blood to the heart.

21 It takes time for the arteries to narrow.

32 Ill-functioning and weakened arteries.

52 Cause it to begin.

Diagram A reduction in the swelling caused by a breakdown of the extra cells and the fat.

2

1 When does fat start to build up within the walls of the coronary arteries?

2 What happens when a clot or spasm clamps a stretch of narrowed artery completely shut?

3 What is the name of the process that causes the narrowing of the coronary arteries?

4 Does the buildup of fat take place in the interior of the artery?

5 What eventually happens when fibrous tissue forms and cholesterol and other debris pile up?

6 According to Ross and Glomset, what causes the irritation in the artery lining, which lets white blood cells enter?

7 What other factors can also set off the process?

8 What effect has the herpes virus been seen to have on the muscle cells and infected cells?

9 Who has shown that it is primarily oxidized LDL that collects in cells?

10 In lab tests, what have kept cells from swallowing oxidized LDL?

3

1 through
2 up
3 up / into / of
4 off
5 up
6 in / down / out
7 in / from / into / up
8 of / of / at / in

4

understood
called
building up
happens
line
swell
congregate
forms
bulges
impeding

5

narrowing
injury
levels
blood
lining
wall
blood pressure
process
virus
sores
enzyme
molecule

EXTENSION EXERCISES

6

gathering
bulge
fight
strike
clamp
deposit
division
irritation
infection
alteration

swelling
form / formation
narrowing
collection
compensation
impairment
a pile up
perception
oxidation
accumulation

7

1 Does fibrous tissue …
2 Is a heart attack …
3 Do both types …
4 Will Jack …
5 Could Mike take …
6 Has Mr. Collins had …
7 Would they lose …
8 Have antioxidants …
9 Can white blood cells …
10 Does fat build up …

8

1 The blood doesn't fight …
2 They haven't narrowed …
3 It doesn't happen …
4 White blood cells don't congregate …
5 It may not be …
6 It can't get picked up …
7 The cells won't swell …
8 The researchers wouldn't like …
9 He couldn't have avoided …
10 He wasn't told …

9

1 f
2 h
3 b
4 g
5 a
6 c
7 e
8 d

GRAMMAR POINT

10

1 was having / received
2 was driving or drove / saw
3 wanted or was wanting / was thinking or thought
4 was giving or gave / were sleeping or slept
5 saw / were limping
6 arrived / were waiting
7 didn't like / were always telling / was
8 told / wasn't getting

IDIOM

Meaning

To say something jokingly or to tease or deceive someone, usually only temporarily

e.g. A. I've just won first prize in the national lottery.
      B. Really!
      A. No, I'm only pulling your leg.

UNIT 14

TEXT BASED EXERCISES

1

22	to make known
24	carried out
26	during the rhythmic contractions
28	distress, inconvenience
29	from a vein
34	without moving
35	to take a snapshot (a photograph)
65	not dangerous
65	if; which of the two
70	blocked

2

1 TRUE
2 FALSE   They can miss evidence of heart disease.
3 FALSE   It fails to detect disease half the time and mistakenly announces it 30 percent of the time.
4 TRUE
5 FALSE   It is the most expensive.
6 FALSE   The results vary from doctor to doctor.
7 FALSE   Only digital angiography accurately determines an artery's narrowings.
8 TRUE
9 TRUE
10 FALSE   It requires one injection during exercise and another at rest.

3

screening	recording
tracings	monitors

measurements   injection
dye   radiation
bypass   flow
interpretations scan

4

a patterns
b rhythm
c activity
d disease
e tracer
f scan
g test
h pictures
i version
j monitors

5

1   typically
2   accurately
3   especially
4   dramatically
5   intravenously
6   incorrectly / nearly / irreversibly
7   quickly
8   visually
9   mistakenly
10 radioactively

6

1 scans
2 narrowings
3 screening / tracings
4 technique / flow

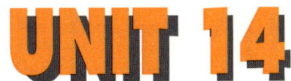

5 recording
6 interpretations

7

1 threaded
2 injected
3 drawn / reinjected / tagged
4 clogged
5 warranted
6 impaired
7 decreased / damaged
8 recorded
9 stressed

EXTENSION EXERCISES

8

1   blind
2   off
3   touch
4   do
5   harm
6   cruel
7   donkey
8   rounds
9   best
10 world

9

She'll have to work hard if she wants <u>to get on</u>.
He <u>gets on</u> very well <u>with</u> his colleagues.
John has some habits that <u>get on his wife's nerves</u>.

The situation is beginning <u>to get out of hand</u>.
I haven't <u>got over</u> the flu yet.
Can you tell me how <u>to get to</u> the station?
They can't wait <u>to get to work on</u> the project.
We hope <u>to get through</u> this work by tonight.
I tried to phone you last night but I couldn't <u>get through</u>.

GRAMMAR POINT

10

1   She had been dancing until dawn.
2   He had been visiting a patient.
3   They had been waiting for it for a long time.
4   He had been eating too much.
5   He had been driving too fast.
6   She had been avoiding everyone.
7   He had been feeling ill.
8   He had been skiing.
9   They had been waiting for an hour.
10 He had been working too hard.

IDIOM

Meaning

> To have a kind, helpful, generous nature

e.g. A. Janet is so difficult to work with.
     B. Don't be taken in. Under that hard exterior, there lies a heart of gold.

UNIT 15

1

1 The effects of the buildup of mental stress on health can be compared to the buildup of pressure in a pressure cooker.

2 Recent studies have shown that mental stress raises blood pressure, squeezes the heart's coronary arteries and makes them go into spasms and increases levels of chemicals in the blood that cause clots.

3 Over the years, these effects can weaken the coronary arteries and the heart muscle.

4 They may not appreciate their danger since the initial stages of heart disease don't reveal themselves with pain or other symptoms.

5 Undetected mini-heart attacks when spasms in the coronary arteries reduce the oxygen reaching the heart muscle and weaken it.

6 No, the hard-driving, competitive businessman who thrives on constant activity and feels in control of his destiny is at no greater risk of heart disease unless he smokes or has other risk factors.

7 Constant pressure and lack of control over work and workloads.

8 They learn stress-reduction techniques, how to overcome hostility and anxiety about time pressure and the importance of group and community activities.

9 It helps them realize how trivial many of their gripes are and can help them control their anger.

10 The sense of being imprisoned by the clock eases.

2

13 Life's irritations and annoyances.

20 Sudden involuntary muscular contractions.

22 A thick coagulated mass of blood.

37 Effects that harm the functioning of the organism.

44 When spasms in the coronary arteries reduce the oxygen reaching the heart muscle and weaken it.

47 Blocked arteries.

53 A temperament characterized by excessive drive and competitiveness.

61 Colleagues whose temperament is characterized by a relaxed, easy-going approach to life.

63 A specialist who studies the interactions between mind and body and their impact on disease and health.

114 Techniques such as meditation, yoga or relaxation exercises that help patients to reduce stress.

3

aggravation	competitiveness	questionnaire
relaxation	isolation	experience
meditation	expectation	reduction
survivor		

4

progression	colleagues	risk
disease	concept	factors
personality	specialist	history
studies	activity	lack
notion	destiny	person

5

1	shown	6	weaken	11	reveal
2	raises	7	lead	12	believe
3	squeezes	8	learn	13	trigger
4	increases	9	suffer	14	reduce
5	cause	10	appreciate	15	set

6

1	up	6	at	
2	in / to	7	of / by / about / in	
3	in / in	8	of	
4	for / by	9	on	
5	of / in / with / of	10	up / of	

7

Dr. Kenneth Pelletier	– a stress expert
recovery programmes for heart patients	– stress-reduction techniques such as daily meditation, yoga or relaxation exercises
Type A personality	– aggressive, competitive impatient and easily angered
Dr. Redford Williams	– a behavioral-medicine specialist
a competitive businessman	– hard driving
workers	– white-collar; blue-collar
Type B personality	– laid-back
psychosocial stress	– unhappiness with job or marriage

EXTENSION EXERCISES

8

a Aggressiveness may be a characteristic of type A personalities.

b Competitiveness doesn't necessarily cause stress.

c Chronic hostility, anger and powerlessness can cause stress.

d Loneliness is an experience which most people find stressful.

e Jack thought he was in for the flu as he had symptoms of tiredness and dizziness.

f Unhappiness with job or marriage are examples of psychosocial stresses.

g Stiffness can be caused by sitting in the same position for too long.

h Everyone noticed Bill's willingness to help.

9

1 He had just finished eating when he started to feel sick.

2 They had just washed the car when the rain started.

3 Steve had just begun his daily meditation when the doorbell rang.

4 Dr. Peterson had just told his colleague that he would stand in for him when he received an emergency call and he had to go out.

5 I had just started to work when I was interrupted.

6 They had just arrived at the airport when they heard their flight being called.

7 We had just got to the bus stop when we saw the bus leaving.

8 Mike had just started a course on coping with anger and hostility when his wife came home and told him she had crashed their new car.

10

1	away	3	with	5	up	7	of
2	up	4	round	6	back	8	up

GRAMMAR POINT

11

1	isn't she	7	aren't there	13	don't they
2	weren't you	8	do you	14	do they
3	has he	9	shouldn't he	15	hasn't he
4	have you	10	couldn't they	16	is it
5	can't I	11	wouldn't he	17	haven't you
6	will it	12	were there	18	won't they

IDIOM

Meaning

To be bold, insolent or presumptuous

UNIT 16

TEXT BASED EXERCISES

1

a   Patients.
b   Prescribing an exercise program for patients with limitations and special requirements.
c   Consultation.
d   Strategies.
e   Text.
f   Exercise plan.
g   Reference.
h   People.
i   Scientific researches.
j   The dividends from keeping fit.

2

a   Obesity is the state of being very overweight.
b   An option is a choice.
c   A precaution is a step taken in advance to avoid damage.
d   Limitations are the restrictions that decide the maximum the patient is capable of achieving.
e   Dialysis is a technique used to purify blood.
f   Strategies are plans.
g   Contributors are those who have written chapters in the book.
h   A reference is a book consulted for specific information but not read straight through.

3

train
illustrate
adapt
comply

quote
prescribe
summarize
opt
refer
limit
divide
require
consult
practise

4

1   special / interesting
2   important / distinguished
3   healthy / simple / appropriate
4   superb / renowned / respective
5   valuable
6   sick / well / growing / scientific

5

1   for / of
2   of / with
3   on
4   for / in / for
5   at
6   of / by / in
7   to / with / of
8   in
9   from / with / from / of / in / of
10 up

EXTENSION EXERCISES

6

unhealthy
unstructured

inappropriate
ineffective
infrequent
insoluble
uninteresting
undistinguished
inexpensive
indirect
unsuited
unscientific
inaccurate
inactive

7

wealthy
responsive
protective
provocative
obese
effective
dangerous
selective
tragic
defective

8

1 It does tell you …
2 The text does include …
3 The final chapter did outline …
4 The figures, tables and illustrations do summarize …
5 A wheelchair-confined patient does need …
6 You do need to design …
7 Their special limitations did pose …
8 Do order today.

9

1 d
2 f
3 b
4 h
5 a
6 e
7 c
8 g

GRAMMAR POINT

10

1 he'll get better treatment.
2 he overeats.
3 you'll miss the meeting.
4 she thinks it isn't really necessary.
5 he calls at the surgery before six o'clock.
6 I decide not to follow the treatment.
7 I'll certainly lend a hand.
8 the doctor will see you in half an hour.
9 you lose weight.
10 I'll have to leave without him.

IDIOM

Meaning

To feel fearful or timid as the time
for action approaches

UNIT 17

TEXT BASED EXERCISES

1

1 They faced certain death within about a year of diagnosis.
2 It slows the development of complications.
3 They must find the root causes.
4 It stems from an autoimmune attack on the pancreas.
5 At the University of Florida, they are trying to determine which components of the immune system are the major agents of attack, what triggers the autoimmune reaction and what allows it to persist.
6 Treatment can be initiated at the very first sign of disease.
7 By the turn of the next century.
8 Hormone-producing cells.
9 No, only the insulin-producing beta cells.
10 As the beta cells are killed and the pancreas stops producing insulin the cells of the body are not helped take up the sugar glucose.
11 Insulin injections cannot mimic the normal pattern of insulin release by the pancreas. Nor can they normalize metabolic functioning well enough to prevent the long-term complications of diabetes.

2

a beta cells	e by-products	h fuels
b attack	f complications	i hormone
c cells	g therapy	j sequence
d diabetes		

3

a devastating	c remarkable
b ideal	d metabolic

e digestive
f normal
g spherical
h major

4

a highly / frequently	d generally / chronically
b recently	e abnormally
c currently	f uncontrollably

5

1	type I	11	ketones
2	death	12	dehydration
3	diagnosis	13	coma
4	pancreas	14	disease
5	ability	15	vessels
6	insulin	16	heart
7	metabolism	17	stroke
8	causes	18	failure
9	breakdown	19	glucose
10	fat	20	attack

6

1	of / up	5	of / in / at / of / of
2	in / of / throughout	6	by / of
3	up / of	7	in / of / down / of
4	from / on	8	for / of

EXTENSION EXERCISES

7

a The new operation should be successful.
b Discomfort should be uncommon.
c Investigators should be working on many projects.
d It should be a rapid task.

e   The technique should be very simple.
f   Severe flexion contracture of the hips should be corrected by total hip replacement.
g   Establishing guidelines should be easy.
h   The treatment should be very economic.

8

1   My doctor recommended that I should change my diet.
2   My doctor suggested that I should work less.
3   My doctor insisted that I should take a holiday.
4   My doctor recommended that I should walk more.
5   My doctor suggested that I should drink less coffee.
6   My doctor suggested that I should relax more.
7   My doctor recommended that I should take up a sport.
8   My doctor suggested that I should worry less.
9   My doctor suggested that I should go to bed earlier.
10 My doctor insisted that I should come for a check-up more often.

9

a   himself
b   themselves
c   itself
d   myself
e   herself
f   ourselves
g   yourself
h   yourselves

10

a   6
b }7/10
c
d   2

e   8
f   9
g   3

h   1
i   4
j   5

GRAMMAR POINT

11

1   I'd study harder.
2   she told you the truth.
3   we'd work better.
4   he'd get a cure for his condition.
5   we asked them.
6   you had time.
7   he excercised every day.
8   we didn't smoke.
9   you invited him yourself.
10 you'd soon feel well.

12

1   If I were you, I'd accept it.
2   If I were him, I'd tell them (what happened).
3   If I were him, I'd take them.
4   If I were them, I'd improve it.
5   If I were you, I'd try it.
6   If I were her, I'd clarify them.
7   If I were them, I'd ask (for help / for it).
8   If I were her, I'd read it.
9   If I were him, I'd start it.
10 If I were them, I'd reveal them.

IDIOM

Meaning

To be fond of sweet
foods and drinks

UNIT 18

TEXT BASED EXERCISES

1

3 Full of great numbers of disease causing microorganisms.
48 Initiate a ceaseless fight.
50 A highly planned attack by the body's immune system.
62 Early-warning cells that constantly monitor the bloodstream and tissues for signs of foreign bodies.
68 The different types of cells of the immune system each having a special task.
70 An obstruction causing many difficulties.
117 Cleverly made new treatments for a large number of illnesses.
127 Treatments that seem likely to succeed.
132 Showing the first signs of a disease.
148 A fundamental part.

2

12 Microscopic organisms
27 Germs
58 Early-warning cells
83 Scientists
85 The immune system
115 Advances
130 Researchers
150 A key component of the immune system
162 Body cells
165 Victims
174 Dr. Anthony Fauci
177 Nature
186 Researchers

3

4 bacteria, viruses, fungi, parasites

37 skin, sweat, saliva, tears, stomach acids, the mucus of the nose and throat
54 early warners
60 remnants of invaders and infected or damaged body cells
63 killers
66 to destroy
83 complex
154 victims

4

1 potentially
2 fortunately
3 extraordinarily / occasionally
4 relatively
5 tirelessly / comfortably
6 usually / eventually

5

a has undergone
b match / enabled / to devise
c is not exaggerating
  have been reported
  announced
  activating
  had increased
d is progressing
  are
  are published
e believes
  would have been
  made
  had come
  be looking

6

1 tough / natural / sticky
2 alarming / vital
3 vulnerable / invading
4 troublesome / serious
5 intricate
6 dormant
7 new

7

1	illness	6	diseases	11	tissues
2	cancers	7	vaccine	12	cells
3	system	8	protection	13	organ
4	allergies	9	epidemic	14	brain
5	disorders	10	bloodstream	15	lungs

EXTENSION EXERCISES

8

a   The respiratory system has a phenomenal ability for bringing oxygen into the body and giving out the unwanted carbon dioxide and water.

b   The circulatory system has a phenomenal ability for transporting materials to all other organs and tissues.

c   The digestive system has a phenomenal ability for digesting and absorbing food and eliminating undigested material.

d   The excretory system has a phenomenal ability for eliminating useless or harmful products which have been made in the body.

e   The nervous system has a phenomenal ability for controlling and co-ordinating the actions of the body.

f   The muscular system has a phenomenal ability for providing the basic means of all movement.

g   The skeletal system has a phenomenal ability for supporting and protecting the parts of the body.

h   The sensory system has a phenomenal ability for receiving information from outside the body.

9

1   it was not until he read about the dangers that he decided to give up

2   it was not until her workload increased that she decided to leave

3   it was not until we went to England that we had the opportunity to speak

4   it was not until her friend needed a transfusion that she decided to become a donor

5   it was not until he dedicated himself to the sport that he started to win championships

6   it was not until he tried the new treatment that he had any relief

GRAMMAR POINT

10

1   had applied / would have got
2   had you asked / would have given
3   wouldn't have lent / had known
4   had told / would have visited
5   wouldn't have broken / hadn't fallen
6   had she attended / would have had
7   had taken / wouldn't have deteriorated
8   hadn't lifted / wouldn't have hurt

11

1   Se avessi saputo che stava arrivando l'avrei incontrato all'aeroporto.
2   Se ieri avesse piovuto, non ci sarebbe andata.
3   Mi avrebbero telefonato dall'ospedale, se ci fosse stata un'emergenza.
4   Se non avesse preso un raffreddore, non avrebbe dovuto perdersi la partita.
5   Se avessi saputo che era in ospedale, sarei andato a trovarlo.

IDIOM

Meaning

To be stupid

UNIT 19

TEXT BASED EXERCISES

1

11 Allowed to develop freely.
34 Other cells of the immune system or of the same kind.
42 A warning signal to attack.
54 The commander of the attack.
91 Thus called.
107 Cells set aside to produce a large number of antibodies.
109 To produce in large quantities to an identical pattern.
118 To destroy.

2

2	general	71	at last
11	more	77	next; at that time
12	in the course of time	80	at the same time
15	easily	84	might
20	still more	168	immensely
27	only	174	for strategic reasons

3

1 a   2 c   3 a   4 b   5 a

4

1 What happens when a flu virus burrows into a cell in the lining of an air passage?
2 What would happen if it were left unchecked?
3 Why does the macrophage probably move from the body tissue into the nearest lymph node?
4 What happens when the macrophage finally runs into a compatible helper T cell?

5 What effects may result when interleukin-I acts on the body's central thermostat?
6 What is the visible result of the stimulation of the defense system?
7 What change takes place in the B cells?
8 What do the infected cells display on their outer membranes that enable killer T cells to recognize them?
9 Why do the killer T cells transmit a signal that causes the cell to chew up DNA from both itself and the virus?
10 Does the body become immune to all viruses after an infection?

5

1	substances	7	viral activity
2	blood vessels	8	immune response
3	bloodstream	9	memory cells
4	infection	10	strain
5	process	11	flu virus
6	fever	12	antibodies

6

1	carries	6	engulf	11	produce
2	enable	7	digest	12	activate
3	survive	8	mature	13	aid
4	secretes	9	calls	14	stick
5	causes	10	begin	15	kills

7

a	4	e	6	h	9
b	7	f	2	i	5
c	10	g	3	j	8
d	1				

8

1	over	3	into	5	out / in	7	down
2	up	4	on	6	up	8	off

EXTENSION EXERCISES

9

a   Capillaries are the smallest blood vessels in the body that connect an artery and a vein.

b   A stethoscope is an instrument used to listen to heart and lung sounds.

c   The oesophagus is the food tube leading from the mouth to the stomach.

d   The kidneys are paired organs which extract nitrogenous wastes from the body for elimination.

e   A protein is a complex organic compound of numerous amino acids.

f   An electrocardiogram is a record of electrical waves from the heart.

g   Insulin is a hormone that controls the oxidation of sugars.

h   An enzyme is an organic substance produced by living cells, that acts as a catalyst in chemical changes.

i   Fibrinogen is a substance in the blood plasma which is changed to fibres to form a clot under certain conditions.

j   A virus is one of the various parasitic agents causing infectious diseases in plants and animals.

10

1   Having broken his leg, he decided to give up skiing.

2   Having had a hard day at work, she went home to relax.

3   Having woken up late, he missed the bus.

4   Having felt ill, Mr. Foster went to see his doctor.

5   Having written the letter, she went out to post it.

6   Having checked that the train strike had been called off, they went to the station.

7   Having driven all day, we were very tired when we arrived.

8   Having been told that he had been promoted, he phoned his wife to tell her the news.

9   Having seen the accident, they telephoned for an ambulance.

10 Having read the book, Carol lent it to her friend.

GRAMMAR POINT

11

1   you die
2   the train hadn't been late
3   you diet properly
4   she is to survive
5   he hadn't had a relapse
6   they are not on duty at the hospital
7   I want to be a doctor
8   he had studied more

12

1   Può darsi che venga oggi, se glielo chiedi.
2   Devi studiare se vuoi passare l'esame.
3   Se mi avesse detto la verità, forse avrei potuto fare qualche cosa.
4   Potrei venire domani pomeriggio se ti va.
5   Se vuoi badare di più alla salute, dovresti mangiare meno cibi grassi.

IDIOM

Meaning

> To pay for something, usually by accepting the total cost

e.g. A. That was a delicious meal.
     B. Let me foot the bill.

UNIT 20

TEXT BASED EXERCISES

1

3 A preparation of a virus used for inoculation.

29 To have more chance of catching the disease.

43 An injected dose of vaccine against influenza.

83 Sudden and relatively permanent genetic changes.

91 Those who offer to do a task.

114 Not functioning correctly.

118 A disease caused by a defect in the immune system.

125 The transfer of bone marrow from a donor to a recipient.

150 Drugs that counteract the release of histamine.

194 An apoplectic attack.

2

10 a piece

16 produce no effect

43 made stronger

47 causing trouble; difficult to deal with

55 deal successfully with

81 examining closely

90 not strong, poor

92 to inject

139 systems

150 only for a time

3

1 Synthesized antigens are used in creating vaccines.

2 Flu viruses mutate rapidly, continually changing their antigens in the process.

3 The malaria parasite penetrates cells so quickly that it is hidden from antibodies.

4 The AIDS virus mutates twice as fast as the flu bug.

5 The AIDS virus can mount a speedy and lethal attack on helper T cells which cripples the immune system before it can counterattack.

6 Even without provocation by the AIDS virus or other infectious organisms, the immune system can sometimes go wrong.

7 Immunoglobulin E antibodies set off an allergic reaction.

8 The immune system mounts an assault against parts of the body, destroying cells or cell components that it mistakenly identifies as alien.

9 When the beta cells which produce insulin are destroyed, the body cannot convert sugar into the energy the cells need to function and unconverted sugar builds up in the bloodstream.

10 Complications associated with type 1 diabetes include heart and kidney disease, poor circulation, eye problems and stroke.

4

antibodies

antihistamines

autoimmune

disagree

disorders

insufficient

incapacitate

ineffective

malfunctioning

overrespond

predominant

provocation

re-engineered

unchanged

unconverted

5

a approach

b techniques

c ingredient

d supply

e growth

f varieties

g reaction

h response

i stages

j condition

6

sufferers

mutation

provocation

response

affliction

inflammation

marker
vaccine
reaction
failure

circulation
arrival
appearance

7

intestinal tract
bacterial meningitis
immunological decoys
multiple sclerosis
nasal sprays

infectious organisms
cancerous cells
allergic reactions
chemical signals

8

1	despite	6	yet	11	because
2	seems	7	for example	12	at least
3	ever	8	as	13	still
4	well	9	strengthened	14	so
5	against	10	also	15	each

EXTENSION EXERCISES

9

1 The marker protein that provokes the immune response is removed from the bug's surface.
2 The antigen is mass-produced.
3 Still other problems are posed by the parasite that causes malaria.
4 A speedy and lethal attack on helper T cells can be mounted.
5 Bits of protein molecules have been synthesised.
6 One such vaccine has been created by a group in Paris.
7 Inflammation and swelling are caused by these changes.
8 The AIDS virus is being scrutinized.

10

1	b	3	a	5	f	7	h
2	e	4	g	6	c	8	d

GRAMMAR POINT

11

1 I want them to go out.
2 We want them to win.
3 She didn't want us to tell you.
4 I want him to accept it.
5 He wants her to become a lawyer too.
6 I want you to tell me the truth.
7 They wanted her to go to the cinema with them.
8 Everyone wanted him to tell them about his experiences.
9 Do you want me to make some coffee?
10 We all wanted it to be the best holiday we had ever had.

12

1 Voglio che egli studi biologia molecolare.
2 Vogliono che io telefoni loro.
3 Vuole che lei aspetti?
4 Voleva che gli prestassi la mia macchina.
5 Volevi che cominciassimo?
6 Voleva che scrutinasse i risultati.

IDIOM

Meaning

To have something in one's past
that one wants to hide

TEXT BASED EXERCISES

1

1 Approximately how many genes does it take to make a human being?

2 In what way does the ability to deactivate specific genes hold great promise for medicine?

3 Are such applications well-developed?

4 What is the basic difference between classical genetics and reverse genetics?

5 Why are additional approaches often needed?

6 In what form does DNA in organisms usually exist?

7 Does DNA make proteins directly?

8 What base difference is there in RNA compared to DNA?

9 Is the function of antisense RNA confined to regulation of DNA replication?

10 What happens when the bacteria transcribe antisense RNA from the sense strand of the transposase gene and the antisense RNA binds specifically with the sense messenger RNA?

2

26 The ordered sequences of the nucleotide bases.

30 The progressive series of changes in organisms.

37 Diseases caused by viruses.

38 Molecules that bind specifically with a targeted gene's RNA message thereby interrupting the precise molecular choreography that expresses a gene as a protein.

43 An approach to genetics that starts with a cloned gene of interest and manipulates it to elicit information about its function.

53 The process of emitting radiant energy in the form of waves or particles.

141 Cell structures which read the encoded information and string together the appropriate amino acids to form the encoded proteins.

197 The process by which a strand of RNA is synthesised.

3

a long-lived
b viral
c classical
d weak
e systematic
f mutated
g broad
h genetic
i observable

4

experiments / experimenter   discovery
generation   radiation
origin   approach
concentration   expression
inhibitors   transcription
products   regulation

5

impossible   long-lived
to turn off   life
new   invertebrate animals
random   weak
realistic   simple

6

1 to fight / seek / destroy
2 to deactivate / holds
3 initiate / pair
4 relies / alter
5 decoded

7

1 contributing
2 pairing / recontructing
3 linking
4 encoding
5 cloning / copying / becoming / turning / modifying

8

1 from
2 with / off
3 of / of / on / of / inside
4 with / among
5 in / at
6 by / by / of
7 on
8 of / in / for

EXTENSION EXERCISES

9

1 Is he perhaps waiting for Mary?
2 Is it perhaps going to rain?
3 Are they perhaps expecting too much?
4 Has he perhaps been delayed?
5 Are they perhaps ill?
6 Is he perhaps going skiing?
7 Was she perhaps feeling tired?
8 Was he perhaps driving too fast?

GRAMMAR POINT

10

1 I wish I knew her name.
2 They wish they didn't have to work late.
3 He wishes he didn't have to go to the dentist.
4 She wishes she could find a job.
5 They wish they didn't have to travel on crowded trains.

6 He wishes he had enough money to buy a new car.
7 I wish I didn't have to study tonight.
8 We wish we didn't have to start work very early in the morning.

11

1 I wish I hadn't driven so fast (or had driven slower).
2 I wish I had remembered to post the letter this morning (or hadn't forgotten).
3 He wishes he had gone to the doctor when the pain started.
4 I wish I had studied Russian.
5 We wish we had eaten less last night (or hadn't eaten so much).
6 John wishes he had known about it.
7 I wish I had bought my house when I had the chance.
8 I wish I had stayed at home yesterday (or hadn't gone out).

12

1 Vorremmo potervi venire a trovare più spesso.
2 John vorrebbe non dovere andare al lavoro oggi.
3 Vorrei che smettesse di nevicare.
4 Vorrebbe potere cambiare lavoro.
5 Vorrei sapere dove sono andati.

IDIOM

Meaning

To have a prickling sensation
in a limb when blood starts
to circulate freely again
after pressure or a cramped position

UNIT 22

TEXT BASED EXERCISES

1

title The 25th anniversary of the Surgeon General's first alarm about the dangers of smoking, indicates that tobacco is still the single most important preventable cause of death, responsible for I out of every 6 deaths in the U.S.

4   Smoking can cause diseases resulting in death such as cardiovascular disease, lung cancer, chronic respiratory ailments and stroke.

5   Highly alarming (literal meaning-large type of bomb capable of destroying a block of buildings).

8   Immediately.

16 In the years from 1940 to 1959.

17 Fashionable.

22 Alarming, unsettling news.

52 In the future years.

61 For a short period of time.

83 What has been said or done is more than sufficient, so that nothing else needs to be said or done.

89 A society that has given up smoking.

2

to look back – to remember; to return in one's thoughts

to give up – to stop; to cut out

to stub out – to extinguish a cigarette by pressing its lighted end against something (a stub: a short piece of cigarette or cigar left when the rest has been smoked)

to stem from – to arise from; to have as its source or cause

to level off – to make or become level

to take up – to adopt as a pastime

to light up – to apply a flame to tobacco

3

1   The U.S. Surgeon General Luther Terry issued a blockbuster report warning about the dangers of smoking.

2   The last twenty five years have seen a revolution in smoking behavior.

3   Smoking is responsible for I out of every 6 deaths in the U.S.

4   Tobacco was previously estimated to have claimed 300,000 lives a year.

5   The average male smoker is 22 times as likely to die from lung cancer as is a nonsmoker.

6   The incidence of lung cancer has been leveling off for men.

7   Only 29% of adults now smoke in the U.S.

8   Nearly half of all living adults who have ever smoked have given up, at least for a while.

9   Level of education is the best predictor of tobacco use.

10 Cigarette use was declining among teenagers, but has now leveled off.

4

ailments
restrictions
population
attack
assertion
campaign

purchaser
school/schooling
puff
escalation

5

1 estimates
2 thirds
3 cardiovascular
4 cancer
5 respiratory
6 smoker
7 times
8 nonsmoker
9 time
10 cause
11 estimated
12 all
13 incidence
14 rising
15 estimate
16 malignancies
17 leading

6

1 of / with / in / against
2 in
3 of / for / out / of / in
4 on / in
5 of / up / down / from / in
6 of / at / for
7 over / in
8 among / by / by
9 in
10 by

EXTENSION EXERCISES

7

1 More lives have been claimed by tobacco than had previously been thought.
2 More high school students have started smoking than had previously been thought.
3 More people have stopped smoking than had previously been thought.
4 More strides have been made in the antismoking campaign than had previously been thought.
5 More men have given up smoking than had previously been thought.
6 More reports have been written than had previously been thought.
7 More women have taken up smoking than had previously been thought.
8 More children are smoking at a younger age than had previously been thought.

8

1 I think so
2 I suppose so
3 I hope not
4 I'm afraid not
5 I expect so
6 I don't think so
7 I don't suppose so
8 I don't expect so
9 I hope so
10 I'm afraid so

UNIT 22

9

1 More college graduates smoked in 1965 than in 1987.

2. More whites smoked in 1965 than in 1987.

3 Less men smoked in 1987 than in 1965.

4 Less blacks smoked in 1987 than in 1965.

5 More high school dropouts smoked in 1965 than in 1987.

6 Less college graduates smoked in 1987 than in 1965.

7 More women smoked in 1965 than in 1987.

8 Less high school dropouts smoked in 1987 than in 1965.

9 Less whites smoked in 1987 than in 1965.

10 More blacks smoked in 1965 than in 1987.

10

a the more likely they are to be overweight

b the more likely they are to drive safely

c the more likely they are to be irritable

d the more likely they are to pass their exams

e the less likely they are of having lung cancer

f the more likely they are to practise sports

g the more likely they are to find a vaccine

GRAMMAR POINT

12

When I was a child I used to *dream* of becoming a doctor. Every night, I used to *lie* in bed and picture myself in a white coat. I used *to study* very hard at school. I was used to *studying* hard, so when I went to university it wasn't a problem. I used to *get* up at half past six every morning in order to catch the 7.15 bus. I never really got used to *getting* up so early. I always used to *arrive* at my lectures still half asleep.

Now I am a doctor, I am used to *working* irregular hours. Before specializing in surgery, I used to *work* in the Casualty Department. I wasn't used to *being* on shifts. In the beginning it was difficult but now I'm used to it.

13

1 Sono abituato a leggere articoli scientifici.

2 Eri solito abitare a Londra, non è vero?

3 A Jack piaceva il suo lavoro, ma adesso si è annoiato.

4 È abituato a risolvere problemi difficili.

5 Erano soliti lavorare molto meno.

IDIOM

Meaning

To have the ability to see in all directions at once and notice all that is happening around one

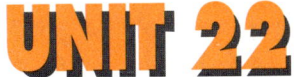

NOTES

UNIT 23

TEXT BASED EXERCISES

1

a backache
b muscles
c shoulder
d allergies

e eyesight
f strength
g fatigue

2

1 They complain about a backache.
2 He has noticed that his young patients seem to break bones much more often these days. Fractures tend to come from just missing a step on the staircase. They don't move their bodies. They don't use their muscles.
3 The minds of Japanese children benefit from one of the world's most rigorous educational systems, but their bodies are woefully neglected.
4 He found pupils yawning in class and complaining about fatigue. Teenagers suffered from stiff shoulders and backaches.
5 41.3 percent of 193 kindergarten teachers throughout Japan noticed that children tend to fall on their faces, instead of sticking their hands out to protect themselves when confronted with a potential danger.
6 Masaki blames postwar prosperity for the decline in physical fitness.
7 In the old days, children had to help around the house cleaning, washing and carrying things which helped to build their back-muscle strength. Now they don't do any of these house chores.
8 In Tokyo, there are only 2.5 square meters of park space for every person, compared with 45.7 square meters in Washington and 19.2 square meters in New York.
9 If found that only 60 percent of the children played outside an hour a day.
10 He says there is a limit to what schools can do to solve the problem because administrators say that the classroom curriculum is so demanding that there isn't time for more physical education.

3

eyesight
backache
outdoor
homework
upswing

postwar
classroom
staircase
afterclass
classmates

4

a stiff
b out-of-shape
c rigorous
d physical
e paper-thin

f potential
g industrial
h drastic
i restrictive
j high-tech

5

1 shoulders
2 backaches
3 strength
4 allergies
5 diet
6 additives

7 pediatrician
8 patients
9 bone
10 fractures
11 bodies
12 muscles

EXTENSION EXERCISES

6

1 Japanese youngsters would probably be better to be more active.
2 Japanese schoolchildren would probably be better to go to bed earlier.
3 Japanese children would probably be better to study less and exercise more.
4 The Education Minister would probably be better to modify the demanding classroom curriculum.
5 Most elementary and junior high schools would probably be better to offer more hours of physical education a week.

6 City dwellers would probably be better to set up special playparks for young children.

7 Japanese children would probably be better to do some of the house chores.

protection
limit / limitation
survey

warning
pollution
schedule

7

| 1 say | 3 says | 5 tell | 7 said |
| 2 told | 4 tell | 6 telling | 8 were telling or told |

GRAMMAR POINT

11

1 to go
2 to pass
3 to apply / to put in
4 to have
5 to be

6 to forget
7 to become
8 to lend
9 to take

8

1 they won't have time for physical exercise
2 I'll give you it
3 they'd be fitter
4 the children would have had more fun
5 the kids will have to be quiet or the neighbors will complain
6 there wouldn't have been such an upswing in allergies
7 they'd be able to run around
8 the schools could offer more hours of physical education a week

WRITING

12

TIRED
INSTEAD
BACKACHE
SCHEDULE
PEDIATRICIAN
STRENGTH
YOUNGSTERS

GLUED
OFTEN
YAWNING
MUSCLES
FATIGUE
SURVEYED
SLIGHT

9

1 to make a start.
2 to make a song and dance.
3 head nor tail of it.
4 make an effort.
5 made a mental not.
6 make both ends meet.
7 made a name for himself.
8 make yourself useful.
9 making headway.
10 make a mountain out of a molehill.

IDIOM

Meaning

Not sensitive.
Not easily upset
or annoyed

10

comparison
notice

complaint
deterioration

UNIT 24

TEXT BASED EXERCISES

performance   blockages
participants   investigation
benefit   speculations

1

2   Putting on.

3   To run in the streets.

5   Methods.

22   Conducted.

27   Factor.

35   Not based on opinion but on an accurate
     assessment.

46   Achievement.

87   To some extent; partly.

2

1   Hard physical exertion is downright unpleasant.

2   A brisk half-hour walk once a day is enough.

3   It strengthens the evidence that exercise can ward
     off cancer.

4   The researchers measured fitness in a
     straightforward way.

5   The subjects were grouped into five different
     fitness levels.

6   You don't have to be a marathoner to greatly
     reduce your mortality.

7   Some scientists speculate that exercise increases
     bowel motility, a factor in avoiding colon cancer.

8   People who exercise just a little bit tend to live
     longer.

3

range   exertion
link   incline

4

a   disease   f   category
b   mechanisms   g   groups
c   protection   h   walk
d   study   i   factors
e   blood flow   j   measure

5

a   hardly / especially / mostly / only
b   sharply
c   periodically
d   greatly
e   plainly
f   literally

6

1   into / on / for   6   in / by / of
2   at / of / of / in   7   for / off
    / at / of   8   in / of / up
3   into   9   of / on / of / of
4   in / on / of   10   off / in
5   in

7

1   participants   9   sedentary
2   health   10   twice
3   allowing   11   included
4   various   12   habit
5   including   13   still
6   weight   14   improvement
7   pressure   15   dramatic
8   history

EXTENSION EXERCISES

8

1 tend to be unfit
2 he tends to get angry
3 I tended to spend my time with my friends so I spoke my native language
4 he tends to become aggressive
5 are tending to smoke less
6 I tend to dream about it
7 tended to be decreasing
8 she tends to avoid answering
9 he tends to exaggerate
10 he always tends to be late

9

a There were 10 of us.
b There were 55 of them.
c There were 4 of us.
d There were 16 of you.
e There were 30 of them.
f There were 100 of you.
g There were 260 of us.
h There were 15,000 of them.

10

1	ghost	9	needles
2	both ends	10	bedside
3	dose	11	skeleton
4	dance	12	cure
5	mental	13	arm / leg
6	leap	14	eyes
7	big	15	foot
8	mountain		

11

1	up	6	up
2	out	7	for
3	up / for	8	out
4	to	9	out
5	up to	10	up

GRAMMAR POINT

12

1	going	6	catching
2	giving	7	attending
3	sitting	8	taking
4	applying / putting in	9	leaving
5	following	10	reading

13

1 Pensò di andare all'estero.
2 Evitava di incontrarlo.
3 Ammise di aver mentito.
4 Ti dispiacerebbe aprire la finestra?
5 Suggerirono di provare un altro metodo.
6 John rischiò di perdere il suo lavoro.
7 Ricordò che gli era stato mostrato il rapporto.
8 Ci siamo divertiti lavorando al nuovo progetto.

IDIOM

Meaning

To speak too readily
or indiscreetly

UNIT 25

TEXT BASED EXERCISES

1

I'd like
see
aren't
thought
assume
are supplied
I've heard
synthesise
believe
provides
to be amplified
sound
use
you've given
looking into

EXTENSION EXERCISES

2

advice   activation
guide   amplification
thought   copy
specification   belief
supply   synthesis

3

a The information was useful.
b The accomodation was excellent.
c The news was bad.
d The people were friendly.
e His behaviour was strange.

f The scissors are blunt.
g His advice was good.
h Her hair is brown.
i The furniture is beautiful.
j The police are questioning a man.

4

1 Isn't the meeting tomorrow?
2 Shouldn't he have left by now?
3 Wasn't it a rather difficult operation?
4 Wouldn't Doctor Baxter like some advice?
5 Didn't we meet them on holiday last year?
6 Aren't these the articles you were telling me about?
7 Isn't this the patient who attends the clinic for treatment?
8 Won't she apply for a job as soon as she graduates?
9 Haven't they forgotten something?
10 Couldn't I do it for you?

5

1 It doesn't feel cold.
2 It doesn't taste stale.
3 They don't look tired.
4 It doesn't taste dry.
5 It doesn't smell (or taste) off.
6 They don't feel warm.
7 It doesn't sound true.
8 They don't look (or feel) old.
9 It doesn't taste hot.
10 It doesn't sound like John.
11 It doesn't smell like French perfume.
12 He doesn't look (or sound) sad.
13 They don't feel (or look) soft.
14 It doesn't taste (or smell) burnt.
15 It doesn't look (or feel) like silk.

7

1 from
2 forward

3 up
4 from
5 up
6 of / off
7 through
8 into / into
9 on
10 off

He does?

7 Were you there last night?
   You were?

8 Has she already left?
   She has?

9 Did they telephone?
   They did?

10 Is it ready?
    It is?

GRAMMAR POINT

9

1 Has he?
2 Would they?
3 Didn't he?
4 Is it?
5 Have you?
6 Hasn't she?
7 Could they?
8 Was it?
9 Doesn't he?
10 Were they?

10

1 Will you see him?
   You will?

2 Have you told him?
   You have?

3 Could they try it?
   They could?

4 Do you like it?
   You do?

5 Are they coming tomorrow?
   They are?

6 Does he work at the hospital?

WRITING

11

ADVICE	REACTION
HEARD	GUIDE
KITS	USEFUL
BELIEVE	THOUGHT
PROBES	WHOLE
CONTROL	SUPPLIED
SPECIFIC	BIOLOGISTS
OWN	COPIES

IDIOM

Meaning

One's feet are sore, causing one pain.
Can also be used for other parts of
the body and for clothing

e.g. My back's killing me.
      My shoes are killing me.

Grateful thanks is due to Mrs June Peterson and Mrs Agnes Sturgeon for their kind assistance in proof reading and to my faithful assistant Cindy.

The author and publisher wish to thank the following for their kind permission to use articles:

SCIENCE: *The Genome Project.*
U.S. NEWS AND WORLD REPORT: *The Path to a Heart Attack; Heart Tests; "The Pressure Cooker Factor"* (adapted); *AIDS risk.*
SCIENTIFIC AMERICAN: *What Causes Diabetes?* (adapted); *Antisense RNA and DNA* (adapted);*The Human Telomere.*
NATURE: *A Nommocnu Impairment.*
JOURNAL OF ORTHOPAEDIC SURGICAL TECHNIQUES: *Lumbar Spinal Osteotomy in Ankylosing Spondylitis* (adapted).
PAIN: *Measuring Pain Quality: validity and reliability of children's and adolescents' pain language* (adapted).
TIME: *Back Surgery Without Stitches; Helping Out a Heart in Texas; The Gene Hunt; Treading on Heredity* (adapted); *Stop That Germ!; Biological Warfare; Deadly Invaders* (adapted); *A-Not-So-Happy Anniversary; Take a Walk-and Live; Safer Blood; Death-Defying Drug Therapy; A Patch of Hope for Smokers.*
NEWSWEEK: *Can Hormones Stop the Clock?; The Tiniest Patients; The Out-of-Shape Generation; Can Sunshine Save Your Life?*
ST. MICHAEL: *Vogue Complete Beauty: Psychological Resilience Test.*
CAMBRIDGE UNIVERSITY PRESS: *Peptides and Proteins by D. T. Elmore: Nomenclature Peptides and Proteins.*
CHURCHILL LIVINGSTONE: *Essential Pathology by Lawler, Ahmed, Hume: Basic Terminology in Pathology.*
WILLIAM HEINEMANN LTD: *Biology by E. Hanauer Mitosis; Hormones and Endocrine Glands Neurons; Blood Vessels.*
HEALTH EDUCATION BOOKLET, DISTIBUTED BY BOOTS: *Causes and Symptoms of Aids.*
MEDICINE AND SCIENCE IN SPORTS AND EXERCISE: *Guidelines for Exercise Training after Cardiac Transplantation.*
W. B. SAUNDERS COMPANY: *Dorland's Medical Dictionary: definition of hormone.*

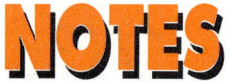

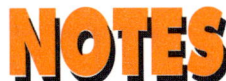

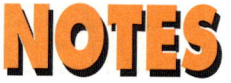
NOTES

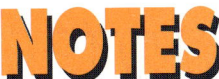

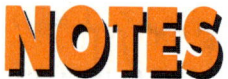

NOTES

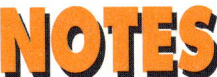

Printed in February 1994 by
Edizioni Minerva Medica
Printing Dept.
corso IV novembre 29-31, Saluzzo (Italy)